Management Strategies in Athletic Training

FIFTH EDITION

Jeff G. Konin, PhD, ATC, PT, FACSM, FNATA

University of Rhode Island

Richard Ray, EdD, ATC

Hope College

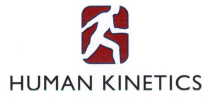

HUMAN KINETICS

Library of Congress Cataloging-in-Publication Data

Names: Ray, Richard, 1957- author. | Konin, Jeff G., author.
Title: Management strategies in athletic training / Jeff Konin, Richard Ray.
Description: Fifth edition. | Champaign, IL : Human Kinetics, [2019] |
  Richard Ray's name appears first in the previous edition. | Includes
  bibliographical references and index.
Identifiers: LCCN 2017033868 (print) | LCCN 2017035167 (ebook) | ISBN
  9781492563051 (e-book) | ISBN 9781492536185 (print)
Subjects: | MESH: Physical Education and Training--organization &
  administration | Sports
Classification: LCC RC1210 (ebook) | LCC RC1210 (print) | NLM QT 255 | DDC
  617.1/027--dc23
LC record available at https://lccn.loc.gov/2017033868

ISBN: 978-1-4925-3618-5 (print)

The web addresses cited in this text were current as of January 2018, unless otherwise noted.

Senior Acquisitions Editor: Joshua J. Stone; **Senior Developmental Editor:** Amanda S. Ewing; **Managing Editor:** Anne E. Mrozek; **Copyeditor:** Annette Pierce; **Indexer:** Karla Walsh; **Permissions Manager:** Dalene Reeder; **Senior Graphic Designer**: Joe Buck; **Graphic Designer:** Dawn Sills; **Cover Designer:** Keri Evans; **Cover Design Associate:** Susan Rothermel Allen; **Photograph (cover):** © Jeff G. Konin; **Photo Production Manager:** Jason Allen; **Senior Art Manager:** Kelly Hendren; **Illustrations:** © Human Kinetics, unless otherwise noted; **Printer:** Versa Press

Printed in the United States of America   10 9 8 7 6 5 4 3 2 1

The paper in this book is certified under a sustainable forestry program.

Human Kinetics
P.O. Box 5076
Champaign, IL 61825-5076
Website: www.HumanKinetics.com

In the United States, email info@hkusa.com or call 800-747-4457.
In Canada, email info@hkcanada.com.
In the United Kingdom/Europe, email hk@hkeurope.com.

For information about Human Kinetics' coverage in other areas of the world,
please visit our website: **www.HumanKinetics.com**   E6881

Projects of this kind are the work of many people—people who bring significant intellectual and technical expertise to providing the highest quality educational product possible. But this book is also the result of the inspired leadership of a very special person. We are both indebted to Joshua Stone for the many ways he encouraged, cajoled, energized, and roused us to our best work. Our names may be on the cover, but Josh's spirit floats above every page. Thank you, Josh.

Contents

Preface

The profession of athletic training continues to evolve and serve in a growing capacity to meet the needs of all populations. As recognized and valued allied health care providers working in interprofessional models of care, today's athletic trainer must continue to possess and demonstrate administrative knowledge, whether to serve in an administrative leadership position or simply to understand the requirements associated with the delivery of athletic training services. This book continues to prepare today's and tomorrow's athletic trainer with the skills necessary to become gainfully and successfully employed regardless of setting and clientele.

Why This Text Is Needed

The role of the athletic trainer has evolved in all settings to require more administrative knowledge than ever before. Athletic trainers will continue to acquire some of the organizational knowledge and skills they need through on-the-job experience, but many entry-level athletic trainers will not get all of the information they need that way. This form of on-the-job training is beneficial and is commonly referred to as *experience* later in life. However, often this knowledge is needed on the first day of employment. The primary purpose of this book is to provide a standard for the kinds of knowledge and skills that every athletic trainer entering the field should master. Because entry-level athletic trainers will confront administrative problems that are growing in number and complexity, they can use this book as a reference to help them cope with such problems while they provide high-quality services to their clients.

This text is also intended to enhance the administrative ability of athletic trainers already in practice. It offers insights into a variety of topics that many athletic trainers beyond the entry level don't consider in managerial or administrative terms. Practicing athletic trainers will learn to apply management theories to the administrative problems they have faced for years and to craft creative solutions to these problems. We have combined decades of academic, clinical, and consultative administrative experience to present a comprehensive resource for all athletic trainers. Furthermore, this book introduces many new concepts to address issues facing practicing athletic trainers that may not have been commonplace in the past. Practitioners who have been in the athletic training profession for many years may find this text refreshing given its contemporary approach to addressing today's management culture.

This text can be used to demonstrate acceptable standards for athletic training administrative practice and as a reliable source for credentialing boards of national and state athletic training organizations to establish valid questions for examinations. The text remains current and provides the greatest depth and breadth of information on athletic training administration available in a single source.

Who This Text Will Benefit

The following are the primary audiences for this text:

- Entry-level students preparing for credentialing by states and the national Board of Certification
- Graduate students either preparing for state and national credentialing or working toward an advanced degree in athletic training
- Athletic training residents seeking to reinforce and apply leadership techniques as part of their residency objectives
- Practicing athletic trainers who are already credentialed, but who wish to develop or update their knowledge and skill in athletic training administration

How This Text Is Organized

This book presents theories underlying the management principles that athletic trainers have historically been forced to learn through experience. Each chapter provides anecdotes, practical suggestions, and case studies to illustrate how management theory applies to the work of athletic trainers. Readers will be able to apply the theories presented in the chapters to real-world situations.

Special Features

The following pedagogical aids are intended to help instructors and students master the content.

- *Chapter objectives.* Each chapter opens with a list of expected learning outcomes. These objectives are broad enough to form the behavioral objectives for an entire course in athletic training administration.
- *Key words.* Key words and important phrases appear in boldface to help readers determine the most important concepts at a glance.
- *Glossary.* Readers will find a glossary of important terms at the end of the book.
- *Sample forms.* Many chapters include sample forms for reference.
- *Key points.* Summaries of the key points of each major section help readers focus on the most important material.
- *Pearls of management.* This feature highlights information that readers should incorporate into their career as an athletic trainer.
- *Case studies.* The case studies are hypothetical scenarios that will help students understand more fully the relationship between the theory and the application of various concepts discussed in the chapter. These cases are accompanied by a series of questions that require students to synthesize the information presented in the chapter and to develop alternative responses to each scenario. The analysis questions are open ended and encourage students to be creative in developing possible solutions. The number of right or wrong answers is not fixed.
- *Key concepts and review.* The most important concepts are summarized at the end of each chapter. This element parallels the chapter objectives for easier review.

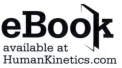
available at
HumanKinetics.com

What's New in the Fifth Edition?

Management Strategies in Athletic Training has been significantly improved in this fifth edition. Like the previous four, this edition is designed to meet

the bulk of the discipline-specific content for an entry-level athletic training curriculum. Each of the chapters from the fourth edition of *Management Strategies in Athletic Training* has been updated, and new chapters have been added that address the history of the profession of athletic training and professional advocacy. Additional new material includes the following:

- Advances in patient charting
- Updated preparticipation physical examination standards
- Updated drug education and testing standards
- Health care financial management
- Providing legal testimony and deposition
- Emergency action planning
- Injury surveillance systems
- Updates on ethical practice in sports medicine
- Updated legal standards
- Updated state regulatory board contact information
- Athletic trainer compensation
- Negotiating skills for accepting a job
- Employment settings for athletic trainers
- Work–life balance
- National Athletic Trainers' Association position statements
- Updates on reimbursement for athletic training services
- Occupational Safety and Health Administration requirements for health care facilities
- *NCAA Sports Medicine Handbook*
- Expansion of information management in athletic training clinical and administrative settings
- Updated information on reimbursement for athletic training services, including the athletic training Current Procedural Terminology codes
- Updated forms

Note to Instructors

If you are an athletic training educator, you might be wondering how you can most effectively use this book as part of a course on athletic training administration. In our experience, students learn this material best when they can apply it to the things they have seen in their short, but interesting, careers. We do not encourage you to lecture from the book or simply transfer the content of the material to a slide presentation for class. Instead, allow students to read the material and develop questions about how they should or could apply the information to real-life problems they've encountered or heard about. Use the questions and exercises in the case studies at the end of the chapters to start class conversations about the material.

Keep in mind that the time you have with your students in the classroom is brief compared to the amount of time that they have on their own. We recommend that you use the time students have on their own for *first-exposure learning*. It may be best to have the students read the assigned chapter and complete the chapter worksheet before coming to class. When they arrive, all you have to do is ask, "Any questions?" and an hour later class is finished. Students may end up spending the entire hour talking about the concepts that they found difficult in their reading as you reinforce and explain these concepts. This method has proven far more effective than lecturing in this kind of course.

Several ancillaries are also available to help you present the material in the text.

- The instructor guide is loaded with useful instructional aids. Each chapter is supported by a repeat of the chapter summary from the book, student activity suggestions, extra case studies, and suggested readings. For instructors who are still uncertain about how to develop their course, a sample syllabus—one that we suggest using as a template—is provided.

- The chapter quizzes include more than 180 questions you can use to generate quizzes or tests.

- The image bank includes most of the figures and tables from the text. Images are grouped first within chapter folders, and you may reuse the images within your own PowerPoint templates to create your own custom presentations.

You can access these ancillaries by going to www.HumanKinetics.com/ManagementStrategiesIn AthleticTraining.

Note to Students

If you are a student using *Management Strategies in Athletic Training, Fifth Edition,* in an athletic training administration course, you might be wondering whether you should use this book just as you would the textbooks you've been assigned in your other courses. We wouldn't recommend it, and here's why: experience. This book was written to help you experience, through reading and doing, what it is like to be an athletic trainer faced with administrative problems. Ask yourself how the concepts in the book can or should be applied in a real-life setting as you read the text. How do they apply to the cases in the book? How do they apply to the athletic training program at your college or university? As you read each chapter, we recommend that you use the margin of the book to write notes to yourself. "Why did the athletic trainer in this chapter go over his athletic director's head? Wasn't that dangerous? Is that something I would have done under the circumstances?" "The book recommends the use of bidding when purchasing supplies. Why doesn't the athletic trainer at our school do this?" Use the questions you develop to guide your participation in class. If you use this approach and aren't afraid to ask questions in class based on your reading, we think you'll find that your athletic training administration class will be one of the most interesting and exciting courses you take on your way to becoming a certified athletic trainer.

Final Word

The fifth edition of this textbook has evolved so that the athletic trainers of the future can better prepare themselves to deal effectively with the many administrative and managerial problems they are likely to face in an increasingly complex and changing health care environment. We hope that after you have read through and experienced the material in this book, you will find yourself prepared for the real world that lies ahead of you. After all, professionals in the athletic training field will require not only expansion and growth in their clinical skills, but also administrative and managerial leadership skills at all levels.

Acknowledgments

As with all of the previous editions of this textbook, many people deserve recognition for their contributions to the revised edition of *Management Strategies in Athletic Training*.

First and foremost, our acquisitions editor at Human Kinetics, Joshua J. Stone, MA, ATC, CSCS, CES, PES, has been the quarterback of this project. Josh deserves all the credit for keeping us on deadline and providing valuable insight into the necessary changes for keeping the material in the textbook current. Amanda Ewing also deserves mountains of credit for attending to every detail that we overlooked. Her level of perfection is second to none. Many other folks at Human Kinetics have worked hard behind the scenes to support our efforts. They include managing editor Anne Mrozek, graphic designers Joe Buck and Dawn Sills, cover designer Keri Evans, art manager Kelly Hendren, technical illustrator Matt Harshbarger, and marketing manager Abby Gailey.

For this edition, new images include athletic training students and student-athletes who graciously agreed to serve as models, allowing us to support the content of the text with visual images. Special thanks goes out to Justin Jacapraro, Paige Alshon, Tiara Higuchi, Sam McMullen, Kristen Robillard, and Brooke Fennell from the University of Rhode Island, and Claire Geyer, Sarah Acerbo, Janelle Prince, Megan DeRoy, Adrienne Fedyna Dembreck, and Ryan Marder from the University of Connecticut.

In this fifth edition, we leaned on some of the best and brightest the profession has to offer to ensure that the content of the written work truly reflects the contemporary practice of athletic training today:

- **Gretchen Schlabach, PhD, ATC,** professor emerita of the athletic training program at Northern Illinois University, provided expertise for the revised chapter 9, Ethics in Sports Medicine.

- **Stephanie Mazerolle, PhD, ATC,** associate professor in the department of kinesiology and director of the professional bachelor's program in athletic training at the University of Connecticut, contributed the content for the new and important section on work–life balance in chapter 4, Human Resources.

- **Greg Janik, MS, ATC,** associate clinical professor in the athletic training education program and head athletic trainer at King's College in Wilkes-Barre, Pennsylvania, provided valuable contributions to the revised chapter 10, Legal Considerations in Sports Medicine.

- **Clark Simpson, MBA, MEd, RKT, LAT, ATC,** president and CEO of Clark Group Associates in Indianapolis, Indiana, contributed to the revision of chapter 8, Revenue for Health Care Services.

- **Michael A. Colello, MS, ATC,** national sales manager for sports at Aegis Sciences Corp. in Nashville, Tennessee, provided valuable insight to the updates for chapter 14, Drug Education and Testing.

- **Marty Matney, MBA, LAT, ATC, LPTA, CEAS,** program manager at Work-Fit in Seattle, Washington, who assisted with the reimbursement content.

- **Valerie W. Herzog, EdD, LAT, ATC,** professor and director of the graduate athletic training program and director of the Office of Graduate Studies at Weber State University in Ogden, Utah, offered to be involved in the revision, and her timing was perfect. In addition to contributing to chapter 1, The Profession of Athletic Training, and chapter 11, Professional Advocacy, which are new to this edition, she served as an additional set of eyes, offering critical editing expertise to all of the chapters and ancillaries in this revision.

The Profession of Athletic Training

Objectives

After reading this chapter, you should be able to do the following:

- Explain the history and governance structure of the National Athletic Trainers' Association (NATA).

- Differentiate between the various NATA committees, including their purpose and functions.

- Explain the functions of the Board of Certification (BOC).

- Explain the evolution of athletic training education, including the roles of the Commission on Accreditation of Athletic Training Education (CAATE) and its predecessors.

- Describe the progress that has been made to improve gender and ethnic diversity within the profession of athletic training as well as recognize where change is still needed.

The profession of athletic training in the United States can trace its origins to 1881, when Harvard University hired its first athletic trainer to work with the football team. Understanding both the development of the profession and the current organizational structures of the governing bodies is important to navigating a career in the field. This chapter outlines the origins of the profession, its progression into health care, and the organizations that manage the national membership, certification, and academic program accreditation.

Evolution of Athletic Training Education

Although many think of athletic training as a relatively young health care profession in the Western world, athletic training has a long and rich history. The first athletic trainers can be traced back to 564 BC in the Greek Olympics and Roman gladiatorial games. They were referred to as paedotribes, meaning masseurs. This was meant to describe people who helped prepare athletes for competition and instructed them in exercise. Later, these paedotribes worked at schools to help prepare young men to be strong soldiers. There is no clear connection between the ancient paedotribes and the athletic trainers in the late 19th century, even though they do share some of the same roles and responsibilities.

James Robinson was hired by Harvard University in 1881 and is the first athletic trainer in the United States who was recognized as such in publications such as newspapers and on the football team roster. However, much of his day was spent coaching and conditioning the athletes with whom he worked, rather than primarily treating and rehabilitating injuries. This was the case for many of the early athletic trainers, although the profession evolved significantly over the next 100 years as athletic trainers moved from conditioning coaches to health care providers. As the game of football became more popular in the United States in the early 1900s, several deaths occurred each year and the athletic trainer's unique role as a health care provider began to emerge. Because few evidence-based practices for preventing and treating injuries existed at the time, the athletic trainers shared with each other what worked best in advising athletes on managing injuries and wounds, nutrition, and conditioning. Athletic trainers (ATs) at the time also repaired and sometimes created new protective equipment and padding to protect athletes from injuries.

In 1890, the first team physician was appointed at Harvard, which allowed ATs to begin working more closely with physicians and learn best practices from them. Early in the 20th century, athletic trainers also worked in sports such as baseball and track and field, performing similar roles as both health care providers and conditioning coaches. Additionally, during World War I, athletic trainers were sought to provide physical conditioning such as stretching, cardiovascular conditioning, and strengthening for soldiers, to help them prepare for the physical demands of combat (Webber 2013).

During the early years of athletic training in the United States, no formal education programs for athletic trainers existed. Similar to other health care professions in the 1940s and 1950s, athletic trainers learned their skills on the job and were mentored by other athletic trainers or physicians. The first undergraduate degree in athletic training was offered by Indiana University in 1948, although it would be many years before there were an adequate number of programs or a defined course of study for the profession. A model curriculum was developed by the NATA Professional Education Committee (PEC) in 1959, but by 1970, only four undergraduate programs in athletic training had been approved by NATA (Ebel 1999). Between 1970 and 2015, the athletic training curriculum evolved, and more than 350 accredited professional programs were developed (Commission on Accreditation of Athletic Training Education n.d.-a).

In 1990, led by the efforts of the NATA Professional Education Committee, the American Medical Association (AMA) voted to recognize athletic training as an allied health profession. This was a momentous occasion for the profession because it officially gave athletic trainers legitimacy as members of the health care team. It also made it possible for the profession to incorporate accreditation of its educational programs by the AMA's Committee on Allied Health Education Accreditation (CAHEA). NATA formed the Joint Review Committee on Educational Programs in Athletic Training (JRC-AT) to develop standards and guidelines for entry-level professional programs. Those involved soon realized that athletic training programs varied quite a bit, creating significant disparities between the knowledge and skills of graduating students (Ebel 1999).

Before 1996, students could choose from several educational routes to become eligible to take the certification exam. Students could graduate from a NATA-approved program, later referred to as a curriculum program. Another option was graduation from an internship program, which required certain course work and offered more flexibility than a curriculum program. Students were expected to spend more time learning in the field than through courses and were required to complete more clinical or internship hours to be eligible to take the certification exam. A third option allowed students who had earned a physical therapy degree to complete a set number of internship hours with an athletic trainer to become eligible for certification (Ebel 1999).

In 1994, a task force within NATA was formed to study the requirements for eligibility for certification and to develop recommendations to reform athletic training education. In 2004, a new accreditation standard was implemented that required all students to graduate with a bachelor's degree from an accredited athletic training program in order to be eligible to take the certification exam. These programs were accredited by the JRC-AT, which was a committee under the Commission on Accreditation of Allied Health Education Programs (CAAHEP), the body that ultimately replaced CAHEA in 1994. The education task force evolved into the Education Council in 1996 to work on issues related to **professional education** and **postprofessional education** and to serve as a liaison with the JRC-AT (Ebel 1999).

KEY POINT

Professional programs lead to eligibility for certification. Postprofessional programs are typically graduate programs (master's or doctoral) for athletic trainers who are already certified.

In 2006, the JRC-AT became independent from CAAHEP and changed its name to the **Commission on Accreditation of Athletic Training Education (CAATE)**. CAATE grew from having just one full-time staff member to having a full-time executive director and several support staff. CAATE also began to award accreditation to postprofessional master's degree programs as well as athletic training residencies. CAATE is independent from NATA, although they work together closely to forge the future of the profession. In 2014, CAATE achieved recognition by the Council for Higher Education Accreditation (CHEA). Each year, CAATE hosts the CAATE Accreditation Conference to support faculty and administrators as they work to implement the accreditation standards and improve their educational programs.

PEARLS OF MANAGEMENT

The Commission on Accreditation of Athletic Training Education (CAATE) sets accreditation standards, and it awards accreditation to professional, postprofessional, and residency programs. CAATE constantly reviews and updates accreditation standards. A school must understand and adhere to accreditation standards and apply for reaccreditation every 5 to 10 years in addition to submitting an annual accreditation report.

Another recommendation of the task force in 1996 was to develop entry-level professional athletic training programs at the graduate level. This would allow graduates with a bachelor's degree in fields other than athletic training to later complete a graduate degree, which would allow them to be eligible to take the certification exam. Programs of this type began to develop, although the vast majority of professional programs remained at the bachelor's level. In 2015, CAATE, in partnership

KEY POINT

The athletic training Strategic Alliance consists of the following:

- Board of Certification
- Commission on Accreditation of Athletic Training Education
- National Athletic Trainers' Association
- NATA Research and Education Foundation

with the other members of the Strategic Alliance (NATA, BOC, and NATA Research and Education Foundation) voted to change the degree required for professional programs to the master's level. The standard states "Baccalaureate programs may not admit, enroll, or matriculate students into the athletic training program after the start of the fall term 2022" (Commission on Accreditation of Athletic Training Education n.d.-b).

National Athletic Trainers' Association

The **National Athletic Trainers' Association** was founded in 1950 with the goal to share ideas and knowledge and establish national standards for the profession. It was intentionally created as a democratic organization that maintained the right of each state and district to determine its members. Brothers Chuck and Frank Cramer had assembled a group to meet and form NATA in conjunction with the First National Training Clinic, a conference for about 125 athletic trainers, which was held in June of 1950 in Kansas City, Missouri. This was the second attempt to create a national organization for athletic trainers. The first National Athletic Trainers Association (note no apostrophe in *Trainers*), was formed in 1938 and was a separate organization from the NATA founded in 1950. The first NATA lasted from just 1938 to 1944 because of financial struggles, World War II, and infighting among its members (Ebel 1999).

Chuck and Frank Cramer, along with their company, the Cramer Chemical Co., provided significant financial support for NATA in its early years. Without the backing of the Cramers, NATA might not have been able to gain enough traction to become self-supporting. By 1955, NATA had 279 members and about $2,000 in savings. With the hard work of many volunteers and visionary leaders, NATA in 1990 had 14,598 members and had grown its assets to over $3 million (Ebel 1999). By 2015, NATA had more than 45,000 members and more than $22 million in assets (National Athletic Trainers' Association 2016).

Each year, NATA hosts the Clinical Symposia and AT Expo, which includes educational programming, an opportunity to talk to vendors about the latest products and services, research presentations, and social events. The conference has grown from 125 attendees in 1950 to a typical attendance of more than 10,000 each year. NATA also sponsors an Athletic Training Educators' Conference every other year for faculty who teach future athletic trainers. In addition, NATA provides educational offerings such as webinars, online courses, and journal quizzes. NATA also produces two of the premier journals in the field, the *Journal of Athletic Training* and the *Athletic Training Education Journal*.

NATA is governed by a board of directors, with one director from each of the 10 districts. The district directors are elected by the members of their district. Following the nominating committee's selection of the top two candidates, the full membership of NATA elects the president. The board of directors elects a vice president and secretary/treasurer, who also serve on the board. The board of directors works closely with the executive director of NATA, which is a full-time staff position at the NATA office in Carrollton, Texas. The executive director oversees a staff of employees who manage the association's business and outreach efforts in areas such as accounting, government affairs, conference planning, marketing, public relations, member services, and business development.

KEY POINT

The National Athletic Trainers' Association is the professional membership organization for certified athletic trainers and others who support the athletic training profession.

Much of the work of NATA is done by members who volunteer to serve on committees (see the sidebar NATA Committees). The committees are supported by the NATA staff previously identified. Over the years, committees have emerged based on current issues. The work of each committee focuses on the greater mission of NATA, which is "to represent, engage, and foster the continued growth and development of the athletic training profession and athletic trainers as unique health care providers" (National Athletic Trainers' Association n.d.-a). The vast majority of the committees are served by representatives from each of the 10 districts and some also have at-large members. NATA members who want to serve on a committee typically contact their district director, who appoints committee members, to express interest in serving on a particular committee. NATA also appoints members to serve as liaisons to external affiliated organizations such as the American Academy of Physician Assistants, the American College of Sports Medicine, and the National Strength and Conditioning Association.

PEARLS OF MANAGEMENT

Athletic trainers who serve voluntarily on committees are approved and appointed by the NATA Board of Directors. Most positions have term limits and can be reappointed for a second term.

Each NATA committee focuses on specific issues, which are sometimes related to certain work settings. For example, the **Secondary School Athletic Trainers' Committee (SSATC)** works on issues specific to ATs who work in that setting. These include identifying best practices for providing care to youth athletes as well as how to improve the marketability of the secondary school athletic trainer. The **Intercollegiate Council for Sports Medicine (ICSM)** focuses on the issues faced by athletic trainers in the collegiate setting, such as complying with National Collegiate Athletic Association (NCAA) rules and guidelines. The committee developed a liability tool kit to help athletic trainers manage and reduce risk in their workplaces.

Three committees are involved with legislative advocacy, each in a different way. The **Government Affairs Committee (GAC)** is made up of representatives from each district who work with each of the states in their district on legislative issues. This includes providing advice on legislative strategies, reviewing proposed bill language, and putting states in touch with other states that have dealt with similar legislative issues. GAC also reviews applications to award grants each year to the states to support their legislative efforts. The **Federal Legislative Council** consists of the NATA president, the NATA executive director, key members of the NATA Board of Directors, some committee chairs, and a NATA staff liaison. This group focuses its efforts on federal legislative issues and coordinates Capitol Hill Day each year, where athletic trainers visit with members of the U.S. Congress in Washington, D.C. The third committee is the **State Association Advisory Committee (SAAC)**, which works directly with the leaders of each state association to support their efforts regarding legislation, and also with general association management. This committee organizes the State Leadership Forum each year, which is typically held one or two days before the NATA conference. Chapter 11 on professional advocacy delves much deeper into what these groups do and how they work together.

The **Committee on Practice Advancement (COPA)** has evolved quite a bit over the past 25 years. It has had different names and was sometimes split

NATA Committees

- *ATs Care Committee.* Provide educational resources and organizational methods relative to critical incident stress management (CISM) at the district and state levels
- *Committee on Practice Advancement.* Supports ATs in emerging settings and works on reimbursement issues
- *Committee on Professional Ethics.* Addresses ethics complaints
- *Convention Program Committee.* Plans and manages annual conference
- *District Secretaries'/Treasurers' Committee.* Supports district secretaries and treasurers
- *Education Journal Committee.* Manages the *Athletic Training Education Journal*
- *Ethnic Diversity Advisory Committee.* Identifies and addresses issues relevant to ethnically diverse members and clients
- *Executive Committee for Education.* Makes recommendations for athletic training education
- *Federal Legislative Council.* Oversees federal legislative efforts
- *Finance Committee.* Oversees NATA finances and investments
- *Government Affairs Committee.* Supports state legislative efforts and awards grants to states to help fund these efforts
- *Historical Commission.* Preserves the history of athletic training, provides athletic training historical education, and serves as a resource to NATA on historical issues
- *Honors and Awards Committee.* Selects award recipients
- *Intercollegiate Council for Sports Medicine (formerly the College/University Athletic Trainers' Committee).* Identifies and addresses issues facing ATs in the collegiate setting
- *International Committee.* Supports ATs working outside of the United States
- *Journal Committee.* Manages the *Journal of Athletic Training*
- *Professional Responsibility Committee.* Supports the legal, ethical, and regulatory standards of the AT Strategic Alliance by encouraging and promoting adherence
- *Public Relations Committee.* Develops tools to promote the athletic training profession
- *Secondary School Athletic Trainers' Committee.* Identifies and addresses issues facing ATs in secondary schools
- *State Association Advisory Committee.* Supports state association management
- *Student Leadership Committee.* Represents student issues and plans student programming at the annual Clinical Symposia
- *Young Professionals' Committee.* Identifies and addresses issues facing newly certified ATs

into two committees, one dealing with reimbursement issues and the other focused on emerging practice settings, such as the military and performing arts. Before reimbursement was a consideration of NATA, the first committee was the Clinical/Industrial/Corporate Athletic Trainers Committee (CIC), formed around 1990. In the mid-1990s, the NATA Board of Directors formed a task force to look at reimbursement issues for athletic trainers, the Reimbursement Advisory Group. This group later became the Committee for Reimbursement and in addressing general revenue generation for athletic trainers, changed its name to Committee on Revenue (COR). Meanwhile, around 2000, CIC expanded its view and changed its name to the Committee on Emerging Practice for Athletic Training (CEPAT). Because the two committees, CEPAT and COR, were doing similar work, plans to combine them were started in 2011. This combining of committees was completed in 2013 and COPA was formed.

COPA now works on both reimbursement and emerging practice settings, with a mission to advance "the athletic training profession in business and employment opportunities, compensation, and brand recognition on athletic trainers as health care professionals" (National Athletic Trainers' Association n.d.-b). Several state associations are meeting with insurance companies to encourage them to pay for athletic training services that are currently within the AT's scope of practice under the **Current Procedural Terminology (CPT)** codes (see chapter 8 for more details on CPT codes). Some states have already seen significant success in these efforts, including Georgia, Vermont, Indiana, and Wisconsin. COPA supports state associations in these efforts through work groups and affiliated organizations associated with COPA. The work groups focus on physician practice, health care administrators, communication, performing arts, military, and worth to value (the remnants of COR). COPA also has support from a variety of NATA groups and committees such as the CAATE, Executive Committee for Education (ECE), PEC, Secondary School Athletic Trainers' Committee, and the Public Safety Athletic Trainers' Society. COPA also plays a vital role in preparing athletic trainers to work alongside other health care providers in an interprofessional manner. Interprofessional practice has traditionally been part of a practicing athletic trainer's operational mode as it requires the ability to work collaboratively with others. Recently in all health care settings, a stronger emphasis has been placed on interprofessional practice. A list of other health care providers and their roles can be found in appendix A.

The **Convention Program Committee (CPC)** plans the NATA Clinical Symposia and AT Expo each year. During this huge annual undertaking, the committee plans many types of sessions, including learning labs, advanced-track sessions, minicourses, and plenary speakers. The committee members also oversee all the sessions during the conference to ensure that the event runs smoothly. A significant portion of the programming at the NATA conference is planned by the **Free Communications Committee**, which is part of the NATA Foundation Research Committee. The committee's role is to review case reports and research abstract submissions to select which will be presented as posters or oral presentations. The Student Exchange Track allows professional-level students to present their research without a competitive peer-review process.

Two committees focus on the newer members of NATA. The **Student Leadership Committee (SLC)** is composed of current athletic training students who are not yet certified. This committee advocates for students' needs, but also prepares a student track of educational and career-mentoring sessions at the NATA conference each year. The **Young Professionals' Committee (YPC)** supports newly certified athletic trainers by addressing issues

such as negotiating for better working conditions, salary, and benefits.

Many athletic trainers have taken jobs abroad in countries such as Canada, China, Japan, Australia, and South Korea as well as throughout Europe. The **International Committee (IC)** and the **World Federation of Athletic Training and Therapy (WFATT)** both support athletic trainers working abroad and forge relationships with similar types of health care professionals in other countries. Canadian Athletic Therapists Association (CATA) and Athletic Rehabilitation Therapy Ireland (ARTI) have officially recognized the certified athletic trainer (ATC) credential, which allows ATs in the United States to take the certification exam in those countries, and vice-versa. Groups in China (Chinese General Administration of Sports [GASC]) and South Korea (Korean Society of Sports Medicine [KSSM]) have expressed interest in developing athletic training degree programs.

Some committees have evolved over time into separate, independent organizations, such as the Board of Certification (BOC), the Commission on Accreditation of Athletic Training Education (CAATE), and the **NATA Research and Education Foundation** (also referred to as the NATA Foundation). The NATA Foundation awards research grants and scholarships to students at all levels: professional, postprofessional, and doctoral. The first scholarship that NATA awarded was the William E. "Pinky" Newell Award in 1971 for $250. NATA then established the NATA Research and Education Foundation, which by 2015 had awarded 64 scholarships for a total of $147,200. The NATA Foundation also awards grants to support research efforts. Since its incorporation in 1991, it has awarded over 260 grants totaling more than $4 million. As mentioned previously, the NATA Foundation also supports the **Free Communications** program at the NATA Clinical Symposia and Expo each year, allowing researchers to share the findings of their studies. In 2015, 432 Free Communications oral, poster, and rapid-fire presentations were given at this conference. The NATA Foundation also supports the National Quiz Bowl, which began in 2009 and awards cash prizes to winning teams.

KEY POINT

The NATA Foundation awards scholarships and research grants and manages the Free Communications portion of the NATA convention.

Board of Certification

Like many other early health care practitioners, athletic trainers haven't always been required to be nationally certified. In fact, a certification exam wasn't even offered until 1970, 20 years after the formation of NATA. An editorial by Lindsey McLean published in the *Journal of Athletic Training* in 1969, "Does the National Athletic Trainers' Association Need a Certification Examination?" played a pivotal role in the development of the certification exam. Thousands of people volunteered their time over several years to help develop exam questions and administer the exam. The delivery of the exam was labor intensive because it included a practical section in which students were required to demonstrate their skills. This required models, examiners, and a great deal of equipment and supplies at each exam site. In 1982, the **Board of Certification (BOC)** was granted administrative independence from NATA and became accredited by the National Commission for Certifying Agencies (NCCA) and has maintained its accreditation ever since. In 2007, the BOC moved to a fully integrated computer-based exam, eliminating the practical portion of the test (Board of Certification 2007). As of 2016, the ATC credential was recognized in 49 states, with almost all requiring it to be maintained in order to practice in that state; Texas still offers a state licensing exam, but it is recognized only in Texas (Board of Certification n.d.).

KEY POINT

The Board of Certification (previously referred to as the NATA BOC) creates and delivers the certification examination in addition to managing continuing education for athletic trainers.

The Board of Certification does a great deal more than just develop and deliver the certification exam. It has conducted an analysis of global practices to determine where the knowledge base and skills of athletic trainers in the United States overlap with those of similar health care providers in other countries. The BOC also supports states in their regulatory efforts and hosts the **BOC Athletic Trainer Regulatory Conference** every other year. The staff communicates with the regulatory bodies in each state to help answer questions, provide interpretations when needed, and share information about athletic trainers who have violated the BOC standards of practice or the laws of that state or both. The BOC also developed the facility principles document, which enables athletic trainers to identify areas of potential risk and make changes where necessary. The BOC also manages the continuing education requirements for athletic trainers to ensure that they stay up to date on the latest advances in the field and that high-quality, evidence-based programming is being provided. Athletic trainers are required to complete 50 continuing education units (CEUs) every two years, maintain emergency cardiovascular care (ECC) certification, and pay an annual certification fee in order to retain their BOC certification.

Appropriate Terminology

Because the athletic training profession has undergone significant changes in so many areas, it is sometimes difficult to keep up with the current terminology. NATA created a terminology work group to clarify the accepted terms for the profession. The first, and most important, are the terms *athletic trainer* and *certified athletic trainer.* The terms *trainer* and *certified trainer* should not be used to refer to athletic trainers because they can be confused with terms used to describe personal trainers, who hold varying levels of education, skills, and expertise. However, *trainer* was commonly used to describe ATs for many years, and some people may still use this word, despite its potential harm to the recognition of ATs as health care providers. This same principle is applied to the athletic training facility and athletic training clinic, which should never be referred to as the *training room.*

There is also confusion regarding how athletic trainers should list their credentials once they are both BOC certified and licensed or registered in their state. ATC is a registered trademark and should not be altered in any way. This means that it is not appropriate to combine your state credential with your national certification such as ATC/L, ATC/R, LATC, or other variations that combine other designations with ATC. The ATC should stand alone after the athletic trainer's name, and the license is listed as a separate acronym—for example, "Sarah Smith, MS, LAT, ATC." Note that the highest credential is listed first. Some might feel that ATC should be listed before LAT, but listing LAT first demonstrates that this credential was awarded after the ATC credential. You must be certified before you can be registered or licensed in your state. Athletic training regulation is discussed in more detail in chapter 11.

One of the most recent changes in terminology is the elimination of the term *physician extender* in 2016. It had been used for many years to describe an athletic trainer who worked in a physician's practice to extend the services of the supervising physician. However, in 2014, the terminology work group decided that this was no longer the best term to describe this practice setting because all athletic trainers work under the direction of or in collaboration with physicians. In addition, the use of the term *physician extender* resulted in dropping the term *athletic trainer* for these practitioners, thereby diminishing the profession's prestige. The terminology work group recommended and adopted the term *athletic trainer in a physician practice*, which keeps the term *athletic trainer* out front. The same approach can also be used for athletic trainers practicing in other settings, such as athletic trainer in a clinic setting or athletic trainer in a performing arts setting. The terminology work group in 2016 continued to evaluate terminology used in the profession to ensure that all of the Strategic Alliance partners use consistent language that best represents the profession.

Women in Athletic Training

Women have made great strides in the athletic training profession over the past 60 years, thanks in large part to the passage of **Title IX legislation**, which was part of the United States Education Amendments of 1972. The purpose of Title IX was to provide educational opportunities to women that were equal to those of men, including scholarships and other funding. Several interpretations and clarifications have been passed since that time, with the most recent in 2003 to better define how equity is determined (Carpenter and Acosta 2005). Title IX made it illegal to discriminate between sexes in school and collegiate athletics that receive federal funding. This resulted in a large increase in the number of women's sports teams, which all needed athletic training services. Dotty Cohen was the first female member of NATA when she joined in 1966, before the passage of Title IX. The number of women in the profession grew by leaps and bounds over the next several decades. By 1990, more than 40% of NATA members were women, and by 2016, 54% were women. In fact, since 1990, more than half of athletic trainers who have become certified have been women.

Julie Max was the first woman to serve as NATA president, from 2000 to 2004, and Marjorie Albohm

KEY POINT

Title IX is federal legislation that states "No person in the United States shall, on the basis of sex, be excluded from participation in, be denied the benefits of, or be subjected to discrimination under any education program or activity receiving federal financial assistance."

was the first woman to serve on the Board of Certification. These women, and many others, laid the groundwork for future generations of women in athletic training. Women now serve on every committee and at every level of NATA. In 2016, the executive directors of both the BOC and CAATE were women.

Women have also made inroads into professional sports that previously excluded them. Ariko Iso was the first female staff athletic trainer hired in the National Football League in 2004 by the Pittsburgh Steelers. In 2012, Sue Falsone made history when she was hired as the first female head athletic trainer in Major League Baseball for the Los Angeles Dodgers. In 2015, the NFL made a commitment to place a female athletic training intern with every NFL team and to hire more female ATs. Just about 18 months later, five full-time female athletic trainers were working in the NFL, and 16 teams selected 22 female AT students to help with their summer training camps (Sitzler 2016).

Work still needs to be done for women to be equally represented in all areas, but changes can be seen in many settings. However, in 2014, only about 18% of head athletic trainers at NCAA Division I universities were women and some professional sports teams still had employed few, if any, female athletic trainers. As of 2016, no female athletic trainers were working in the National Basketball Association.

Ethnic Minorities in Athletic Training

Minorities in athletic training are underrepresented when compared to the population of the United States. This issue has been examined and discussed publicly in the profession since 1968. In the 1980s, NATA created the Ethnic Minority Advisory Council to study the issues affecting minorities choosing to study athletic training in college as well as barriers to entering and staying in the profession. This committee was later renamed the **Ethnic Diversity Advisory Committee (EDAC)**, which has continued these efforts. EDAC offers grants of up to $5,000 for educational institutions to enhance ethnic diversity within the profession. At the NATA conference each year, EDAC sponsors several educational sessions, a town hall, and a social and honors a member with the EDAC Bill Chisolm Professional Service Award, which recognizes "an individual who has contributed to the development and enhancement of ethnically diverse athletic trainers" (National Athletic Trainers' Association n.d.-c).

KEY POINT

Bill Chisolm was an athletic trainer and coordinator of the athletic training program at Brooklyn College from 1970 to 1992, where he was highly respected as an educator and role model. He served NATA as a member of the Ethnic Minority Advisory Council.

Despite gradual increases over the years, by the end of 2015, still only 13% of the certified members of NATA were ethnic minorities. However, in the same year, more than 20% of the student members were ethnic minorities. Progress is being made to increase both gender and ethnic diversity, but the leaders of the profession should not be satisfied until people from all walks of life have equal representation and feel welcome and supported in the athletic training profession.

Summary

The athletic training profession has evolved extensively over the past 100 years. Athletic trainers are now represented by a well-established, professional membership organization: National Athletic Trainers' Association. Professional education programs are moving exclusively to the master's degree level and are accredited by the Commission on Accreditation of Athletic Training Education upon demonstration of meeting rigorous educational standards. Graduates of these programs are eligible to take the certification exam, offered by the Board of Certification, which also establishes continuing education standards. The NATA Research and Education Foundation awards scholarships for students as well as grants for researchers. All four of these members of the AT Strategic Alliance are devoted to advancing the athletic training profession and preparing athletic trainers to provide exceptional client care.

Learning Aids

Case Study 1

Renee recently graduated with a master's degree in athletic training and is eager to get involved in the profession. For the past two years, she has been working mornings in an outpatient rehabilitation clinic and afternoons at a high school. Her long-term goals include working with a collegiate soccer team and eventually landing a job as an athletic trainer with a major league soccer team.

Questions for Analysis

1. Which NATA committees might be most beneficial for Renee to communicate with regarding her professional goals? Explain why each would be a good choice.

2. Does Renee possess skills or characteristics that would benefit the association if she chose to voluntarily serve on a committee? If so, what skills and characteristics do you think Renee possesses? Which committees, if any, might Renee be able to contribute to in a positive way?

3. Do you have additional advice for Renee with respect to her professional advancement?

Case Study 2

Jaclyn is a graduate assistant at a midsized university. When she first arrived, the director of the sports medicine department asked her to help revise a clinical policy and procedure on the prevention and management of exertional heat illness. Having just recently been certified as an athletic trainer, Jaclyn didn't have much firsthand exposure to draw from aside from her clinical experiences as an athletic training student. Nonetheless, the director had enough confidence in her knowledge and work ethic to task her with this important project.

Questions for Analysis

1. Where should Jaclyn look first if she uses NATA as a starting point to research this topic?

2. Would you suggest that Jaclyn communicate with a specific NATA committee to inquire about the existing standard of care? If so, which one?

3. If you were Jaclyn, would you feel confident in actively participating in this process, or would you prefer it be delegated to a staff athletic trainer with more clinical experience? Explain your answer.

Key Concepts and Review

Explain the history and governance structure of the National Athletic Trainers' Association (NATA).

NATA was founded in 1950, with a representative on its board of directors from each of the 10 districts. The board of directors works closely with NATA staff in Texas, including the executive director.

Differentiate between the various NATA committees, including their purpose and functions.

NATA includes several committees, some that represent particular work settings, such as the Secondary School Athletic Trainers' Committee, and others with specific functions such as the Government Affairs Committee. Others represent particular groups of members and their needs, such as the Ethnic Diversity Advisory Committee and the Student Leadership Committee.

Explain the functions of the Board of Certification (BOC).

The Board of Certification develops and administers the national certification exam for athletic trainers. In addition, the BOC manages the continuing education for athletic trainers and supports states in their regulatory efforts. It also hosts the BOC Athletic Trainer Regulatory Conference every other year.

Explain the evolution of athletic training education, including the roles of the Commission on Accreditation of Athletic Training Education (CAATE) and its predecessors.

Similar to other health care professions, athletic training began as a trade, where ATs learned from one another and through workshops and internships. Over the years, the body of knowledge was organized into courses, which were later organized into academic majors. For graduates to be eligible to take the certification exam, they must graduate from a CAATE-accredited program, which will eventually include only master's degree programs.

Describe the progress that has been made to improve gender and ethnic diversity within the profession of athletic training as well as recognize where change is still needed.

Significant progress has been made since the 1980s in the athletic training profession to increase representation of ethnic minorities and women. Title IX was part of the United States Education Amendments of 1972 and made it illegal to discriminate based on gender within any aspect of an educational program or activity that is supported by federal funds. This resulted in a proliferation of women's sport teams, followed by female athletic trainers to care for their injuries. Women now represent about half of the certified athletic trainers in the United States. However, the percentage of athletic trainers who represent ethnic minorities still does not match their representation in the U.S. population.

Principles of Management

Objectives

After reading this chapter, you should be able to do the following:

- Define the concepts of power, authority, and leadership.

- Understand the historical trends in management and how they might apply to athletic training.

- Understand the various managerial roles that athletic trainers assume.

- Understand the various strategies that athletic trainers can employ to improve their managerial effectiveness.

Many practicing athletic trainers can relate to challenges faced when working with administrators in their organization. Although they typically lack formal education or training in management theory, athletic trainers need to be conversant in major theories of organizational behavior to make maximum use of the power, authority, and leadership that are normal components of their personal and professional profiles.

Foundations of Management

Athletic trainers are often responsible for managing programs that have large budgets and staffs. Until recently, intuition and on-the-job experience have been athletic trainers' only tools for attempting to solve administrative problems. Formal study of the principles underlying sound management practice should help athletic trainers perform their jobs better.

The emphasis on the conceptual and theoretical aspects of management is important. Too often, athletic trainers who assume management roles continue to behave like health care providers and neglect to behave like managers. This role confusion is understandable. After all, if you have been a practitioner for 10 years and suddenly assume a new position with new responsibilities, you have to make an adjustment. Managerial responsibilities are different from client care responsibilities. When you take care of a client, your only responsibility is to the client. Managerial duties, on the other hand, require you to consider the needs of not only the clients but also the employees, the department, and the organization. You must consider the needs of various external stakeholder groups. In short, you will need to expand your worldview and begin thinking like a manager. An understanding of the major theories of management will help athletic trainers make the transition.

In some cases, schools employ just one athletic trainer, immediately thrusting the individual into a managerial role. It is not uncommon for recent athletic training graduates and newly certified athletic trainers with no previous employment experience to accept such positions. More often than not, a staff athletic trainer who has proven to be the most effective clinician, whether in a college or university setting or a clinic-based environment, is asked to serve as the director of athletic training and sports medicine and to assume the administrative and managerial responsibilities for the program. He or she may have no previous formal or informal training for this role. This phenomenon is referred to as the **Peter Principle**, which states that in a hierarchy, every employee tends to rise to their level of incompetence (Peter and Hull 2011). While promotion of an athletic trainer to managerial leadership does not in and of itself mean the person will fail as a leader, taking on a position that requires a very different set of skills—and that tends to affect a greater number of staff members—is a challenge that can easily be underestimated.

PEARLS OF MANAGEMENT

Athletic trainers can perform their managerial responsibilities best when they exercise leadership with the authority provided by their superiors. Both leadership and authority represent a certain kind of power that all athletic trainers have as a benefit of their position and expertise.

KEY POINT

The Peter Principle states that in any organizational hierarchy, an individual will rise to his or her level of incompetence. This means that taking on additional responsibilities may come about in the absence of appropriate preparatory training and education.

Power

Scholars who devote their careers to the study of power do not agree on a precise definition, but the one most inclusive of the research done on the subject was put forth by Bass (2008) and remains commonplace today. **Power** is the potential to influence.

Why is it important for students of athletic training administration to be able to define, recognize, and use power? Power is the glue that binds people or groups in a relationship. It is the basis for both authority and leadership. Athletic trainers have significant power in their relationships with coaches, administrators, clients, and other health care professionals. Athletic trainers can exercise power over those above them, below them, and at the same level in an organization. The two primary modalities for the exercise of organizational power are **position power** and **personal power**.

Position Power

Athletic trainers, by virtue of their positions, have resources they can use to influence the behavior of others in their organizations. Someone who supervises athletic training students, for example, can influence their behavior through the use of rewards and punishments, such as grades, financial aid, work–study money, desirable team assignments, and internship placements. In an organization that follows a medical chain of command, the athletic trainer can use the power provided by that policy to change the behavior of a coach who may want to usurp the athletic trainer's medical authority.

In 1981, the ability to influence the behavior of a superior was originally termed **counterpower** (Yukl 2012). Counterpower is a tool that most athletic trainers need because they are typically viewed as support personnel who are less important than other organizational decision makers. Without counterpower, athletic trainers would be little more than technical consultants to more powerful coaches and athletic administrators, unable to influence the actions of those two important groups.

Personal Power

The athletic trainer's ability to influence others in the organization often depends more on personal characteristics and personality attributes than it does on formal authority. Indeed, athletic trainers who use charisma and personal appeal to influence others in their organizations are more likely to receive acceptance and support for their ideas. Coercive power and authoritarian methods, on the other hand, are more likely to produce mere compliance, decreasing satisfaction and performance levels among the staff members whom these athletic trainers supervise (Yukl 2012).

One of the most effective elements of athletic trainers' personal power is their reputation as experts. People are likely to follow the recommendation of someone they perceive as an expert (Fisher 2015). Athletic trainers make judgments every day based on their expertise in sports medicine. Athletes and other physically active clients who follow the treatment plan outlined by an athletic trainer probably have faith in the athletic trainer as an expert. When they fail to follow their treatment and rehabilitation plans, they may have lost faith in the expertise of the athletic trainer supervising their programs. In these cases, the athletic trainer must resort to position power as the basis for achieving compliance. Unfortunately, using the external motivators of position power is rarely as effective as using the internal motivators of personal power.

It should also be noted that one's expertise in health care is often influenced by one's "bedside manner" and interpersonal skills. It has been said that people do not care how much you know, until they know how much you care. This statement can be directly applied to an athletic training setting. That is, if an athletic trainer is extremely knowledgeable with her assessment and rehabilitation skills but is abrupt and curt with a client, the client may not place trust in the interaction and may not be motivated toward compliance. On the other hand, if an athletic trainer is courteous, does not appear to be rushed, and finds time to allow the client to ask questions regarding his injury, the client will likely place a higher level of trust in the athletic trainer and comply with whatever advice he receives. We see these types of exchanges whenever we visit a physician's office. Regardless of the prestige displayed by wall plaques in a medical office, the provider–client exchange will likely determine the client's level of satisfaction and the client's ultimate perception of the provider's expertise.

Authority

Authority is the aspect of power, granted to either groups or individuals, that legitimizes the right of the group or individual to make decisions on behalf of others. If power is the glue that binds people or groups together in a relationship, then authority is the applicator through which power is exercised. Without authority, athletic trainers would lack position power. One example of authority granted to collegiate athletic trainers was the National Collegiate Athletic Association's major conference approving a rule in 2016 that gave school medical professionals (e.g., athletic trainers and physicians) complete authority and autonomy from others in determining when an athlete may return to play following a concussion (Chicago Tribune 2016).

Another characteristic implicit in this definition of authority is that it involves decision making and is therefore action oriented. Like its parent, power, authority can be observed only when it is exercised. Athletic trainers are called on to make many administrative decisions during the course of a typical day: Should I order more tape? How should I arrange the team physician's injury clinic schedule? How many athletic trainers will I need to cover the wrestling tournament? Athletic trainers exercise the authority that they have been granted when they answer these questions with action. Indeed, many of their administrative problems stem from hesitation to use their authority.

One notable exception exists to the action orientation normally associated with authority. Some situations call for the athletic trainer to exercise authority by making a conscious decision *not* to act. While athletic trainers will face many dilemmas in any single job, each one should be assessed individually on its merits before being acted on. The common statement "It's not worth the battle" sums up a situation that is best left alone and not pursued further. Another common statement, "It is better to say nothing than say the wrong thing," summarizes the best approach on many occasions. The athletic trainer's use of authority can be a powerful tool to prompt the accomplishment of a task. Authority provides a new athletic trainer an immediate power base to help her accomplish tasks. This circumstance is sometimes referred to as the **honeymoon effect**. Newly hired people in athletic training programs are often granted more authority to make decisions than they will be six months or a year after arrival. The honeymoon effect is an important factor in rejuvenating programs. Without it, new athletic trainers would have less effect because they wouldn't be able to implement new ideas as easily.

Athletic trainers who serve in leadership roles should be careful not to overuse their authority. Doing so may yield the requested level of task-related compliance absent sincere and dedicated efforts. Athletic trainers who rely too heavily on their authority are likely to find that their staff responds with mere compliance and minimal effort. The athletic trainer who constantly reminds his assistants that he is the boss might be successful in extracting a modest amount of work from the assistants, but he is also likely to experience a high rate of turnover. Athletic trainers who rely heavily on authority are also likely to find that their subordinates try to avoid them. The threat, perceived or real, that an authoritarian supervisor will impose negative sanctions against subordinates is a common theme, even for athletic trainers who have no rational basis for their perceptions.

Leadership

Leadership is the process of influencing the behavior and attitudes of others to achieve intended outcomes. There are nearly as many definitions of leadership as there are scholars who have studied the topic—more than 130 distinct definitions exist (Helmrich 2016). One of the few common denominators among this host of definitions is the assumption that leadership involves an intentional influence process by a leader over followers (Yukl 2012). In addition, leadership is success oriented. If a "leader" attempts an action and doesn't gain the support of followers, has leadership really taken place?

Why is a discussion of leadership important for athletic trainers? The exercise of leadership is the keystone of managerial success. Without the ability to influence attitudes and behaviors toward a predetermined goal, the athletic trainer is an ineffective agent for change in her organization. Unfortunately, we often think of leaders as people on the national or international stage. Churchill, Gandhi, and Roosevelt were certainly effective leaders. The more common form of leadership, however, is a local phenomenon. Leaders surround all of us in our homes, churches, and communities and in the sports medicine settings in which we work. Without leadership, the organizations that employ us would stagnate and cease to be effective in providing needed services to clients.

Athletic trainers can better appreciate the importance of effective leadership and the effect it can have on their managerial success by understanding the two types of leadership found in most social structures, including organizations that employ athletic trainers. Leadership can take two distinct forms (Surbhi 2015):

1. Transactional leadership
2. Transformational leadership

Transactional Leadership

Transactional leadership involves the simple exchange of one thing for another in a relationship between two people. An athletic trainer pays her assistants in exchange for work. An athletic director agrees to send an athletic trainer to a conference in exchange for covering a state high school basketball tournament. Most administrative activities in organizations in which athletic trainers work involve the transactional form of leadership. However, if your leadership style focuses solely on transactional behaviors, you will not get the most out of your team. A program or organization in which only transactional leadership takes place will probably not thrive.

Transformational Leadership

Organizational renewal and program improvement require transformational leadership. **Transformational leadership** transcends the day-to-day administrative requirements of operating an athletic training program by elevating standards through the creative use of change and conflict. The athletic trainer who can successfully prepare budgets, hire staff, purchase supplies, and schedule personnel is an effective transactional leader. The athletic trainer who recognizes the need to reduce the incidence of eating disorders among his athletes and who implements programs that successfully accomplish this task exhibits transformational leadership.

Transformational leadership usually involves change in the organization. This change is likely to engender some degree of conflict. Consider the example of setting up an eating disorders program. Such programs cost money. Instructional materials must be developed or purchased. Group facilitators and therapists must be contracted for. Funding will have to come either from existing programs or be raised specifically for the project. Making decisions about these issues often brings athletic trainers into conflict with coaches and athletic administrators who are in competition for scarce financial resources. The athletic trainer who is a skilled transformational leader will be able to manage the conflict to meet the needs of coaches, athletic administrators, and the athletes with eating disorders. As you can see, the transformational aspect of leadership is both challenging and essential if an athletic training program is to meet the changing needs of its clients.

Transformational leaders are typically charismatic, but their effectiveness is closely related to them "walking the walk." They exhibit high ethical and moral standards in all aspects of their lives. They also demonstrate genuine interest in developing their employees. They put the needs of their staff above their own to help them feel satisfied at work. This is accomplished by taking the time to get to know each member of the staff to determine what their goals are and how to best motivate them. Transformational leaders help to develop leadership qualities in others so that everyone can move up together. They trust their employees to take on significant projects that offer intellectual challenges. These leaders work with the team to develop goals for the future as well as the plan to achieve those goals. By placing the focus of success on the individuals in the organization, those individuals will then work harder for the organization. Transformational leaders have more satisfied employees and experience lower attrition rates than those who focus more on transactional leadership practices (Surbhi 2015).

Modern Management Theories

Starting the 1950s, many theorists have devoted entire careers to the study of management. One such theorist was Kurt Lewin (Gillies 1994). His field theory of human behavior posits that employee actions in the workplace are the product of three interacting variables: employee personality, workgroup structure, and sociotechnical climate. Lewin believed that influencing employees to change their behavior (and thereby improve productivity and efficiency) involved three phases:

1. *Unfreezing.* Creating motivation for a change in behavior, either by applying pressure or by reducing threats associated with the change
2. *Changing.* Modifying behavior by either mimicking a role model or learning new behaviors through a discovery process
3. *Refreezing.* Integrating the new behavior into the workplace with constant reinforcement from others

Imagine a situation in which a relatively young and inexperienced university athletic trainer repeatedly made the mistake of leaving the athletic training students assigned to him in unsupervised situations. As this athletic trainer's supervisor, you would be responsible for enforcing the program policy of requiring supervision of students at all times. Using Lewin's theories, you might employ a three-stage strategy to make sure that this happened.

First, you would attempt to unfreeze the athletic trainer's behavior. You might accomplish this in several ways, including education and familiarization with institutional and accrediting agency rules. You could also employ threats of sanctions. ("Student supervision is one of your most important jobs. I can't recommend a raise or a favorable performance review if you continue to leave the students unsupervised.")

Next, you would attempt to change the athletic trainer's behavior by providing him with a copy of the institutional and accrediting agency rules. You might also ask him to shadow you for a day in your work environment so that he can learn how you successfully integrate your clinical and educational roles. The final step in the process would be to refreeze the appropriate behavior by praising the athletic trainer when you see him providing supervision of student clinical activities. Better yet, you might ask a few of the students to thank him for sharing his time and expertise.

As far back as 1960, social psychologist Douglas McGregor proposed a new conception of human nature in the workplace with his Theory X and Theory Y. Theory X represented the traditional view of humans at work. Under Theory X, workers were assumed to be inherently lazy, avoiding work whenever possible. Theory X assumes that workers prefer to be directed by others and that their primary concern is financial reward rather than self-improvement. Because of these qualities, Theory X postulates that workers must be coerced to perform their jobs well. Theory Y, on the other hand, holds that work is a natural activity and is as necessary as rest or play. If a person is committed to a task, she will require little direction to accomplish her goals. The belief that workers naturally learn to seek out and accept responsibility is also a tenet of Theory Y. Finally, Theory Y hypothesizes that most people have the capacity to solve organizational problems and that this ability is not the sole province of managers.

Most of us can probably think of supervisors we have worked for who were from either the Theory X or the Theory Y school of thought. Athletic trainers who anticipate moving into a management role should contemplate which set of assumptions they agree with most closely. If your management style is predominantly Theory X and your supervisees are predominantly Theory Y, workplace friction is likely to be a problem. Similarly, if you are new to your supervisory role and your staff was previously led by a supervisor with a contrasting set of assumptions about the nature of work and workers, you should expect a difficult period of transition.

The most interesting and important trend in management theory and practice in modern times is the application of W. Edwards Deming's management principles to the industrial workforce in post–World War II Japan. Deming's ideas form the cornerstone of the **Total Quality Management (TQM)** movement, which is still popular in organizations all over the world. Deming taught the importance of a clear focus on the mission of an organization and the need for management to demonstrate continuous commitment to this mission and to communicate it to everyone in the organization. He believed that trust and rewarding innovation were two important elements of organizational improvement. Education and self-improvement for people at every level of an organization are fundamental. Total Quality Management is a popular management philosophy in health care organizations. Athletic trainers who work in hospitals are likely to find themselves involved in TQM at an early stage in their careers.

The Japanese took Deming's ideas and integrated them with the particular characteristics of their culture to create one of the most powerful, efficient, and productive workforces in history. This development was based on six central managerial concepts (Gillies 1994).

1. The primary trait desired in potential employees is the quality of their character. The training they will need to perform their jobs can be delivered in-house.

2. Employees develop a close personal identification with the organization because they are employed for life. Although lifelong employment as a national norm is eroding in Japan, the concept of making an employee feel part of an organizational family is a sound one.

3. The Japanese believe that career progress should be steady but slow. Employees should

work in many departments before moving into managerial positions.

4. Decision making in Japanese companies is a collective process. Members of the work group all have input into organizational decisions. The group is more valued than the individual.

5. A culture of continuous improvement based on the needs of clients is of overriding importance.

6. Japanese companies practice the Asian cultural tradition of saving face by supporting and moving unproductive employees around the organization until they become successful.

Three Management Roles

Management is the element of the leadership process that involves planning, decision making, and coordinating the activities of a group of people working toward a common goal. Athletic trainers' regular management activities include scheduling, purchasing, hiring, evaluating, developing programs, accounting, and many others. In his classic text on the science of management, Fayol (1949) defined the following five elements of management: (1) planning, (2) organizing, (3) command, (4) coordination, and (5) control. Gulick and Urwick (1977) added staffing, directing, reporting, and budgeting to Fayol's original list.

Mintzberg (1973) described three major types of roles that all managers, including athletic trainers, assume from time to time:

1. Interpersonal
2. Informational
3. Decisional

PEARLS OF MANAGEMENT

Athletic trainers in managerial positions have to assume three types of roles as part of their jobs: interpersonal, informational, and decisional. Each type of role is complex and is made up of multiple components.

Interpersonal Roles

Every athletic trainer who manages a department or program will probably be forced to assume three different **interpersonal roles** at one time or another. The first is the **figurehead role**. As the person who has been granted formal authority for a particular program, the athletic trainer will be called on to perform certain routine functions such as providing signatures, speaking publically, and answering requests for information. The figurehead role is often the most visible managerial task that the athletic trainer will undertake. Although it is probably not as vital to the long-term health of the program as other managerial roles, the figurehead role is important because of the public relations value that it can yield.

The second managerial role the athletic trainer must assume is that of a leader. We have already discussed transactional and transformational leadership.

The third managerial role the athletic trainer must assume is that of liaison. The **liaison role** is an important part of the athletic trainer's success or failure as a manager. Athletic trainers must work with a variety of people to run a successful athletic training program (figure 2.1). Although vertical liaison with coworkers above and below him in the organization is commonly understood to be a function of the athletic trainer, horizontal liaison with professional peers is vital to developing and maintaining goodwill between the athletic training program and other departments of the organization and between the program and outside entities. Mintzberg (1973) hypothesized that social equals tend to interact with one another more often than they do with superiors or subordinates. Thus, athletic trainers need to develop relationships with athletic trainers at other institutions, health professionals in the community, coaches, consulting

physicians, and parents. All these people will have an effect on the athletic trainer's managerial success.

Informational Roles

The first **informational role** an athletic trainer plays is that of both a **monitor** and a **disseminator** of information. The athletic training program is constantly bombarded by information from a variety of sources on a variety of topics. Journals and trade publications present news of technological advances in preventing and treating athletic injuries. Newsletters and memoranda route organizational news and policy changes. Progress reports and clinical notes arrive in the mail from team and consulting physicians. The first response of the effective athletic trainer-manager is to filter the information. Is it appropriate to share a memo with the staff? Who needs to know about the complications of someone's knee surgery? Athletic trainers in a variety of employment settings decide these and similar choices daily.

After deciding what information should be passed along and to whom it should be passed, the athletic trainer must decide how to deliver it in a timely, efficient, and effective manner. Some items can be posted on a bulletin board where the staff can scan the information at their leisure. Other items require more explanation and documentation and should therefore be put in writing and delivered individually. This process is especially important if the information is confidential or if it is necessary

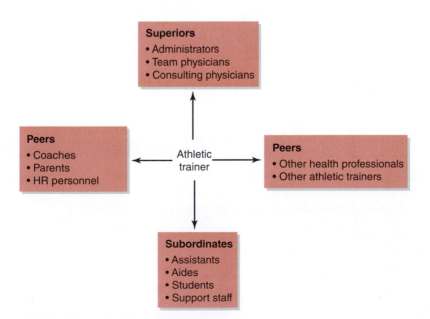

Figure 2.1 Liaison relationships of the athletic trainer.

to document that the information was actually passed along. For example, if an athletic trainer is not performing up to the standards set by the organization, it would be important to communicate these concerns in writing to keep them confidential and to document that the institution had warned the athletic trainer of dissatisfaction with her work.

Oral Communication

To be effective in the role of monitor and disseminator of information, the athletic trainer must both understand and be skilled at communicating with everyone in the organization. Oral communication is one of the primary modes of disseminating information in an organization. Three elements influence the process of oral communication (Drafke 2002):

1. The meaning of the sender
2. The meaning of the receiver
3. Interference between the sender and receiver

Unfortunately, these three elements often interact in a way that impedes effective communication. How often have you said something to someone only to learn that the person was offended either by the way you said it or by the context in which the message was delivered? This becomes even more of an issue with electronic communication, such as e-mails and texts.

Interference in the communication process is a common problem. Noisy or distracting work environments can cause interference. Interference is also inherent in the methods used to transmit a message from one person to another. For example, because a written message does not usually allow for immediate feedback or clarification, the potential for interference using that method is quite high. Face-to-face communications, on the other hand, allow for greater interaction between the parties and therefore have a much lower potential for interference. Information filtered through a third party is the method most likely to result in corruption of the original message, because it is subject to interference at more than one step of the process. Because of the potential for altered meaning caused by interference in various communication methods, Drafke (2002) ranks the following methods in terms of their effectiveness:

1. Face-to-face communication
2. Telecommunication
3. Written communication
4. Communication through a third party

A note on Drafke's ranking is appropriate. As previously mentioned, written communication serves an important purpose in helping to document that communication actually occurred. Although sitting down with a colleague to discuss an issue in a quiet, calm environment has certain advantages, much of the benefit of this method is lost if the environment becomes noisy or uncomfortable. Written communications also have the advantage of allowing the sender to make careful choices about the words used to convey the message. A good strategy is to work through issues in a face-to-face meeting, but then follow up with an e-mail to document what was agreed to. This takes advantage of the strengths of both types of communication.

Listening Skills

An important aspect of successful two-way communication involves what is referred to as active listening. Athletic trainers spend abundant amounts of time listening to others: coaches, athletes, and

---

Methods for Effective Communication

As a monitor and disseminator of information, you need to use appropriate communication tools. Keep in mind important issues such as efficiency, necessity for documentation, and confidentiality when choosing a method. Several methods of communication can be effective:

Bulletin boards   Telephone calls

Staff meetings   Electronic mail

Individual meetings   Text message alerts

Letters and memos   Web pages

Newsletters

Levels of Listening

1. *Analytical.* Listening for specific kinds of information
2. *Directed.* Listening to be able to answer specific questions
3. *Attentive.* Listening for general information in order to obtain an overview
4. *Exploratory.* Listening because of one's own interest
5. *Appreciative.* Listening for pleasure
6. *Courteous.* Listening as a result of feeling obligated
7. *Passive.* Listening in an inattentive manner

staff. Active listening involves a total effort and attention given to a message (Konin 1997). Of greatest significance is that the listener does not have a preconceived outcome for the verbal exchange and instead approaches the conversation with an open mind. One key to verifying successful active listening skills is to simply repeat back a portion of the conversation to the other party. For example, if an athlete asks you whether you think he will be ready to return to play within the next week, you can respond by saying, "Do I think you will be ready to play within the next week? There is a good possibility that if your healing continues at the pace it has been going thus far and you remain compliant with your exercises, you may be able to play before the end of the week." If your response was merely, "I'm not sure," the athlete may not feel as though you listened or even cared about what he was saying. Smith (1975) has described levels of listening skills that can be adapted for athletic trainers to use as a guide for improved communication. Different circumstances may warrant the use of different approaches and techniques for active listening.

PEARLS OF MANAGEMENT

Active listening requires one to provide undivided attention to the messenger without having a preconceived thought about what one wants or expects to hear.

One level athletic trainers often use is **analytical listening**. This happens every time an athletic trainer takes a medical history from a client and listens for specific kinds of information to be conveyed. For example, if you were taking a medical history from a soccer player who recently injured her knee, you would listen for key words such as *pop* or *twist* and associate such words with a ligament

or meniscus injury. This is not preconceived listening because you may also hear other words such as *grinding* or *squeaking*, and you might associate such terms with a patellofemoral malalignment. Therefore, you are technically being open minded in your listening approach.

Nonverbal Communication

The most important modifiers of an intended message are usually nonverbal elements of that message. Nonverbal cues can function in a variety of ways to alter a message. Gestures and body position can reinforce an oral message, or they can contradict it. See the sidebar for a list of nonverbal communication cues that you should be aware of (Drafke 2002).

The **spokesperson role** is the third informational role that athletic trainers assume. Mintzberg (1973) points out that effective managers must keep two important groups informed. The first group includes the organizational decision makers, also known as **internal influencers**. Internal influencers are people who either are members of or have close ties to an organization and who have the power to help shape policy and practice. Here are examples of internal influencers in various settings where sports medicine programs operate:

- *High school.* Coaches, team physicians, athletic directors, principals, central office administrators, board of education members
- *College and university.* Coaches, athletic administrators, other university administrators, team physicians, trustees
- *Clinic.* Clinic owners, hospital administrators, referring physicians, hospital trustees, supervisors
- *Professional athletics.* Coaches, general managers, other club administrators, owners, team physicians

Nonverbal Communication Cues

- *Clothing and grooming.* Neat, well-fitting clothes and grooming that conforms to cultural norms often send a message of competence and control.
- *Territoriality.* A culturally accepted distance is usually 24 to 40 inches (60 to 100 cm) in the United States when addressing a colleague. Meetings that take place in the manager's office are often intended to be more formal, serious, or important.
- *Posture and facial expression.* Crossed arms or a body orientation facing away from a person indicates anger, impatience, or boredom. A fixed gaze with a scowl indicates anger or disagreement. Avoiding eye contact often indicates guilt or embarrassment. Long, uncomfortable stares may be seen as intimidating.
- *Gestures.* Finger tapping expresses boredom. A closed fist or a pointing index finger can indicate anger. A polite handshake indicates receptiveness.

The second group an athletic trainer should communicate with in his role as spokesperson is the organization's public. Like internal influencers, the members of the sports medicine program's public will vary by setting. Common to each setting are clients (physically active patients, athletes, student-athletes), suppliers, community supporters (members of booster clubs, parents, fans, members of alumni groups), consulting health professionals, and the news media. The athletic trainer will communicate with each of these groups from time to time, taking on the role of the organization's expert in sports medicine. The expert spokesperson role is a source of considerable personal power for the athletic trainer.

Decisional Roles

The last group of roles that athletic trainers must assume as part of their managerial responsibilities is probably the most important; it is made up of **decisional roles**. Decisional roles require the athletic trainer to use both personal and position power by exercising authority. The effective athletic trainer-manager will also use decisional roles to exercise transformational leadership by planning strategies to serve clients better.

KEY POINT

The four decisional roles are entrepreneur, disturbance handler, allocator of resources, and negotiator.

The first decision-making role assumed by the athletic trainer is an **entrepreneurial role**. Although most of us envision an entrepreneur as someone who creates new businesses, the term refers here to an athletic trainer who designs and initiates changes for her programs and organizations. If the athletic trainer fails in this entrepreneurial role, the sports medicine program will probably stop improving. One of the ways athletic trainers can become entrepreneurs for the sports medicine program is by focusing on small, solvable problems and new opportunities and initiating improvements in both areas. All athletic trainers could probably come up with a list of 10 to 15 concrete steps that would improve their programs. Athletic trainers could also improve their programs by taking advantage of some of the opportunities they face. The key is the ability to make decisions about which changes to implement based on what is feasible.

Being entrepreneurial does not require one to possess a Master of Business Administration degree. People possessing entrepreneurial-like skills can be described as having the five Ds: desire, diligence, (grasp of) details, determination, and discipline. Furthermore, generally speaking, entrepreneurs are highly competitive, tend to possess a liking for social environments, and believe strongly in organization and planning. A strong argument can be made that these same characteristics are necessary for success in any athletic training setting.

The second decision-making role involves the athletic trainer as **disturbance handler**. Disturbances requiring the attention and intervention of the athletic trainer usually revolve around conflict. The role of conflict manager is often a difficult and uncomfortable one for athletic trainers for several reasons. First, conflict usually involves change. Controlled change is a necessary ingredient for healthy program and organizational growth. Unfortunately, such change often occurs with human costs attached.

The third decision-making role played by an athletic trainer is **allocator of resources**. The athletic trainer generally has formal authority to determine how time, money, supplies, equipment, and personnel should be deployed. If the athletic trainer-manager does not have this authority, frustration and managerial apathy are likely to result. The final managerial role that an athletic trainer assumes is the role of **negotiator**. The athletic trainer negotiates on behalf of the organization he represents. Thus, the negotiator role is a combination of several roles, including the figurehead, the resource allocator, and the spokesperson (Mintzberg 1973). Although someone closer to the top of the organizational structure usually ratifies most arrangements negotiated by the athletic trainer on behalf of the organization, the athletic trainer must be granted enough authority to enter into meaningful discussions with another party. Typical arrangements negotiated by athletic trainers include prices for supplies and services, sponsorship for various activities, involvement with development and fund-raising efforts, and grants for specific programs.

Improving Managerial Effectiveness

Leaders usually, but not always, exercise authority by making legitimate requests. In response, staff might commit, comply, or resist. Athletic trainers can use many methods to decrease the likelihood of resistance and increase the possibility of commitment (Yukl 2012). When making requests of subordinates, athletic trainers should take the following positive steps to ensure commitment.

- *Be courteous and respectful.* Avoid emphasizing differences in status, intelligence, financial responsibility, and other factors related to rank. Statements such as "I'm the boss," "You work for me," or "Do it or else" might accomplish short-term

employee compliance but is not the best approach to building long-term relationships.

- *Radiate confidence.* If the leader communicates doubt through verbal or nonverbal cues, the staff is unlikely to comply with enthusiasm. By saying "Don't worry; I'll get this mess straightened out," a leader can instill confidence in an employee's mind.

- *Use simple language.* When instructions must necessarily be complicated, be sure that subordinates understand *them*. Inexperienced leaders often make the mistake of using excessively technical terminology as a way to demonstrate their position power.

- *Make reasonable requests.* Test requests for legitimacy by consulting with coworkers above you or at the same level in the organization. Referring to formally approved policies, rules, and negotiated agreements can help legitimize requests.

- *Provide rationale.* Providing reasons for your request will help reduce the perceived status gap between you and your staff. It is always best to have facts, statistics, or data to support proposals, policies, or other requests.

- *Use the chain of command.* Following established lines of communication decreases the possibility of message distortion. Make requests in writing whenever possible. Failing to follow a chain of command of communication can lead to confusion and difficult circumstances, not to mention the perception of disrespect and insubordination.

- *Use authority regularly.* If you make legitimate requests regularly, your staff will be less likely to resist. If you continuously back away from issues that require decisions based on authority, employees will grow accustomed to that mode of decision making.

- *Exercise authority to confirm task accomplishment.* If you do not demand compliance for legitimate requests, future noncompliance is more likely. If you ask an employee to do something and the employee doesn't do it, and then you take no action, all employees will soon figure out that you are a pushover and a weak leader.

- *Be open minded.* Staff members who consider their leader a heartless automaton with no concern for their ideas or feelings are unlikely to respond to requests with enthusiasm. If you listen to your employees' concerns with genuine interest and act on those concerns whenever possible, you are much more likely to gain their trust and respect.

PEARLS OF MANAGEMENT

Successful athletic trainer-managers will be able to elicit commitment from their subordinates and coworkers if they are courteous, confident, and open minded. Athletic trainers must also use simple language, make reasonable requests, and explain their requests. Finally, they must use their authority regularly, especially to confirm task accomplishment.

Summary

The role of the athletic trainer in a health care arena requires skills beyond those that incorporate only a clinical knowledge base. Athletic trainers in all practice settings need to understand the concept of leadership and the principles associated with power and authority. Athletic trainers will often take on managerial roles and tasks in the absence of prior formal preparation or training. Strategies that include timely and effective communication, efficiency, and attention to detail can contribute to an athletic trainer's managerial style. Communication is a critical part of ensuring teamwork and productivity. Rapidly changing technology has enhanced the options available for communication. Additionally, interpersonal skills remain important for both verbal and nonverbal human interactions. How one communicates as a leader and a manager can be just as important as the content of the message itself. Being an effective manager and leader also requires the ability to plan, organize, and coordinate multiple tasks simultaneously. Ultimately, an athletic training manager possesses the responsibility for decision making that determines the outcomes of circumstances. Athletic training managers should make such decisions while incorporating a reliable foundational process, taking into consideration all stakeholders who would be affected by a managerial decision.

Learning Aids

Case Study 1

During the second half of a National Collegiate Athletic Association (NCAA) Division III tournament soccer game, the goalkeeper of the host team was involved in a collision and fell to the ground in pain. Julie, the school's athletic trainer, evaluated the injury on the field and determined that the goalkeeper, who was unable to run or cut and could walk only with a pronounced limp, had suffered a grade 2 ankle sprain. Julie decided to remove the player from the game based on three factors: The athlete could not perform without significant dysfunction, the team had another game in a few days and the athletic trainer wanted to begin immediate treatment in preparation, and the team was winning the game by two goals and appeared to be in control.

As Julie helped the goalkeeper from the field, the coach jogged out to meet them and asked the athlete how he felt. When he replied that his ankle was injured but not too badly, the coach said it was the athlete's decision whether to keep playing. Julie interjected, telling the coach that she thought further play would jeopardize a rapid recovery. The coach looked again at the athlete and said that the decision was his. The athlete replied that he would try to continue. Julie again tried to express her opposition, but the athlete was already limping back to the goal and the coach was leaving the field.

Julie was confused, upset, and incensed that the coach would usurp her authority in the matter. The athletic department had a medical chain-of-command procedure that clearly authorized the team physician, or the athletic trainer in the physician's absence, to make decisions about playing status for injured athletes. Julie wasn't sure what she could have done to change the outcome.

Questions for Analysis

1. How do the concepts of power and authority apply to this case? Who had power, and how was it used? What was the basis for this power? Who had authority, and how was it used?

2. What might Julie have done differently (either before or during the incident) to prevent the situation?

3. What should Julie do now? What are some ways she can improve managerial effectiveness? Is there only one correct solution, or do several possibilities exist?

Case Study 2

After interviewing for a job in a large Texas high school, Mateo, a certified athletic trainer with 17 years of experience, decided he would accept the job offer. His primary reason for accepting the job was that he was burned out in NCAA Division I athletics. He thought that the high school position would give him contact with athletes, an aspect of his work that he enjoyed, without the headaches of running a major university sports medicine program.

Mateo arrived in Texas in June to allow plenty of time to organize his new program before the athletes came back in August. During the first week on the job, he began to realize that he should have asked a few questions during his interview. Although the sports medicine program had an adequate budget, Mateo could not order equipment or supplies without the written permission of his athletic director. When Mateo presented a list of supplies needed for the next year, the AD approved only half the items. In addition, he told Mateo that he would have to purchase them from the local sporting goods dealer. Mateo complained that he needed all the items on the list and that if he purchased everything from the local vendor, the sports medicine budget would be spent before Christmas.

Another problem Mateo faced during the first few weeks concerned a drug and alcohol education program he proposed for student-athletes. Mateo wanted to involve all the coaches and team captains in a preliminary workshop and then develop programs for individual teams. When he presented his plan, the AD smiled and said, "That kind of thing has been tried before and it didn't work. I don't see why it would work now. Besides, we don't have any serious problems like that in our school."

When the athletes arrived in August, Mateo quickly gained a reputation as a caring and competent athletic trainer. Injured athletes came to know him as someone who would take good care of them and who could help them return to action as soon as possible. The coaches also appreciated Mateo's talents and expertise. They liked the way he communicated with them and appreciated his hard work in keeping their teams healthy.

Questions for Analysis

1. In what ways did the honeymoon effect work for Mateo in his new job? In what ways didn't it work?

2. Which of Mateo's early leadership actions were transactional? Which were transformational?

3. Which management roles did Mateo assume during his first few months on the job? Which were most important in helping him establish relationships with the various groups at his new school?

4. Mateo is obviously having trouble working with his new athletic director. Which strategies should he consider in attempting to work out his differences? Given the personality style of the AD, what are some likely outcomes of Mateo's conflict management attempts?

5. If you were in Mateo's position, would you have handled anything differently? What alternative actions would you have taken?

Key Concepts and Review

Define the concepts of power, authority, and leadership.

Power is the potential to influence. Athletic trainers hold two forms of power: personal and positional. Authority is that aspect of power, granted to either groups or individuals, that legitimizes the right of the individual or group to make decisions on behalf of others. Leadership is the process of influencing the behavior and attitudes of others to achieve intended outcomes. Leadership takes two forms: transactional and transformational. Transactional leadership involves the exchange of one thing for another between two people in a relationship. It makes up the majority of managerial tasks that athletic trainers perform. Transformational leadership raises the standards of the program or organization through the creative use of conflict and change. It is essential for the ongoing health and development of a sports medicine program. Its focus is on developing people and building long-term relationships and trust.

Understand the historical trends in management and how they might apply to athletic training.

Various trends in management theory occurred in the 20th century. The primary goal of scientific management was to increase productivity. Modern management theories include Lewin's field theory, McGregor's Theory X and Theory Y, and Deming's Total Quality Management.

Understand the various managerial roles that athletic trainers assume.

Management is the element of the leadership process that involves planning, decision making, and coordinating the activities of a group of people working toward a common goal. Athletic trainers play many managerial roles, which can be generalized into three groups: interpersonal, informational (which includes elements of both verbal and nonverbal communication), and decisional roles.

Understand the various strategies that athletic trainers can employ to improve their managerial effectiveness.

Athletic trainers can improve their managerial effectiveness by using nine techniques: making polite requests, making requests in a confident tone, making clear requests, making legitimate requests, explaining the reasons for the request, using proper channels, exercising authority regularly, insisting on compliance, and being responsive to concerns of subordinates.

3

Program Management

Objectives

After reading this chapter, you should be able to do the following:

- Understand and develop vision and mission statements for a sports medicine program.

- Understand the principles underlying sports medicine strategic planning.

- Develop and link sports medicine policies, processes, and procedures.

- Communicate and develop ownership in a sports medicine program among inside and outside stakeholders.

- Understand the principles of effective meeting and conference planning and management.

- Understand the principles of effective sports medicine program evaluation.

Whether you are employed in a high school, college, professional, industrial, corporate, or clinical setting, you are bound to face organizational changes at some point in your career. These changes force us to examine our sports medicine programs from time to time to see whether they are still consistent with both the planning of our patient care and the mission of the institution that employs us. The concepts discussed in this chapter will help athletic trainers plan, implement, and evaluate sports medicine programs, as well as make the necessary and timely changes required to effectively manage a program.

Vision Statements

The first step an athletic trainer must take when planning sports medicine programming is to develop a brief, succinct description of what the program should eventually become—a **vision statement**. The vision statement should be both ambitious and compelling (Block 2016). It should spell out the athletic trainer's hopes and aspirations for the program. An example of a vision statement for a fictitious hospital follows:

> *The Memorial Hospital Sports Medicine Outreach Program shall provide injury prevention, care, and rehabilitation services of recognized excellence to the high school students of Ashton County. Memorial Hospital is committed to becoming the leader in sports medicine services in the Ashton County area.*

The vision statement contains four distinct elements:

1. The statement identifies the provider of the service: Memorial Hospital.
2. It identifies the service to be provided: injury prevention, care, and rehabilitation.
3. It identifies the target clients: the high school students of Ashton County.
4. It includes a quality declaration that identifies aspirations for how internal and external audiences will receive the program.

Although these elements might seem self-evident, they are important because of the way they function in the next step—the mission statement. The vision statement should become the ultimate standard by which the program is judged. Without a clearly articulated vision statement, developing the program mission and evaluating the effectiveness of the program become much more difficult. As programs evolve over time, managers must consider modifying the goals associated with the program's vision statement, or in some cases changing the vision statement to adapt to necessary changes in the program.

Four Elements of the Sports Medicine Program Vision Statement

1. Name of the service provider
2. Description of the service to be provided
3. Identification of the target clients
4. Quality declaration

Mission Statements

After the athletic trainer has explored and identified her vision for the sports medicine program, she should expand on this vision and create a mission statement. A **mission statement** broadly defines an organization's core purpose and function. It is a statement of purpose and normally remains unchanged for an extended period of time. Gibson, Newton, and Cochran (1990) have suggested the following components of a mission statement. Adapted for a sports medicine program, they include

- the particular services to be offered, the primary market for those services, and the technology to be used in delivery of the services;
- the goals of the program;
- the philosophy of the program and the code of behavior that applies to its operation;
- the "self-concept" of the program based on evaluation of strengths and weaknesses; and
- the desired program image based on feedback from internal and external stakeholders.

The mission statement for a sports medicine program should help an athletic trainer accomplish three things (Gibson, Newton, and Cochran 1990). First, the mission statement should help the athletic trainer direct resources toward accomplishing specific tasks. This aspect is especially important because athletic trainers are often called on to perform a variety of tasks for a divergent group of supervisors. Athletic trainers need a framework within which they can make decisions about the relative importance of one task versus another.

The second function of the successful mission statement is to inspire athletic trainers to do a good job. The mission statement should communicate that the work they do is important and needed. The athletic trainer should believe in the precepts described in the mission statement. A well-written mission statement assists the athletic training staff in better understanding the organization's core values, which in turn has the potential to increase staff commitment and retention.

Finally, the mission statement should be action oriented and should stimulate a change in behavior. The statement should require the formation of program goals and objectives. Ideally, it should challenge the athletic trainer to conduct a periodic evaluation of the effectiveness of the sports medicine program.

Based on these principles, the mission statement for the Memorial Hospital Sports Medicine Outreach Program might read as follows:

The Memorial Hospital Sports Medicine Outreach Program delivers traditional athletic training and sports medicine services to the student-athletes of the three high schools located in Ashton County. The services that we will deliver are of three primary types: injury prevention (taping, bracing, padding, orthotics construction), management of musculoskeletal injuries, and rehabilitation of musculoskeletal injuries. In addition, whenever possible, we will strive to integrate education about musculoskeletal injuries so that our clients can learn to lead healthier, injury-free lives. We are committed to using whatever technology is available and affordable in the delivery of these services. We will remain committed to the continuous upgrading of the equipment used in the delivery of sports medicine services so that our clients will receive the most modern care available in the area.

The purpose of the program is fourfold. First, we hope to allow easy access to sports medicine services for high school student-athletes. Second, we hope to encourage a philosophy of sport that places a high value on health and wellness. Third, we hope to enable injured student-athletes to return to their sports as soon as is medically safe. Finally, we hope to achieve a substantial reduction in the risk of musculosketal injury for high school students in our service area.

The underlying philosophy for the outreach program is the same as that for all other programs of Memorial Hospital; that is, the needs of the patient shall always be the first consideration for all members of the hospital staff. Furthermore, we expect the athletic trainers who will provide these services to maintain the highest standards of quality consistent with the Board of Certification's Standards of Professional Practice and the credentialing statutes of this state.

We are committed to ongoing evaluation of our outreach program so that our clients can be assured of the highest quality in sports medicine care. Furthermore, we are committed to address-

ing problems and concerns in a timely manner so that we can continue to meet the needs of our clients and employees.

Finally, the Memorial Hospital Sports Medicine Outreach Program aspires to be a program of recognized excellence. We intend to support the program with the human and financial resources necessary to accomplish the stated goals of the program. We desire to establish Memorial Hospital as the primary and most outstanding outlet for the delivery of sports medicine services in the area.

Planning

The athletic trainer has long been thought of as a jack-of-all-trades. Although athletic trainers' roles have become more specialized since sports medicine clinics began in the late 1970s, most athletic trainers still handle a variety of job-related activities (see figure 3.1). Because the athletic trainer's job has so many aspects, he must develop planning skills.

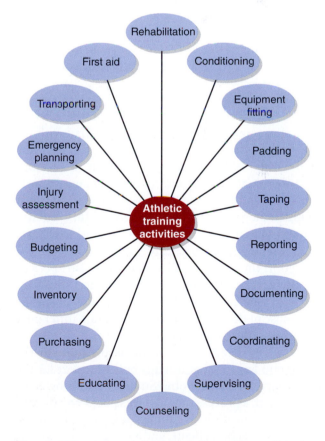

Figure 3.1 Job-related activities of the athletic trainer.

Planning is an athletic trainer's best hope for accomplishing sports medicine program goals. Without planning, she leaves the ultimate success or failure of the sports medicine program to chance.

PEARLS OF MANAGEMENT

Athletic trainers must engage in two kinds of planning to help their programs fulfill their mission: strategic and operational. Both are essential if a sports medicine program is to be successful.

Strategic Planning

Strategic planning is a process that identifies a course of action to be taken to bring about a future state of affairs. Although those at the top of an organizational structure usually conduct it, strategic planning at the program level can have many benefits.

First, strategic planning requires an athletic trainer to examine the sports medicine program and ask two questions: Why does this program exist? What should the business of this program be? These questions are fundamental. Because all organizations and their programs change, the questions must be asked and answered regularly, or athletic trainers might find that their sports medicine programs no longer serve the purposes for which they are most needed.

The second reason for ongoing strategic planning at the program level is to determine whether the sports medicine program is consistent with the overall mission of the institution or organization. This issue is especially important in institutions or organizations subject to rapid change. Sports medicine clinics based in hospitals are especially vulnerable to the shifting missions of their institutions. The mission of a professional athletic team often changes dramatically when a new coach is hired. If the sports medicine program isn't periodically reviewed for mission congruence, problems will arise because the administration might view the purpose of the sports medicine program differently than the athletic trainer does.

The third reason for strategic planning at the program level is that it helps build support for the sports medicine program. Strategic planning is, by definition, a process that involves people at all levels of the organization. By asking students, staff athletic trainers, coaches, clients, and administrators to take part in the strategic planning process, an athletic trainer will forge relationships with important allies with an increased sense of ownership in the sports medicine program. Furthermore, input from stakeholders can provide a breadth of knowledge compiled from an external perspective that may be overlooked by those directing and implementing a program.

Finally, strategic planning should be a tool for improvement, helping to determine the relative strengths and weaknesses of the program and to transform it positively. In addition, the strategic planning process will help direct operational plans that are more action oriented. Proponents of strategic planning suggest incorporating a strategic planning process that is performed regularly (at least every few years) and involves input from all stakeholders. Some organizations make the mistake of performing a strategic planning process only in the wake of adverse experiences or concerns.

Many conceptual models could be used to develop a strategic plan for the sports medicine program. Steiner (1979) describes a model that takes into consideration major outside interests and major inside interests that should always be considered within a strategic planning process.

Major Outside Interests

When developing a strategic plan, the first groups whose interests must be considered are those outside the institution or organization. Of these groups, the interests of clients should take precedence. Other important interests include those of parents; the local community; vendors; professional associations like the National Athletic Trainers' Association (NATA) and the National Collegiate Athletic Association (NCAA); and local, state, and federal governments. Professionals who manage athletic training education programs must be familiar with the Board of Certification (BOC) requirements and the standards of the Commission on Accreditation of Athletic Training Education (CAATE). In some cases, an athletic trainer will need only simple information from one of these groups. For example, if a program is in a state that monitors the credentials of athletic trainers, it is obvious that the program will need to be staffed by athletic trainers with the credentials required by law. Conversely, some of the information that the athletic trainer will need in order to develop the strategic plan might be more difficult to gather. For example, as important vendors of medical services, local physicians might have a substantial interest in how the sports medicine program is planned. Only by meeting with those physicians and involving them in the planning process can an athletic trainer be assured of their enthusiastic endorsement of the program being planned.

Major professional associations and the government are two important sources of information for assessing what outside interests are necessary for developing the strategic plan for the sports medicine program. Professional associations such as NATA, the NCAA, and the National Federation of State High School Athletic Associations (NFHS) are important because they are often the source of professional credentials that act as gatekeepers for practitioners in sports medicine and they mandate quality standards for sports medicine programs. The NCAA and the NFHS set the rules for each sport, including safety rules that affect athletic trainers and sports medicine programs. Both of these organizations have established rules for administering physical examinations that have a marked effect on sports medicine programs.

Clients   The most important group in the strategic planning process is the program's client base. Without patients, athletic trainers and sports medicine programs would be unnecessary. The athletic trainer can incorporate clients' perceptions into the strategic planning process in several ways, including the use of written questionnaires, telephone surveys, and suggestion boxes.

If the athletic trainer needs detailed insight, it might be necessary to involve clients as members of planning committees. Another method for securing detailed feedback from clients on the quality of services and their desire for future services is the focus group technique. This technique involves gathering a group of approximately 10 clients who are representative of the total population of clients. A trained facilitator meets with the group and asks a series of open-ended questions about program quality and the clients' desires for the future. This process is generally repeated with several different groups as a reliability check. The information is then collated and used to help build the strategic plan.

Gathering valid and reliable information from clients is not a task for the untrained. The literature is full of poorly written and poorly analyzed client-based questionnaires. Sampling methods and statistical analysis of the data must meet modern scientific norms. Athletic trainers can turn to several sources of assistance for this phase of the strategic plan. Most colleges and universities have faculty members with expertise in social science research who are willing to consult. Many larger educational institutions have full-time planners available to assist with projects like these. Most large hospitals have either full-time planners or contracts with management consultants to help in the development of the strategic plan. The skills required to adequately and appropriately collect reliable, valid, and valuable data should not be overlooked. One should be prepared to budget for potential consulting fees if the services of external reviewers or even internal faculty members are used. In any case, the amount of money budgeted on the front end may be well worth the investment compared to the potential costs associated with less-than-helpful data compiled as the result of inexperienced planning.

Accreditation   Among the most important outside interests a sports medicine program must consider is standards-setting groups that provide health care organizations or their programs with **accreditation**. Accreditation is a statement by a standards-setting organization that the sports medicine program meets certain performance standards. Although athletic training service programs associated with high schools, colleges, and universities are generally not accredited (except as part of their institution's overall accreditation by one of the regional educational accrediting agencies), sports medicine programs housed in clinics and hospitals will be

Methods for Gathering Feedback on Sports Medicine Services From Clients

- Written questionnaires
- Web-based surveys
- Telephone surveys
- Suggestion boxes
- Involvement on planning committees
- Focus groups
- Exit interviews

subject to the scrutiny of the accreditation process typically associated with those settings. Accreditation is usually voluntary, but strong incentives for a health care organization to become accredited are often in place. In some cases, the state license that an organization needs in order to operate is dependent on its accreditation status. Access to third-party reimbursement and managed care contracts is often easier if a health care organization is accredited by an appropriate standards-setting body.

Although the process for obtaining accreditation is similar for most standards-setting bodies (see the later section on program evaluation), the important element to remember during the strategic planning process is to build the goals, programs, and practices of the sports medicine program with accreditation standards in mind. Be aware that accreditation standards are usually minimalist in design. In other words, a particular standard usually describes the absolute minimum level of performance the sports medicine unit must achieve to satisfy the requirements of the standard. The danger in building a program around the accreditation standards is that the program might do things well, but at a minimally acceptable level. If outstanding performance is the goal, athletic trainers will have to look well beyond the minimal requirements of most accreditation standards. Those who plan clinic- and hospital-based sports medicine programs should consult two important accrediting agencies: the **Joint Commission** and **CARF International**.

The Joint Commission is the oldest and largest health care standards-setting body in the nation. It accredits approximately 15,000 health care organizations in the United States and has offered accreditation for ambulatory care facilities, including hospital-based and independent rehabilitation clinics, since 1975. Advantages of Joint Commission accreditation include the following:

- Provides objective evaluation of the program's performance
- Stimulates quality improvement
- Enhances community confidence
- Helps meet Medicare certification requirements
- Enhances access to third-party reimbursement
- Helps meet facility licensing requirements

Another accreditation agency that athletic trainers who work in clinics and hospitals should consider as they plan their programs is CARF International.

CARF International is a nonprofit agency that establishes standards of quality for rehabilitation services. Established in 1966, CARF International accredits approximately 38,000 programs. The agency offers accreditation for organizations that typically house sports medicine programs through its Medical Rehabilitation Division. Accreditation by CARF International is intended to

- offer consumer protection and enhance consumer confidence,
- involve consumers in developing standards for rehabilitation,
- promulgate common performance standards for rehabilitation programs,
- identify rehabilitation programs that have met national performance standards,
- improve government relations with the rehabilitation industry by offering evidence of effective use of public money for rehabilitation purposes, and
- provide rehabilitation facilities with tools for improvement.

Athletic training in settings such as high schools, colleges, and professional sports teams should use the Board of Certification's Facility Principles document (also available as an online resource) to determine whether the facility is meeting safety and compliance standards and best practices. The online resource allows athletic trainers to answer questions about their facility and produce a report showing where issues still need to be addressed. Maintaining compliance with these standards is an important step in reducing risk and liability.

Major Inside Interests

More and more athletic trainers who understand the importance of strong leadership skills are being promoted to top management positions within organizations and institutions. Top managers, including team owners, university administrators and trustees, and boards of education have certain expectations for the sports medicine program, so it is important that the athletic trainer involve a representative sample of these people as part of the planning team. Without the active support of these groups, the strategic plan for the sports medicine program is likely to fail.

Coaches make up another major inside group. Including coaches in the planning effort is wise because they have a legitimate need to be involved in, or at least informed about, the health care of their athletes. The success of the team and their success as coaches often depend on the overall health of their athletes. In addition, coaches exert a powerful influence on the attitudes and behaviors of the athletes on their teams. The final reason to involve coaches in the planning process is that they form an important power base in any athletic program. A successful coach can become one of the most powerful people in the entire organization. Using this power to build alliances with the sports medicine program makes sense.

The most important inside group to tap in developing the strategic plan is the institution's athletic trainers. They are the professionals inside the organization with the most sports medicine expertise. As such, they are the best sources of information about how to develop the program, but they must be involved in the proper manner. Too often, meetings intended to develop strategic directions for sports medicine programs can become complaining sessions about problems with working conditions, salary, and professional standing in the institution. These issues are important, but if they become the focus of the athletic trainers' roles in the strategic planning process, the resulting plan will be little more than a shopping list of their demands—an outcome that is unlikely to foster administration support or improved care for injured athletes and other physically active patients. Athletic trainers must constantly ask themselves during the planning process, "How can we improve the quality of service to our patients?" Questions that deviate significantly from this are unlikely to have strategic value.

One method of appealing to inside-interest stakeholders is to present information comparing your own sports medicine program to peer sports medicine programs. Peer institutions can be defined in several ways. They may be similar to your program in geographical location, thus drawing from a similar clientele. They may be in a different geographical location but serve the same type of client population that your program serves. They may also have a facility similar to yours in size or even care for similar total numbers of athletes and teams. By providing a comparative analysis showing how your organization stacks up against peers, you can often present a compelling case for your program's growth and development. One word of caution: You should be prepared to find that your program fares better than its peers in some categories. While it is

a benefit to be aware of such findings and this may even be a positive attribute for internal stakeholders to know about, upper-level management may interpret this information as reasons to limit investment in your growth.

Benchmarking is the term for associating a recognized comparison of one's own program to the best in the industry. Different aspects of services, outcomes, and deliverables can be measured in terms of metrics and used to assess a program's overall performance level as well as components of the program. As a result, improvements can be made related to quality of care, timely delivery of services, and perhaps cost savings. Historically, benchmarking for the athletic training profession has been accomplished through informal networking among colleagues. In the future, more formal approaches should be considered to justify athletic training services, outcomes, and costs in the health care arena.

The Database

Compiling data and then interpreting it during the strategic planning process helps athletic trainers devise alternative action plans and estimate their potential value for meeting the goals of the sports medicine program. First, the past performance of the program is analyzed; trends in patient loads, injury rates, clinic profits or losses, and athletic trainer performance evaluations are considered, along with other information. Next, the program's present situation is analyzed. Data about staffing levels, budget, client population size, number of sports to be served, demands and expectations of outside and inside interests, and applicable laws that affect the program will be needed. Finally, a **forecast** for the future is developed. The process of forecasting involves using factual information, trends, and data in an effort to predict circumstances. Forecasts are highly informed guesses that should always be backed up with documented evidence. Athletic trainers should consider the predicted rise in the cost of medical goods and services and the future availability of professional staff, support employees, and consulting medical personnel when preparing the forecast. In addition, they should consider advances in technology, because the available technology often drives the practice of sports medicine.

SWOT Analysis

The last data collection procedure to be accomplished in the strategic planning process is often referred to as a **SWOT analysis**. SWOT is an acronym for strengths, weaknesses, opportunities, and threats. Because the SWOT analysis identifies strengths and weaknesses already present in the sports medicine program, it is most appropriate for programs that are already established (see appendix B). A broad spectrum of participants should conduct the SWOT analysis. Interpretation of the data is subject to the biases of the interpreter, so only the involvement of a representative group of both outside and inside interests will yield useful results.

The SWOT analysis often reveals important sources of both opportunities and threats for the sports medicine program. Many of the techniques used in this strategic planning process can be interchanged with those used in the process of program evaluation. See the section on program evaluation for more information. A SWOT analysis has also been referred to as a **WOTS UP analysis**, representing the same categories of assessment, with UP standing for underlying planning, indicating that it is used for strategic planning purposes.

Operational Planning

After developing a strategic direction for the sports medicine program, an athletic trainer must translate the strategies into practice through use of **operational plans**. Whereas strategic plans are meant to provide program direction over a long period, say five years, operational plans define the activities of the program for a much shorter period, usually no more than two years. The importance of functioning operational plans for the sports medicine program should not be underestimated. In the end, the goal is to effectively translate the strategic vision for the program into a useful operational plan. Three often misunderstood types of operational plans are policies, processes, and procedures.

Policies

A **policy** is an organized plan that addresses a specific program or action. By definition, policies are broad statements of intended action promulgated by boards empowered with the authority to govern the operation of the organization.

Policies are not intended to answer detailed questions about how the sports medicine program operates. They are intended as road maps to guide an athletic trainer in developing and operating a sports medicine program in accordance with the desires of the policy board. Athletic trainers will rarely be empowered to dictate institutional policies unless

Sample Policy Statement

Memorial Hospital acknowledges its role in the following activities:

- Reducing the incidence of injury among high school student-athletes
- Making competent medical care readily and easily available to the student-athletes of Ashton County

In addition, Memorial Hospital recognizes that a program delivering sports medicine services to the three high schools of Ashton County will help it fulfill its mission to be the leader in sports medicine in the Ashton County area. Consequently, the Board of Trustees of Memorial Hospital has established the following policies:

1.0 Provide sports medicine services at the site of athletic practice and competition for the three Ashton County high schools.

1.1 Provide sports medicine coverage using only personnel who have been trained and credentialed as experts in sports medicine, including certified athletic trainers.

1.2 Maintain an injury database to determine the risk of injury to athletic participants.

1.3 Provide hospital-based management of injuries requiring follow-up care.

1.4 Provide education on the prevention of injuries and the development of healthy lifestyles to the students of the three Ashton County high schools.

1.5 Assist in the prevention of athletic injuries by providing physical examinations and screening services for the students of the three Ashton County high schools.

they sit on the governing boards of institutions. They should, however, be consulted in the development or modification of policies that affect the sports medicine program (Neal and Konin 2017). A well-managed organization with a sports medicine program should have policies in place that express the intended behaviors of the program. The athletic trainer is obviously a crucial ingredient in advising those in authority on the development and implementation of these policies. An example of a policy statement for the Memorial Hospital Sports Medicine Outreach Program might look like the statement on page 32.

Processes

Processes are the next step down from policies on the hierarchy of operational plans. **Processes** are

Processes of the Sports Medicine Program

- Injury prevention
- Injury recognition
- Injury management
- Injury rehabilitation
- Organization and administration
- Education and counseling

the incremental and mutually dependent steps that direct the most important tasks of the sports medicine program. Each process should relate to at least one, and possibly many, of the policies that govern the program. Each policy will undoubtedly have several supporting processes.

Procedures

Procedures provide specific interpretations of processes for athletic trainers and other members of the sports medicine team. They are not abstract. They should be written in clear and simple language so that different people will interpret them in the same way. Procedures are the lowest level of the planning hierarchy. The sidebar Linking Policies, Processes, and Procedures is an example of how policies, processes, and procedures are linked for the Memorial Hospital program.

Practices

Even the most well-considered procedure often leaves room for an athletic trainer to make professional judgments about how to handle particular administrative tasks. The ways in which administrative tasks are actually accomplished are known as **practices**. Practices should never contradict the directions provided for in the procedure they are intended to support. For example, a sports medicine

Linking Policies, Processes, and Procedures

Policy 1.0

The policy of Memorial Hospital is to provide sports medicine services at the site of athletic practice and competition for the three Ashton County high schools.

Process for the Injury Rehabilitation Subfunction

The sports medicine team, including the physician, athletic trainer, and physical therapist, shall work together to provide student-athletes with a rehabilitation program appropriate for their injuries. Consideration will be given to the location of the rehabilitation program (home, school, or hospital), the equipment required to attain the desired rehabilitative effect, the insurance coverage provided by the student's family, and the insurance coverage provided by the school.

Procedure for Discharge From Rehabilitation

Physical therapists or athletic trainers shall discharge student-athletes from rehabilitation only after consulting with the attending physician. Discharge shall occur when the critical long-term goals, established when the student-athlete was admitted, have been met. All discharged student-athletes shall be given oral and written instructions in the long-term care of their injuries. The names of all discharged student-athletes shall be placed on the mailing list for the Memorial Hospital Sports Medicine Newsletter. All discharged student-athletes shall be called at both six months and one year postdischarge by an athletic trainer to check on the status of their injuries.

clinic might have a written procedure requiring that all therapeutic modalities be calibrated and safety inspected once per year. This sound procedure is consistent with professional standards. The athletic trainer-administrator still has several decisions to make. Which vendor will he contact to service the equipment? What time of the year will he choose to have the equipment serviced? Should he send all the equipment out at once, send half of the inventory at one time, or stagger the schedule for each piece of equipment? The decisions he makes are examples of practices. Practices are important because they allow the athletic trainer to make decisions based on changing conditions without violating the letter or spirit of the policies and procedures manual.

The sports medicine program should assess its practices from time to time for congruence and conformity to the procedures they support. In addition, the practices in the sports medicine program must be consistent with professional standards and state and federal laws. For example, sports medicine programs operating in NCAA colleges and universities must use practices consistent with the guidelines included in the *NCAA Sports Medicine Handbook* and all athletic trainers should follow the recommendations outlined in the NATA Position Statements.

Handbooks

Policies, processes, and procedures are usually communicated to employees in the form of a policies and procedures handbook. This document is important. Not only does it educate employees regarding the procedures they are to follow, but it also serves as a legal foundation for action if they do not. Poorly written or incomplete procedure handbooks are frequently the basis for employee action against employers because they are often viewed as a kind of contract. It is important to ensure that all parties held accountable for the policies and procedures not only are provided with and asked to read the handbook, but also are asked to sign a document stating that they have in fact read all of the information, understand the policies and procedures, and agree to abide by them.

Large organizations, such as hospitals and universities, commonly have more than one handbook. One contains all of the organization's policies (remember that policies are statements passed by the board in control of the organization). Another contains procedures intended to apply to all employees of the organization, regardless of which department employs them. Human resources procedures are typically codified in procedure manuals of this type (see figure 3.2). The last kind of manual contains procedures specific to a certain subunit or department of an organization. It typically includes procedures that apply only to the kinds of activities that take place in that department. See figure 3.3 for an example of such a manual for a hospital-owned orthopedic and sports medicine clinic. Examples of procedures drawn from two settings—a dress code from a university sports medicine program and a procedure for 10-hour work shifts from a sports medicine clinic—are highlighted in the following sidebars.

Communicating and Developing Support for the Plan

Unfortunately, all the effort an athletic trainer expends developing the sports medicine program plan will be wasted unless other people inside and outside the organization accept it. One of the most difficult aspects of planning for the delivery of sports medicine services is developing a sense of ownership in the people who make up the major organizational power bases. Plans developed without such ownership are unlikely to remain politically viable for long. The ability to translate plans into action and develop support for the program is the ultimate measure of political skill. The concept and process of incorporating stakeholders into a form of shared ownership are often referred to as buy-in. Achieving buy-in for a sports medicine program plan is a key step toward successful implementation.

Types of Organizational Players

Block (2016) has developed a support-building strategy that could be useful to athletic trainers as they attempt to develop ownership for their sports medicine programs. The strategy is based on the **agreement–trust matrix** (see figure 3.4). The first step in the process is to identify people who will have an influence on the eventual success or failure of the sports medicine program. After these people have been identified, they can be assigned to one of four categories.

The **allies** of the athletic trainer exhibit a high level of agreement with the plans for the sports medicine program. In addition, they are people whom the athletic trainer trusts. They not only are supporters of the sports medicine program but also

CONTENTS

PROCEDURE TITLE

Absences, Excused
Absences and Tardiness, Unscheduled
Adoption Assistance
Benefit Accrual Hours
Bereavement
Bulletin Boards
COBRA
Collective Bargaining Agreement
College Savings Plan (529 Plan)
Confidential Information
Confidentiality of Information on Computer Systems
Counseling, Corrective Action
Credit Union
Death in Family
Disability Insurance
Dismissal
Diversity
Dress Code and Personal Appearance
Dual Relationships Between Hospital Employees and Patients
Educational Assistance
Employee Assistance Program
Equal Opportunity
Family and Medical Leave, Unpaid (FMLA)
FERPA
Flexible Spending Accounts
Flexible Staffing
Floating Holiday Time
Gifts and Tips
Grievances
Health Requirements and Services for Employees
HIPAA
Holidays
Insurance, Dental
Insurance, Life and Accidental Death
Insurance, Medical
Insurance, Supplemental Life
Insurance, Vision
Intellectual Property
Introductory Employees
Job Posting

Jury Duty
Lay-Off Procedure
Leave of Absence
Mission
New Employee Orientation
Overtime, Rest, and Meal Periods
Paid Time Off
Part-Time Employees
Patient Care, Staff Requests Not to Participate in Aspects of
Pay, Shift, and Weekend Premium
Payroll Check Distribution
Payroll Deductions
Performance Reviews
Personnel Records
Preemployment Alcohol and Drug Screening
Professional Development
Prescription Drug Plan
Promotion Guidelines
Recruitment Cash Bonus
Relatives, Employment of
Release Time
Resignations
Retirement
Retirement Savings Plan (401K)
Sabbatical
Salary
Seniority
Sexual Harassment
Social Security
Solicitation and Distribution of Literature
Staffing, Supplemental
Time Clocks
Travel Assistance
Tuition Reimbursement Program
Vacation
Weapons
Work Schedule
Workplace Violence
Workers' Compensation
Workers' Compensation Supplement

Figure 3.2 Table of contents for a human resource procedures manual for a midsize not-for-profit hospital.

CONTENTS

AUTHORIZATION AND INTAKE

Medical supervision of rehabilitation services
Receiving and processing referrals for rehabilitation services
Prior authorization

Reimbursement
Intake process
Privacy and confidentiality

DOCUMENTATION AND COMMUNICATION

Communicating the status of the hospital outpatient
Communicating the physical therapy ambulatory and transfer needs of the hospital patient with nursing and other ancillary services

Communicating the status of patients seen under contract

RECORD KEEPING

Patient records—The patient folder
Department records

Record retention policy

PATIENT CARE

Assignment of patients
Outpatient registration
Patient scheduling
Priority of care for hospital patients
Dispensing of crutches, braces, and other patient care items
Broken appointments and cancellations
Discharge planning for rehabilitation patients
Quality assurance
Home visit program
Participation of the patient and family in the treatment plan
Assessments of patients
Orientation
Initial assessment
Case management—Neurorehabilitation

Initial team meeting
Individual program plan
Therapeutic progress report
Client referral
Follow-up
Waiting list
Physical aggressive behavior and self-injurious behavior
Recipient rights
Peer review
Input from persons served
Outcomes
Accessibility
Education of clients and care givers regarding universal precautions and infection control
Nonvoluntary discharge

DEPARTMENT MANAGEMENT

Hours of operation
Charging for services
Preventive maintenance
Approval process for new and revised procedures
Pricing for patient charge items
Ordering supplies and equipment
Authorizing and training vehicle operators
Maintenance and inspection of van

Handling vehicle incidents and accidents
Access to outpatient rehabilitation
Utility management
Robbery emergency plan
Hostage crisis plan

(continued)

Figure 3.3 Table of contents for a procedures manual for a hospital-owned orthopedic and sport medicine clinic.

Adapted by permission from *Rehabilitation services procedure manual* (Holland Community Hospital, Holland, MI).

PERSONNEL

Flexible staffing
Dress code
Time, mileage, and productivity logging
Orientation
Continuing education
Comp time for professional salaried exempt employees

Vacations and leaves of absence
Ten-hour shift option
Rehabilitation department staffing
Therapist staffing pool
Verification of credentials

SAFETY

Handling incidents
Handling patient arrests
General safety rules

Emergency plan
Power failure

INFECTION CONTROL

Personnel policies—General information
Contract personnel policies
Three-minute surgical scrub
Debridement
Linen disposal
Wound cultures
Dressing removal
Burn patient management
Special handling of physical therapy equipment
Isolation patients receiving whirlpool

Reusable sterile supplies, Care and storage of
Disposable sterile supplies, Care and storage of
Disinfection of whirlpool tanks
Departmental routine cleaning
Routine cleaning by Environmental Services
Disinfection of bandage scissors
Disinfection of hyperbaric extremity chamber
Treatment protocol for hyperbaric chamber
Management of catheterized hydrotherapy patients
Fluidotherapy

PHYSICAL THERAPY

BAPS
Biofeedback
Compression—Jobst pump
Compression—Wright linear pump
Conditioning—Treadmill
Contrast bath
CPM
Cryotherapy—Cold packs
Diathermy
Electrical stimulation—High voltage
Electrical stimulation—Low voltage
Electrical stimulation—Medium frequency
Electrical stimulation—MENS
Electrical stimulation—TENS
Fluoromethane spray

Gait training
Hot packs
Hydrotherapy—Hubbard tank and whirlpool
Hyperbaric oxygen unit
Hyperstimulation analgesia with pulsed IR laser
Isokinetic testing
Massage
Myofascial release
Paraffin bath
Phonophoresis
ROM splint fitting
Traction—Cervical, manual
Traction—Cervical, motorized
Tilt table
Ultrasound

Figure 3.3 *(continued)*

have an established record of honesty and truthfulness. **Opponents** of the athletic trainer should not be viewed as enemies. They are people whom the athletic trainer trusts to give an honest opinion of the sports medicine program or its components, but who have opposing views to those of the athletic trainer. Opponents can often serve a useful purpose—their challenge can lead to critical examination of the sports medicine program, resulting in stronger strategic and operational plans (Friedman and Greenhaus 2000).

Bedfellows are those who agree with the plans of the athletic trainer for the sports medicine program but have a history of untrustworthy behavior.

Topics on Which the NCAA Has Issued Sports Medicine Guidelines

The most recent versions of these guidelines from the *NCAA Sports Medicine Handbook* are available online.

Sports Medicine Administration

Medical Evaluations, Immunizations, and Records

Dispensing Prescription Medication

Lightning Safety

NCAA Alcohol, Tobacco, and Other Drug Education Guidelines

Emergency Care and Coverage

Medical Disqualification of the Student-Athlete

Skin Infections in Athletics

Prevention of Heat Illness

Assessment of Body Composition

Nutrition and Athletic Performance

Nontherapeutic Drugs

Nutritional Ergogenic Aids

Menstrual Cycle Dysfunction

Weight Loss—Dehydration

Blood-Borne Pathogens and Intercollegiate Athletics

The Use of Local Anesthetics in College Athletics

The Use of Injectable Corticosteroids in Sports Injuries

Cold Stress and Cold Exposure

"Burners" (Brachial Plexus Injuries)

Concussion or Mild Traumatic Brain Injury (mTBI) in the Athlete

Participation by Student-Athlete With Impairment

Pregnancy in the Student-Athlete

The Student-Athlete With Sickle Cell Trait

Protective Equipment

Eye Safety in Sports

Use of Trampoline and Minitramp

Mouth Guards

Use of the Head as a Weapon in Football and Other Contact Sports

Guidelines for Helmet Fitting and Removal in Athletics

Catastrophic Incident in Athletics

Dietary Supplements

Depression: Interventions for Intercollegiate Athletics

NCAA Legislation Involving Health and Safety Issues

NCAA Injury Surveillance System

Summary

Banned Drug-Classes

Dress Code Procedure

All members of the university sports medicine staff shall be professionally attired at all times during their work shift. Staff members and students shall wear a university-approved name badge at all times when on duty. The first badge shall be provided at university expense. The cost of replacement badges is the responsibility of the staff member. While on duty, athletic trainers (staff and students) shall wear a uniform shirt approved by the head athletic trainer. Each staff member will receive two uniform shirts per year. Additional uniform shirts are the responsibility of the staff member. All staff members shall wear a uniform jacket when covering outdoor events during cool weather. The jackets are the property of the university and may be checked out from the clothing locker in the main athletic training room storage room. The following clothing is prohibited at all times, regardless of setting:

- Blue jeans
- Sweatshirts
- Unkempt clothing
- Clothing with holes

Direct questions regarding this procedure to the head athletic trainer.

Ten-Hour Work-Shift Procedure

Memorial Hospital offers its employees the option of working either five 8-hour shifts per week or four 10-hour shifts per week. Because each department can accommodate only a certain percentage of its employees on a 10-hour shift, each employee is required to apply for this privilege with his or her supervisor. Interested employees should complete the request for 10-hour shift form and submit it to their supervisor. The supervisor shall make every reasonable effort to accommodate an employee's request, consistent with the need to keep the department adequately staffed at all times. The supervisor shall respond in writing to the employee's request within 10 days. Supervisors are instructed to consider the following elements when deciding whether an employee should be granted 10-hour shift status:

- The minimum number of employees required to service patients during peak, minimal, and average loads
- The minimum number of employees required to implement the department's emergency plan
- The degree to which the employee requires supervision consistent with hospital policy and state law
- The number of employees already granted 10-hour work-shift status; the number of employees should not normally exceed 25%

Employees who have questions regarding this procedure should consult with their supervisors.

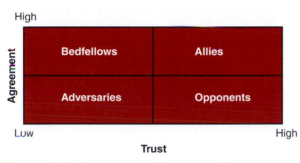

Figure 3.4 Agreement–trust matrix.

The empowered manager: Positive political skills at work, P. Block, Copyright © 1987 Jossey-Bass. Adapted with permission of John Wiley & Sons, Inc.

Bedfellows are generally quick to ally themselves with the sports medicine program, but they tend to be manipulative and to operate "behind the back." Bedfellows are often quick to support ideas in the conceptual stage, but they often fail to deliver when they are asked to contribute to get a program up and running.

People with whom the athletic trainer has attempted negotiation that has been fruitless are known as **adversaries**. They not only disagree with the athletic trainer's plan for the sports medicine program but are untrustworthy and dishonest as well. The athletic trainer must be able to distinguish between adversaries and opponents. A common pitfall occurs when opponents who are honest, trust-worthy people with different viewpoints are labeled as adversaries. Opponents can make the sports medicine program stronger. Adversaries often gain strength through confrontation because that tends to legitimize the alternative vision they have for the sports medicine program. Negotiation will not alter their vision of how the program should function. If an athletic trainer has done a good job of including a wide spectrum of people in the planning effort, the number of adversaries should be relatively small. Negotiating with those who oppose a plan is often best done one-on-one, rather than in a group setting.

Gaining Support From Organizational Players

Block (2016) suggests specific strategies for developing support among the four types of organizational players.

ALLIES

- Confirm the fact that the person agrees with the sports medicine plan.
- Profess appreciation for the quality of the relationship.
- Admit faults and shortcomings of the sports medicine plan.
- Request the support and continued counsel of the ally.

OPPONENTS

- Profess appreciation for the quality of the relationship. Emphasize the trust and honesty that have characterized the relationship.
- Explain the plan for the sports medicine program along with arguments that support its implementation.
- Define your interpretation of the opponent's views in a nonthreatening manner.
- Attempt to engage the opponent in a problem-solving process to find common points.

BEDFELLOWS

- Confirm the fact that the person agrees with the sports medicine plan.
- Convey your concern about the person's willingness to be open and honest. Express a willingness to share a portion of the blame and to find a way to improve the trust relationship so that the program can move ahead.
- Clearly state your expectations for the person's behavior toward the sports medicine program. What is it that you want the person to do?
- Ask the person what expectations he or she has for you in order to improve the relationship.
- Attempt to establish a consensus for future working relationships with bedfellows.

ADVERSARIES

- Explain the plan for the sports medicine program with arguments that support its implementation.
- Define your interpretation of the adversary's views in a nonthreatening manner.
- Explain actions you have taken or will take to implement the sports medicine plan so that everything is out in the open.
- Avoid making demands that are unlikely to be met.

Meetings and Conferences

Two important planning subfunctions about which competent athletic trainer-administrators should be knowledgeable are planning for effective meetings and conferences. Every athletic trainer will be involved in meetings from time to time during their professional career. Although the opportunity to plan for conferences comes less often and to fewer athletic trainers, the responsibility to coordinate this activity properly is important because of the expense and the number of people commonly affected by the typical conference.

Planning for Meetings

One of the most common methods for developing and communicating organizational plans is the meeting. Meetings in sports medicine settings can take many forms. The most common is the staff meeting, in which personnel from a work group unit (for example, the athletic trainers employed by the university athletic department or the rehabilitation professionals employed in an outpatient clinic) gather to discuss issues critical to the function of the unit. Athletic trainers can also be involved in other kinds of meetings. For example, athletic trainers who work together in a particular school district will undoubtedly have to meet—probably more than once—with the staff from each school and the clinic or hospital if applicable to coordinate the athletic training services. Regardless of the type or setting, meetings are often viewed as exercises in frustration. Many of us have participated in meetings that accomplished nothing. We often walk away afterward fuming, "Did anything useful happen in there? What a waste of time!" (Lencioni 2004).

Although dull and unproductive meetings might be common, they are not inevitable. Tropman's (2003) research with meeting experts throughout North America revealed that four qualities characterized successful meetings:

1. The group was able to reach decisions in the meetings.
2. The group rarely needed to meet to undo or revise decisions that they had already made; they made high-quality decisions the first time.
3. The decisions made were important and meaningful to the organization.
4. The meetings were enjoyable, and the members felt that they had spent their time well.

PEARLS OF MANAGEMENT

Athletic trainers can experience more success in their meetings if they organize well, divide the meeting into three parts, control their own meeting behavior, avoid new business and reports, look to the future, and make high-quality decisions.

1. Prepare for the Meeting

Although it sounds obvious, many meetings fail because nobody prepares for them. Meetings are like a play—they need a script, actors, props, and practice. The script is the agenda (see figure 3.5). The actors are the meeting participants. Some will have more noticeable roles than others, but all are necessary if the meeting is to be successful. The props are the materials needed to conduct business during the meeting. These usually include various documents and might include equipment such as a whiteboard, flip chart, or computer projector. The last element—practice—is something that most meeting managers disregard. All of us in athletics know the importance of practice. Practice helps eliminate mistakes and prevents random elements from interfering with performance. Practice in the context of a meeting might include checking with several key members of the meeting group to get their read on important issues to be discussed or decided during the meeting. Practice certainly involves the preparation that each participant makes for the meeting by becoming familiar with the items on the agenda. It may be helpful to request agenda items from meeting participants in advance and provide a deadline by which items must be added.

2. Divide the Meeting Into Three Parts

Too often, participants in a meeting play a role that requires them to speak only once. One method to organize a meeting and maximize the participants' time and input is to divide the meeting into three parts:

1. Announcements
2. Decisions
3. Discussion

If this formula is rigidly adhered to, all meeting participants will be able to give appropriate input at the right times. Meeting managers who deviate from this formula run the risk of allowing the meeting to stray from its original purpose.

3. Control Your Meeting Behavior

Most people who hate meetings (which is most people) are particularly annoyed by the behavior of other meeting participants. We are quick to see the faults in others but slow to recognize our own shortcomings. This issue is important for athletic trainers who participate in meetings. Behavior in a group setting is infectious. Optimism or pessimism can sweep through a meeting room if the climate is right. You should carefully analyze your own meet-

---

AGENDA

Sports Medicine Outreach Program Planning Committee Meeting

Feb. 5, 2018

ITEM	FACILITATOR
1. Announcements	
a. High school contract negotiations	Monique
b. New supply bid procedures	Bill
2. Decisions	
a. Budget allocations	Jose
b. Staff travel reimbursement	Bill
c. Comp time for ATCs covering night events	Monique
3. Discussion	
a. Which physicians should we recruit?	Monique
b. How should we market the program?	Jose and Monique

Figure 3.5 Sample meeting agenda.

ing behavior as a first step toward trying to improve the meeting behavior of others.

4. Avoid New Business

A common item on most meeting agendas is new business. The intent of the new business section is to allow meeting participants to bring issues or concerns to the table for discussion and decision. The problem with this time-honored practice is that nobody in the room, with the exception of the person who introduced the issue, is prepared to address the topic with any intelligence. New business, therefore, violates the first principle—prepare for the meeting. People can't organize for something they don't know anything about. A good rule to follow when conducting a meeting is to discuss everything on the agenda and don't discuss anything not on the agenda.

5. Avoid Reports

Too often, staff members waste valuable time listening to reports in a meeting when the information could more effectively be delivered and analyzed in writing beforehand. Written reports can be referred to in the decisions section or the discussion section of the meeting. If participants receive written reports in advance of the meeting, they have the opportunity to digest the information and formulate well-considered questions at their own pace rather than make snap judgments on a tight time schedule. Written reports should be brief and contain only the most important elements of an issue or proposal. Participants can be referred to reports that are more inclusive if they want more information, but short executive summaries will encourage them to read and prepare for the meeting. It is common practice to approve all of the reports in a single vote by placing all on the consent agenda and accepting them as a group.

6. Look to the Future

One of the most frustrating aspects of most meetings is the sense of hurried decision making. Most meeting groups gain exposure to issues too late in the decision cycle. Athletic trainers involved in planning meetings can avoid this problem by carving out time—during either the announcements or the discussion period—for consideration of future issues. This preview helps those in the group prepare their thinking for when the issue is finally presented to them in a formal way. Facilitating informal discussion of issues is a difficult technique to master.

The meeting chairperson must be well versed in the organization's issues and be able to package the information for the group so that members can process it appropriately. This future-oriented discussion is different from the new business section discussed earlier. In the new business section of a meeting, one of the participants typically makes a formal motion that will require the group to make a binding decision. Future-oriented discussion is just that—discussion. The group need not make immediate decisions, although they may choose to brainstorm about the way they might handle future challenges.

7. Make High-Quality Decisions

Making high-quality decisions is difficult. Most meeting groups fail because they cannot make decisions at all—of any quality. They simply fail to decide. Those who do make decisions often have to go back and undo or revise their decisions. The important elements involved in making high-quality decisions in a group setting include gathering and communicating all pertinent information, processing the likely outcomes of various alternatives, developing a list of pros and cons for the alternatives, considering the perspectives of all the stakeholders, and deciding to decide. The chairperson of the meeting is critical in this regard. Decisions do have to be delayed when these elements are not satisfied. When the chair can orchestrate all these elements, however, it is time to make a decision. Revisiting the decision after its implementation to evaluate its effectiveness and learn lessons for the future is important, but this process should not interfere with making a decision in the first place.

Planning for Conferences

One of the most common—and most expensive—continuing education methods for all kinds of professions is the conference or symposium. Every athletic trainer will be involved several times in his career as a participant in conferences, and some will coordinate or serve on conference planning committees from time to time. Conference planning is an important leadership skill that will enhance the administrative skills package of any athletic trainer in any employment setting. To an extent, conference planning is similar to meeting planning, except the magnitude of the planning process and number of responsibilities are greater. The following elements are important steps in planning conferences. Although they are presented sequentially, many will overlap with each other, and depending on the situation, the order of the steps may be modified to meet a specific need.

Conference planning must be done correctly to prevent expensive mistakes. Conference planning involves working with a steering committee, establishing a theme, planning a program, identifying and recruiting speakers, and making space and other physical arrangements.

18 to 24 Months Before the Conference

The following activities are the first to be accomplished in the planning of a conference. Generally, the larger the conference, the earlier this planning should begin.

Appoint the Conference Coordinator　The conference coordinator typically serves as chairperson of the steering committee (see the next section). The following are a few qualities this person should possess.

- *Organized.* The primary duty of the conference coordinator is to coordinate the various members of the steering committee in their work. The conference coordinator must be able to synthesize information from a variety of sources to ensure that critical planning elements are accomplished.

- *Decisive.* The conference coordinator is expected to make decisions—sometimes with the support and agreement of the steering committee and sometimes on the spur of the moment. When crises arise during the conference—as they usually do—the coordinator must be decisive enough to make good decisions quickly based on the information available at the time.

- *Visionary and detail oriented.* The coordinator must be able to keep the goals of the conference in mind at all times and must be able to guide the various subcommittees in their work toward accomplishing those goals. On the other hand, the conference coordinator must also monitor the hundreds of details that are part of a successful symposium and be able to step in and make decisions when required.

- *Flexible.* The coordinator will learn throughout the planning process that many aspects of the plan will undergo change. In some cases, the

changes will be unexpected, and in other cases the coordinator will be required to make changes in the conference planning process. It will benefit the coordinator to be prepared to accommodate changes by being flexible and developing alternative plans.

Establish the Steering Committee　Planning a conference is usually not a solitary activity—it is a team effort. Conferences have so many elements that they would quickly overwhelm one person, no matter how well organized and efficient. Because most athletic trainers plan conferences on a volunteer basis as part of their professional service activities, or on a paid basis as only one part of their job responsibilities, the work should be spread around so that no one person is excessively burdened. The members of the conference steering committee often serve as the chairpersons of subcommittees charged with one narrow aspect of the conference (for example, marketing and promotions, entertainment, audiovisual, or registration). Only people who possess the following qualities should be chosen for the steering committee:

- *Knowledgeable.* Each member of the steering committee should have enough experience and expertise to understand the issues involved in the conference. Ideally, steering committee members should have previous experience in conference planning. They should have the necessary skills to carry out the functions that they will manage in planning the conference. For example, the member of the steering committee who chairs the finance subcommittee should have experience in business or in managing budgets. Similarly, the audiovisual subcommittee chair should have computer and similar technical skills.

- *Interested, committed, and available.* Conference planning can take a long time. Some steering committees meet for two years or more before the conference. Even after the conference has ended, details remain to attend to. Steering committee members must be committed to sticking with the project from start to finish. In addition, potential committee members must have enough time to dedicate to their planning responsibilities. All prospective members of the committee should reflect on their commitments during the conference planning time before agreeing to serve to ensure that they will be able to fulfill their responsibilities.

- *Team oriented.* Some people work well in groups. Others don't. The steering committee is a team—a group of people working toward a common goal. Although each member of the steering committee may be responsible for a different aspect of the conference, all these elements are intimately connected. Committee members must be able to communicate and work effectively with others to deliver an effective experience for conference participants. It is likely that areas of planning will overlap between different groups, necessitating team collaboration. Collaboration between committees is essential. For example, audiovisual committee members may choose to include cutting-edge technology to create the best possible presentation images. However, the finance committee members may not approve of this because of budgetary limitations.

• *Responsible and dependable.* The chair of the steering committee will be frustrated and the committee will be demoralized if one or more committee members fail to do the jobs assigned to them. The committee chair should learn as much as possible about prospective steering committee members before extending an invitation to serve. Those with a proven record of responsibility should be further considered. Those who have a reputation for letting people down or leaving tasks uncompleted should be removed from consideration.

Establish the Conference Theme, Objectives, and Target Audience
People attend conferences for a variety of reasons, but underlying each of these reasons is the desire or need to learn more about a particular topic. The best conferences have a theme that is supported by several objectives. The more narrowly focused the conference theme, the more likely the conference is to appeal to an audience with a specific learning objective. For example, a conference with the topic of knee injuries is much broader than one dedicated to the topic of advances in the surgical management of ACL injuries. The former is likely to attract a larger, more diverse audience, but is unlikely to provide as much depth as the latter.

Often planning for conference topics takes into consideration what is currently of greatest interest among attendees. Some conferences by necessity are targeted to large audiences—sometimes with thousands of attendees (for example, the annual conferences of NATA or the American College of Sports Medicine). These conferences usually have broad, nonspecific themes, such as Athletic Training in the Next Millennium or New Horizons in Sports Medicine. Large conferences like these commonly include several smaller, more-focused sections that cover a single topic or a group of related topics.

In any case—whether the conference is large or small, with a broad or a narrow focus—specific learning objectives for the conferees should be established in advance. Each learning objective should relate in some way to the overall conference theme. Learning objectives should be assessed as a way of determining the degree to which the purposes of the conference have been accomplished.

Set a Date and Establish a Time Line
The date of the conference is critical to its eventual success or failure. The following are a few questions planners should consider when choosing a date:

• *Is this conference traditionally held on a specific date?* Some annual conferences attract the same target audience year after year. People often schedule their yearly calendars around these traditional conference dates. Moving the date of a conference that is traditionally held during a specific week may alienate some members of the target audience, but it may draw in new attendees who have other annual commitments during that time. It is also helpful to know when reporting for continuing education credit is due, as typically there will be a fair number of athletic trainers who have not yet met their requirements for recertification or licensure.

• *Are members of the target audience available?* Although predicting the availability of all members of the target audience is impossible, the steering committee should know the audience well enough to avoid obvious conflicts. For example, a conference targeted to high school athletic trainers is unlikely to draw many attendees if it is held on a Friday evening in the fall. A survey sent to a random sample of the target audience asking for the most convenient dates for the conference is a good way to determine the availability of potential conferees. Holding a conference at the same site and close to the date of another event that large numbers of the target audience will attend is another way to ensure that potential conferees may be available. However, if a large event held locally is of interest to your audience to the point that it detracts from your ability to attract attendees, overall participation may diminish and revenue generation could be affected.

• *Are the facilities available?* If the conference is tied to a specific location, then the date for the conference could be influenced by the availability of the facilities. The earlier the date for the conference is established, the more likely it is that the desired location and facilities will be available. It is also important to keep in mind that earlier booking sometimes translates to higher fees, whereas booking closer to the conference date—before a facility has been rented—provides some leverage for bargaining but is slightly more risky.

Once the date has been established, the steering committee should establish a time line for each of the tasks involved in planning the conference. In addition, each subcommittee should develop its own time line that will allow it to accomplish its duties in a manner consistent with the master time line. See figure 3.6 for a sample time line.

15 to 17 Months Before the Conference

After the planning committee is in place, preparations for the conference begin in earnest. Specific members of the committee should be appointed to manage each of the following functions.

Establish the Program   Along with the speakers, the program will be the heart and soul of the conference. The various presentation topics included in the conference should make up a minicurriculum designed to help attendees accomplish the learning objectives established for the symposium. Several methods are available for delivering the conference curriculum:

- *Lectures.* Traditional format in which a single person or a panel of experts addresses the audience. This method can accommodate a large number of attendees at once.
- *Keynote.* A type of lecture usually delivered to the entire assembly of attendees, often at the beginning of the conference, dealing with a topic central to the conference theme.
- *Workshops.* Sessions led by an instructor, usually involving smaller numbers of attendees, that allow for a higher degree of audience participation.
- *Laboratories.* A kind of workshop that emphasizes hands-on skill building, often using instructional aids, tools, or specimens.
- *Panel discussion.* Typically follows a series of two or more speakers and is moderated by a facilitator who poses questions to the panelists and directs questions from the participants to the speakers.
- *Point–counterpoint.* Typically involves two speakers with opposing views on a topic. One speaker presents the topic from one point of view, followed by the second presentation from an opposing viewpoint. Point–counterpoints may also be followed by panel discussions.

These teaching methods can be used individually in developing the program or can be combined. For example, a conference might begin with a keynote address, after which conferees can choose between concurrent sessions composed of lectures followed by breakout sessions on topics related to the lecture subject matter. Some conferences are made up exclusively of lectures but offer pre- and postconference workshops, sometimes at additional cost. Conferences that have a small target audience are often delivered exclusively in workshop format. No matter what format is used, plan adequate time between educational sessions for meals and breaks.

Establish the Budget   Conferences are expensive. After the desired format of the conference has been established, create a realistic budget that supports the conference objectives. Consider the following factors when establishing the conference budget:

- *Expenses.* Have all likely costs been included (see the later section on miscellaneous services)? Does the budget include a contingency for cost overruns?
- *Income.* Has the registration fee been established at a level sufficient to pay the costs associated with the conference? If not, have other sources of income, including exhibitor fees and sponsorships, been included at a level that is reasonably achievable? Do the registration, exhibitor, and sponsorship fees represent a reasonable value given the audience resources and content of the conference?

Identify the Location and Secure the Facility   Once you have identified the target audience, established the program, and fixed the budget, you can choose the conference location. Two critical factors in this decision are geographic location and facility type.

1. *Geographic location.* Several factors influence the choice of a geographic location for a conference:
   - *Nature of the target audience.* If the audience is national or international in scope, the conference will most likely have to take place in or near a city with a large airport. If the audience will be large, a city with a large conference center and many hotels in reasonable

TASK	TARGET DATE
1. Speaker thank-yous and honoraria sent	Late July
2. Exhibitor request forms sent	Late July
3. Exhibitor prospectus prepared	July/August
4. Exhibitor contract prepared	July/August
5. Tour companies researched and solicited	July/August
6. Speaker database created	August
7. Shuttle bus and security proposals solicited	August
8. Speaker and registration gift selection begun	August
9. Advance registration form prepared	September
10. Housing form prepared	September
11. Media sales company proposals solicited if necessary	September
12. Speaker and registration gift selected	September
13. Cancellation insurance application mailed	September
14. Liability insurance application mailed	September
15. Times for free communications and poster presentation sessions confirmed	Late September
16. Letter that proceeding publisher sends to speakers approved	Late September
17. Registration flier prepared	September/October
18. Speaker database to proceeding publisher distributed	Mid-October
19. Related-organizations' letters of program invitation for following-year convention sent	Late October
20. Preliminary program prepared	October/November
21. Shuttle bus company and security selected	November
22. Tour company contract signed	November
23. Exhibitor registration form prepared	November
24. Proceedings publishers' letters to speakers sent	November
25. Summary of room-block categories prepared	November
26. Exhibitor room-block request form prepared	November
27. Room-block memo to special housing groups sent	Late November
28. Preliminary program to Marketing Department sent	December 1
29. Exhibitor registration form sent to printer	December
30. Brochure sent to vendors	December
31. Speaker registration, housing, and A/V speaker forms sent	December
32. Exhibitor forms for confirming packet (e.g., registration, housing) prepared	December
33. Moderator and panelist information e-mail sent	December
34. Awards lunch menu and catering coordination begun	January
35. Welcome reception menu and catering coordination begun	January
36. Memo and meeting space request form mailed to committee and task force chairs	January
37. Final program preparation begun	January

(continued)

Figure 3.6 Sample time line for a large international conference held in July.

Courtesy of the National Athletic Trainers' Association.

38. Shuttle bus contract and security contract signed	January
39. Memo to next city convention and visitors bureau about exhibit arrangements for prepromotion sent	January
40. Media sales company selected	January
41. Memo to host city convention and visitors bureau and convention personnel needs for kiosks and city information sent	January
42. Reconfirm or order if necessary adequate inventory of logo golf-type shirts for office volunteers	January
43. Badge holder order placed	January
44. Ribbon order placed	January
45. Catering planning begun	January
46. Committee and allied groups meeting confirmation e-mailed	Ongoing as of January
47. Exhibitor packets e-mailed	February
48. Exhibit booth assignments begun	February
49. Complimentary exhibit booth invitations and materials mailed	February
50. Host committee dinner arrangements completed	March 1
51. Meeting plans drafted for convention center, hotel(s), decorator	March
52. Reminder memo sent to speakers with incomplete paperwork	March
53. Rooming lists begun	March
54. Final program to desktop publisher sent	Mid-March
55. Production of staff guide begun	March
56. A/V and speaker release forms received from speakers	March
57. Convention event tickets ordered	March
58. Final shuttle arrangements determined	March
59. Items for registration packets reviewed and follow-up action taken	March
60. Moderator meeting and guidelines memos and resumes sent	Late March
61. Invitations and complimentary registration e-mails to liaison organizations and association CEOs sent	April 1
62. Attendee registration confirmation and information e-mail sent	April 1
63. Speakers' names sent to gift company for imprinting	Early April
64. Final rooming list to housing service sent	April 1
65. Special event invitations e-mailed	April
66. On-site registration form prepared and printed	April
67. Security arrangements finalized	April
68. Speaker final arrangements e-mail sent	April 15
69. Meeting plans to convention center, hotel(s), and decorator sent	May 1
70. Convention plant and flower order placed	May
71. Convention materials shipped to convention center	Mid-June
72. Postconvention bills paid	July
73. Rebates for hotel determined	July-September

Figure 3.6 *(continued)*

proximity to the conference center will be required. Some cities are more expensive places to host conferences than others. The affordability of the city for the target audience is an important consideration in deciding where to host a conference.

- *Time of year.* Most cities have a peak season and an off-season. Hotel and meeting space costs are higher during the peak season.
- *Recreation and entertainment.* Some conferences include recreation as an important adjunct to the program. Warm-weather sites or locations with interesting cultural attractions can boost conference attendance or encourage attendees to bring their families.

2. *Facility type.* The two most important considerations in determining the kind of facility in which to host a conference are length of the conference and the number of likely participants. Conferences longer than one day that draw attendees from more than a few hours away require a facility with sleeping rooms and restaurants. Large conferences require meeting facilities with large ballrooms for lectures and several smaller rooms for workshops and other breakout sessions. The convention and visitors bureau or the chamber of commerce of the city in which the conference will be held will provide information on the facilities available in the area. (These organizations will also provide, often at no charge, other items designed to improve the experience of the conferees, such as reduced room rates, free Wi-Fi, and so on.) When conference meetings become larger in scope so that increased meeting space is required and more participants are likely to use hotel rooms for overnight stays, leverage to negotiate lower conference room rental fees, reduced or no costs for rented audiovisual equipment, and other perks may be negotiated with hotel conference managers. The following kinds of facilities are most often used for conferences:

- Large hotels in urban areas
- Suburban hotels with conference facilities
- Conference centers
- Colleges and universities

12 to 14 Months Before the Conference

The pace of the planning effort picks up significantly about one year before the conference. The conference will begin to take shape after three elements have been planned: speakers, meals and entertainment, and registration.

Recruit Speakers Although all the elements included in this discussion are crucial to the success of a conference, nothing will have a greater effect on the success or failure of the conference than the quality of the speakers. Establishing and sticking to a reasonable speakers budget is important, but if the speakers are not good, the conference will fail. For recruiting speakers, Watkins (2003) recommends the following:

- *Determine the desired outcome of a presentation before choosing a speaker.* Make sure that the speaker understands the objectives the committee has established for his or her presentation, and make sure that the speaker will tailor the presentation to accomplish those objectives. If the speaker has a canned presentation that he or she is unwilling to modify to meet the objectives of the conference, the presentation is unlikely to be effective.

- *Investigate the speaker's reputation.* Learn as much as possible about a speaker's effectiveness before extending an offer to be part of the program. Websites, articles, and books written by the speaker, and testimonials from those who have heard the speaker, are helpful. Keep in mind that the most expensive or well-known speakers are not always the most effective for a given purpose.

- *Research the speaker's ability to engage the audience.* Public speaking requires expert content level and delivery at a minimum. However, keeping an audience engaged in learning and sustaining engagement over an extended period of time often involves a form of entertainment on the part of the speaker. An experienced public speaker takes the time to review course evaluation feedback in order to improve. Over time, incorporating such feedback benefits the speaker's presentations and ultimately the audience's receptiveness to the delivery of the material.

- *Have a backup plan.* A variety of events can conspire to cause a speaker to be late for his or her presentation. Inclement weather, transportation delays, communication errors, illness, and simple irresponsibility are common reasons. Careful planning can minimize the effects of some, but not all, of these circumstances. Develop a risk management plan to minimize the likelihood that a speaker will be a no-show. In addition, try to have a backup speaker available, typically from the local area, who can be ready to step in at short notice. All this is part of the flexibility associated with the planning of meetings.

Speakers who agree to present at the conference should be asked to sign a contract specifying the date, time, location, and topic of their presentation. The amounts of honorarium and reimbursable travel expenses should be included in the contract.

Plan for Meals and Entertainment   All people, including all conference attendees, need to eat. Most people also like to be entertained. The steering committee must plan for both of these important elements. Several factors must be considered in this part of the conference plan:

- *Time*. Build in enough time for meals and recreation. If conferees are on their own for meals, make sure that an adequate number and variety of restaurants in various price ranges are nearby and that participants have enough time to eat and return to the conference punctually.
- *Meal functions*. Meals are sometimes included as part of a conference program. A speaker may be a part of some meal functions, and awards ceremonies are occasionally part of others, depending on the nature of the conference. Meals included as part of the program are usually, but not always, included in the registration price. Most conference facilities that provide food and beverage services require that conferences contract for these services rather than bring in food or drink from the outside to serve the participants. It is important to know whether a contract includes such requirements because the fees will likely be higher than for external catering.
- *Registration*. Some entertainment or recreational events may require preregistration. A minimum number of participants may be needed to keep costs at prenegotiated levels.
- *Information*. Provide conferees with information on local restaurants, entertainment, and recreational venues. This information is usually available from the convention and visitors bureau or the chamber of commerce, sometimes at no charge.

Plan for Registration   The steering committee must decide in advance how it will handle registration for the conference. Most conferences encourage preregistration (and offer discounted prices if people register early) because planners can then allocate resources appropriately. Preregistration also helps cement the prospective attendees' commitment to

attend the conference. Additionally, preregistration helps to reduce the number of late or same-day registrations, which can add costs for copying, room space additions, postcontractual meal additions, and so on. The steering committee will have to decide whether it will allow on-site registration, and if so, whether the price will be different from that for attendees who register before a predetermined deadline. The registration form should include all the information the planners will need to accommodate the needs of the attendees and to plan for the proper arrangements for each aspect of the conference (see figure 3.7). A mix of registration methods will enhance the convenience of the conference participants. Usual methods for preregistration include submitting the registration form online, through the mail, or by fax.

6 to 11 Months Before the Conference

Eleven months before the conference, the planning committee should begin recruiting exhibitors, negotiate and sign contracts for other services, and compile all documents required for fulfillment of continuing education units (CEUs) and continuing medical education (CME) units. For new conferences, potential exhibitors can initially be approached while exhibiting at other conferences.

Recruit Exhibitors and Sponsors   Many groups have a stake in the success of a conference. Obviously, the conference planners, sponsoring organization, and conferees hope that the symposium is a success. Businesses that sell their products to the target audience may wish to use the conference as a tool for marketing those products. Conference planners can take advantage of this desire by charging companies to display their products at the conference. This is an excellent way to keep the cost of attending the conference down while also meeting the needs of the businesses that support the profession. Businesses are typically invited to support the conference in one of two roles:

- *Sponsor*. Sponsors are businesses that provide either a sum of money or a gift in kind that supports one or more aspect of a conference. For example, conference planners may solicit funds from various businesses related to sports medicine to support the costs associated with an individual speaker. Planners may solicit other sponsors to pay for a meal function or other social event. Sponsors should receive public recognition at the conference and an expression of gratitude for their contribution.

Advance Online Registration Form

Annual Meeting & Clinical Symposia
National Athletic Trainers' Association
1620 Valwood Parkway, Suite 115, Carrollton, TX 75006
214.637.6282

Please complete this form in full and press the SUBMIT button at the bottom of this form. Use the tab key to maneuver between the fields. Do not use the enter key.

This form can only be used with a credit card.

Mailing Info: Registration packet will be mailed after May 1 to this address.

Last Name: * [   ] First Name: * [   ] Member Number: [   ]

Address: * [   ]

[   ]

[   ]

City, State, Zip * [   ]

Work Phone: [   ] Home Phone: [   ]

Spouse (if attending): [   ]

Child(ren) & Age(s) (if attending): [   ]

Emergency Contact Name & Relationship: [   ]

Emergency Contact Phone: [   ]

　　　* Required

Badge Info: Name badges will be prepared from this information.

Nickname for Badge: [   ]

Credentials (Limit 3): [   ]

Institution: [   ] City, State: [   ]

Figure 3.7 An example of an online conference registration form.

Courtesy of the National Athletic Trainers' Association.

● *Exhibitor.* Exhibitors are companies that are invited, for a fee, to display their merchandise at the conference. Exhibitors are commonly assigned to a booth (the larger or more prominently placed the booth, the higher the fee) in an exhibit hall near, but not infringing on, the rooms where the sessions will be held. If exhibitors will be invited to participate, breaks should be built into the conference schedule to allow and encourage the conferees to visit the exhibit hall.

Contract for Miscellaneous Services Even the simplest conference incurs many expenses, each of which must be planned for. Each item of sub-

stantial cost should be agreed to in advance in the form of a signed contract. Most vendors that supply the conference will have their own contracts. Conference planners should review contracts carefully for acceptable terms. Most conferences require the following services:

● Audiovisual equipment
● Pipe and drape (the curtains used to create exhibit booths and demarcate other spaces)
● Transportation
● Security
● Printing

- Mailing and marketing
- Meeting room space
- Hotel sleeping rooms
- Food and beverage functions

Many of the items listed can be negotiated based on the size of the conference. For example, late checkouts can be requested for course participants when the meeting might end on a day after the typical 11:00 a.m. checkout time. Also, as noted earlier, audiovisual equipment, catering, and room space are all negotiable.

Speaker Information Important pieces of information are collected from the speaker to meet compliance issues for awarding course credit to participants, as well as to assist course directors who are planning and running the event. Information that is needed may include, but is not limited to, a biographical sketch to introduce the speaker, a current resume or CV, audiovisual needs, speaker travel information, and any other special needs. It is also important to secure a conflict of interest form and ask a speaker to disclose financial arrangements that could relate to the topic of the presentation (see figure 3.8).

Continuing Education Units The Board of Certification (BOC) establishes criteria for continuing education for athletic trainers to maintain certification status. Organizations and individuals that offer continuing education courses have the opportunity to become **approved providers** of continuing education for athletic trainers through the BOC. Becoming an approved provider requires the completion of an application process that demonstrates compliance with the standards set forth; this is an effort to ensure that a level of quality is in place for course offerings. Applicants are asked to provide examples of course agendas, cancellation policies (the policy a provider has in place for participants of courses that are cancelled; such a policy is needed in order to receive recognition as an approved provider by BOC), a manual of policies and procedures, and other relevant components of continuing education management. Additional requirements for courses have an evidence-based practice (EBP) designation.

Being an approved provider also entails responsibilities for each course offering. Much of the preparation occurs months before the course is delivered. Templates for certificates of attendance and completion need to be developed, and course evaluations need to be developed and issued for all participants. A roster with the name, contact information, and certification number of participants needs to be maintained for potential auditing purposes. The BOC website is thorough and explains all of the details of the requirements for approved providers. To attract other types of health care providers, you might need to pursue approval from other professional organizations as well. Other professions may require course approval on a statewide basis.

KEY POINT

Conference organizers who wish to become approved providers of athletic training continuing education programs should visit the Board of Certification website and click on the Approved Providers tab.

3 to 5 Months Before the Conference

The final planning activities to be completed include conference marketing and the preparation of learning materials. Conference planners usually accomplish these tasks a few months before the beginning of the conference.

Market the Conference A conference will fail if people do not attend. The marketing process is one of the elements that will inform potential conferees and encourage them to attend. In many ways, a conference brochure is like a person's resume: A good first impression is attractive to the consumer, whereas a poorly designed and cheap-looking advertisement for a course may lead to the perception that the offerings lack quality. For this reason, consider saving money on the marketing aspect of the conference very carefully. Even the best speakers can't make up for lost revenue as a result of an insufficient number of participants. You can use a variety of methods to market a conference. Some require access to a database of names and addresses of the target audience. Conferences marketed to health care professionals are generally more successful if the conferees can earn required continuing education credits by attending. Marketing should begin well before the conference because most professionals plan their travel schedules far in advance. Methods for marketing a conference include the following:

- *Direct mail.* Either the postal service or e-mail can be an effective way of reaching potential conference attendees. Professional organizations to which the members of the target audience belong often sell mailing lists.

CONTINUING EDUCATION PRESENTER CONFLICT OF INTEREST FORM

Name: _____   Credentials: _____

Email: _____   Phone: _____

Address: _____

Activity title: _____   Activity date: _____

Live presentation

Webinar

Recorded program

Correspondence program

Activity hours: _____

By way of my signature below, I, _____ (print name) acknowledge that I have no existing or known conflict of interest pertaining to the material and content that I have agreed to present. For the purposes of this agreement, a conflict of interest may include, but is not limited to, a financial relationship with a commercial interest discussed in my presentation. A commercial interest herein is defined as any entity promoted within the presentation whereby the audience participants may have interest in, in such a way that the presenter would further benefit or profit from. Such interest may also include an immediate or other family member who maintains similar interests in an entity promoted by the presenter.

Please confirm that you, as the presenter, have no conflicts of interest related to this activity.

❏ *I am confirming that I have no known conflicts of interest to report.*

If you believe that you have known and/or potential conflicts of interest, please confirm and complete the required information.

❏ *I am confirming that I believe I have a conflict of interest. (Complete requested information below.)*

Description of conflict of interest		Self conflict	Family member
Company Name		❏	❏
Check the appropriate relationship below	**Describe general terms of the relationship**		
❏ Royalty			
❏ Salary			
❏ Intellectual Property			
❏ Consulting Honorarium			
❏ Stock/Bond (other) Ownership			

If you have more than one conflict of interest to report, please duplicate this form and complete the requested information.

Signature: _____   Date: _____

Figure 3.8 Speaker information and disclosure form.

Developed by Jeff G. Konin.

- *Web-based advertising.* If the conference will be advertised online, the website that presents the advertisement must be one that substantial numbers of the target audience visit frequently. A mass e-mail message containing a link to the online advertisement is a useful strategy.

- *Social media.* Promoting the conference through social media outlets is also effective and affordable. No cost is associated with this and additional sharing of messages through the various social media outlets can expand the overall reach of the program to potential participants.

- *Print advertising.* Advertisements placed in professional and trade publications that are commonly read by members of the target audience can be effective. Some journals and newsletters will list the conference in a free calendar of events section, but such publications may charge a fee for regular advertising space. If the conference targets a local audience, the local newspaper may be a good choice for informing prospective conferees. A press release sent to the local newspaper describing the conference may or may not result in a story, but planners always have the option of buying space for an advertisement. Keep in mind that from a financial perspective, print advertising could be much more costly than electronic promotion.

Prepare Learning Materials A practice common to most conferences is providing attendees with a packet of learning materials. These materials vary in content and scope. Some are simply reprints of the speakers' PowerPoint notes. Others include abstracts of each presentation. A book containing the abstract or outline of each speaker's presentation is known as **proceedings**. Conference participants very much appreciate proceedings that are complete. Pages omitted or left blank because speakers have not turned in prepared outlines detract from proceedings. Although the task can be somewhat cumbersome, conference planners must provide speakers frequent reminders of deadlines so that participants will have access to handouts in a timely manner.

When preparing learning materials, conference planners should consider these three methods for distributing them:

1. *Online and through an app.* Placing the abstracts or outlines online or distributing them through an app allows attendees to download and print the parts of the conference proceedings that they find useful. This method offers considerable cost savings and is the most common way that proceedings are distributed. This also allows the conference organizers to continually update the materials as the speakers submit them.

2. *Hard copy.* Depending on its scope and quality, a hard copy of the proceedings may be included in the registration fee or sold to conferees for an additional charge. Large conferences sometimes contract with publishing companies to provide this service. Because of the cost to produce these, this is becoming much less common.

3. *CD, DVD, or USB storage device.* Another method of disseminating conference proceedings is to place the presentation outlines and documents on a CD, DVD, or USB storage device (jump drive) that can be distributed at the beginning of the conference. This method allows participants to follow the presentations on a laptop or notebook computer without requiring Internet access at the conference. It also allows speakers to provide outlines and accompanying documents without concerns for size limitations. If a conference chooses to distribute print materials, a large cost can be associated with producing and copying those materials. The cost of producing CDs or DVDs for a large number of participants is less than a hard copy, but still typically more costly than placing them online. The time required to make the number needed depends on whether they are made by hand or prepared by a business service.

Conferences as Fund-Raising Events

Conference planning requires careful thought, and it helps to have experience to ensure a profitable, high-quality program. A combination of experience, careful planning, and some luck determines the success or failure of a conference. One method of minimizing risk and attempting to raise funds for organizations, such as student athletic training clubs, is to offer a continuing education course. All of the previously described key elements of operating a successful course also apply to managing a successful fund-raising event. With careful planning, you can take a steps to reduce overhead costs and affect revenue generation.

Typically, these types of events are targeted toward local participants, possibly preceptors of a program and clinicians in the geographical region. Thus, e-mail distributions and physically dropping off brochures are options that can significantly reduce costs. Courses can be given in just a day so that hotel stays are not required. Meeting space can be "borrowed" at minimal to no cost through use of a classroom or meeting room at the school, or a conference or meeting room at a local clinic or hospital facility. Audiovisual equipment can also be borrowed from the school or local facilities.

Perhaps two of the largest costs to consider are food and the speakers' honorariums and travel expenses. When hosting a continuing education course as a fund-raiser, consider seeking sponsorships from local and other businesses that your program regularly supports through annual purchase of athletic training supplies. Often these businesses are happy to provide funding to support continental breakfasts or snacks and beverages in exchange for displaying their banner and distributing their brochures. In some cases, the business may also offer to sponsor the speaker.

Contracting one speaker who possesses enough expertise to provide all of the content for a course is much easier and less expensive than having multiple speakers. In some cases, speakers will generously waive their honorarium to support the fund-raising effort, although conference planners should not expect a speaker to waive travel costs such as gas, airfare, airport parking, or meals associated with travel. Speakers who support a fund-raising conference by waiving their honorarium may or may not want this acknowledged, and meeting facilitators and moderators should be cognizant of their preference. Whether or not the speaker waives the honorarium, giving a gift that serves as a keepsake of the meeting, one related to the location or the host group, is a kind gesture. Gifts may be items that remind speakers of the city or the university they visited to assist with the fund-raiser, and such gifts may have more lasting meaning than an honorarium.

Program Evaluation

Athletic trainers are regularly called on to assess various aspects of a sports medicine program. How is Bill's knee rehabilitation coming along? Is he on schedule? Was the drug education seminar we hosted last week effective? Will the behavior of the athletes change as a result? Questions like these help determine the quality of the program. Unfortunately, even the most thorough and well-conceived strategic and operational plans don't always produce the desired results. To maximize the value of a sports medicine program, athletic trainers must engage in **program evaluation** regularly.

KEY POINT

Sports medicine program evaluation is a critical, but often ignored, part of the athletic trainer's managerial responsibilities. Program evaluations can be either formative or summative. Evaluations typically use goals, objectives, criteria, and outcomes, based on patient charts and other data sources.

The athletic trainer should answer two underlying and related questions when evaluating a sports medicine program:

1. What would the likely effects be if the sports medicine program ceased to exist?
2. How are those who have access to the program better off than those who do not have access to the program?

Each of these questions is crucial; the answers will help the organization determine whether it is committing an appropriate amount of human and financial resources to sports medicine. Answers to these questions, and indeed to questions about every area of the program evaluation, should be supported by documented evidence.

Evidence of sports medicine program quality can and should be derived from several sources. Patient files, injury and treatment summary statistics, and client testimonials are examples of useful data. Educational programs should evaluate student graduation and certification rates. Surveys of satisfaction among clients and alumni can provide valuable evidence of perceived program quality because they allow respondents to reflect for a time before providing feedback. None of this evidence is sufficient in isolation. Considered together, however, it can help provide an overall assessment of the effectiveness of the sports medicine program. Although the athletic trainer will certainly have to render judgments based on professional experience, others who judge the program will need tangible proof that the sports medicine program is accomplishing its mission.

Types of Evidence to Support Sports Medicine Program Effectiveness

- Patient files
- Injury summaries and statistics
- Treatment summaries and statistics
- Client testimonials
- Athletic training student graduation and certification statistics

- Critical incident reports
- Staff accomplishments
- Client surveys
- Alumni surveys
- Surveys of employers of alumni

Chart Auditing

Patient chart auditing is one of the most common methods for evaluating the effectiveness of a sports medicine program. The patient chart should contain a detailed history of the patient's problems, treatment goals, specific interventions, and reactions to those interventions (see chapter 7). As such, it is an excellent data source from which to draw conclusions regarding the effectiveness of the sports health care the program provides. Although many chart-auditing techniques exist, internal and external techniques are most common.

Members of the sports medicine staff typically perform an **internal chart audit**, which serves as an important component of a Total Quality Management process for the sports medicine program. Chart auditing is an internal check to ensure that certain quality standards are being upheld in the treatment of injured patients. The procedure might examine several factors. For example, the director of a sports medicine clinic might be concerned that a large number of anterior cruciate ligament (ACL) patients are having a portion of their reimbursement requests denied because they are exceeding the allowable number of visits. One way to find out why this is happening is to pull the charts of all ACL patients for the preceding year and look for common elements. Was there a common surgeon? Were one or two clinicians seeing most of the patients who had their insurance claims denied? Were the patients mostly older industrial workers or younger physically active people? After staff members have identified a pattern, they can develop and implement a plan to address the causes of the problem.

Computerized patient databases make internal chart audits fairly painless. Searching for every patient with an ACL injury, for example, and discovering common elements between patients are simple tasks when using injury tracking and patient management software. When records are not computerized, the process must be performed by hand, which can be extremely time consuming.

Internal chart auditing should be performed in a peer review format; in other words, clinicians should not review their own charts. The results are more objective and more beneficial when a peer reviews another provider's charts with a fresh set of eyes. The provision of constructive feedback by a peer reveals strengths and weaknesses in overall delivery of care and serves as a thorough assessment of outcomes in relation to interventions.

A second kind of chart-auditing process is known as an **external chart audit**. External chart auditing is used by accreditation agencies to ensure that a sports medicine program is upholding commonly held standards of practice in patient care. (See the earlier section on accreditation and the later discussion of external evaluators in the section Summative vs. Formative Evaluation.) Third-party reimbursement agencies also use external chart audits to determine the appropriateness of claims for reimbursement. One of the most common instances of external chart auditing occurs when practitioners bill Medicare for the services they provide to qualifying patients. Either a **carrier** or an **intermediary** evaluates these claims, which must be extensively documented to qualify for reimbursement (Esposto 1993). When an intermediary or carrier evaluates a Medicare claim, it looks for a record of the patient's progress and a rationale for reimbursement. The chart must contain information sufficient to document that the services were directly related to a treatment plan established by the physician or other health care provider. The chart must also document that the services provided were reasonable and necessary. The Medicare guidelines for determining what is reasonable and necessary include the following:

- The treatment must be accepted as standard for the effective remediation of the patient's condition.

- The patient's condition must be such that only the services of the particular health care provider could be used to provide the care.

- There must be a reasonable expectation that the patient's condition will improve in a specific period.

- The treatment plan must be reasonable with respect to the amount, duration, and frequency of treatment.

Another way to perform external chart auditing is to hire experienced consultants who offer expert reviews in a manner preferable to the client. The fee paid to the consultant is often based on the number of hours of work required. Although this may seem like an unnecessary expense, the use of an experienced reviewer adds value to the audit. Furthermore, using external consultants for chart audits as part of an ongoing plan, as opposed to implementing an external review only after problems or concerns have been identified, will likely improve quality control. In particular, external consultants can help an organization plan for upcoming accreditation reviews.

Summative vs. Formative Evaluation

Outcomes assessment, accountability, and overall reporting of results have become more important during program evaluation. For an athletic trainer, it is important to be able to differentiate between the two more common types of program evaluations: summative and formative. **Summative evaluations** typically describe the effectiveness or accomplishments of a program, whereas **formative evaluations** are used for program improvement purposes. The summative evaluation includes, but may not be limited to,

- a summary statement of program effectiveness,
- a description of the program,
- a statement of documented achievement of program goals,
- unanticipated outcomes of the program,
- comparisons with other similar sports medicine programs (benchmarking),

- a summary of the resources used, and
- a summary of revenue and expenses.

The formative evaluation includes, but may not be limited to,

- identification of potential problems in the sports medicine program,
- discussion of areas that need strengthening,
- recognition of program strengths,
- ongoing assessment of program objectives,
- opportunities for areas of improvement, and
- threats to potential future changes to be implemented

Good program evaluation is expensive in terms of both overt and covert costs. Ideally, athletic trainers should use rigorous experimental research designs incorporating control or nontreatment groups for every program evaluation. This method is the best way to determine whether a sports medicine program is having the intended effect. Unfortunately, only athletic trainers with the appropriate graduate school training will have the research and statistical skills necessary to carry out such experimental designs. In addition, athletic trainers often find it impossible to carry out evaluation projects of this scope and complexity because they take too much time away from their other duties. The athletic trainer should strive to include as much comparative information as possible in the program evaluation to help other stakeholders appreciate the quality of the program compared to other programs of its type.

One way in which athletic trainers can provide evidence of quality in comparison to sports medicine programs at similar institutions is to use other athletic trainers as **external evaluators**. This is a process that is all too often underutilized by athletic trainers in clinical settings. This is similar to using external reviewers for chart auditing, and can be done on a larger programmatic scale. For example, athletic trainers trained in program evaluation are employed to judge the quality of athletic training education programs for schools requesting accreditation. External evaluators can also be useful for reducing bias. Athletic trainers will find it difficult, or even impossible, to be objective about their own programs. Asking expert third parties, who have little to lose or gain, to assess the program helps lend credibility to the evaluation results. External reviews can also be performed solely on specific policies that are in place, such as emergency action plans or drug education and testing programs. For the purposes of internal reviews, scientific reporting is not necessary. In fact, to the contrary, the more practical the information and the greater the potential for immediate application, the more favorably a report will be received.

Before the external evaluator arrives, the institution must commit itself to allowing reasonable access to the people and information the evaluator will need to make accurate judgments and generate useful suggestions for improvement. A competent external evaluator will want to have access to all the evidence. In addition, a good external evaluator will interview the athletic trainers, team physicians, athletic administrators, coaches, athletic training students, athletes, and other physically active patients to gain a broad-based perspective of the quality of the sports medicine program. After the site visit, the evaluator should prepare a report that lists perceived strengths and weaknesses of the sports medicine program and specific steps that the institution could take to improve the program. It is helpful to provide external reviewers with as much information as possible in advance of a site visit. This information should include, but not necessarily be limited to, all department and organizational policy and procedure manuals, the website URL, and especially the goals that the organization wants to achieve with the aid of the external review.

Goals, Objectives, and Criteria

Program evaluation should be based on an analysis of the goals and objectives of the athletic training program. Evaluation of goals and objectives should use measurable criteria established in advance of the evaluation. **Goals**, general statements of program intent, are derived from the mission statement. Two or more objectives support each goal. **Objectives** are more specific than goals and identify how the program intends to achieve a particular goal. **Criteria** are highly specific, and typically quantifiable, statements that provide the yardstick for determining whether a particular objective has been accomplished. Examples of a goal and supporting objectives and criteria might include the following:

Goal: The Memorial Hospital Sports Medicine Outreach Program shall provide easy access to sports medicine services for high school student-athletes.

Objective 1: High school student-athletes will have access to Outreach Program staff within 24 hours of the onset of injury.

Criterion for objective 1: Of the high school student-athletes responding to the Outreach Program annual patient satisfaction survey, 80% will indicate that they were seen within 24 hours of the onset of their injuries.

Objective 2: High school student-athletes will incur minimal travel time in accessing the services of the Outreach Program staff.

Criterion for objective 2: Of the high school student-athletes responding to the Outreach Program annual patient satisfaction survey, 90% will indicate that they traveled less than 5 miles (8 km) from their homes to be seen by an Outreach Program staff member.

Frequency of Program Evaluation

How often should a sports medicine program be evaluated? Although there is no universal answer, some guidelines apply regardless of the setting in which the sports medicine clinic is housed:

- *Collect and collate evaluation evidence continuously.* If data are collected only immediately preceding the evaluation, sufficient time may not be available to complete the task. Gathering the evidence is the most time-consuming aspect of program evaluation.

- *Perform a mini-evaluation every year.* This approach has two advantages: The athletic trainer will have to compile evidence of program effectiveness for a reasonable time frame, and the evaluation will identify program weaknesses that require immediate attention.

- *Conduct a complete evaluation of the sports medicine program every three to five years.* This schedule will allow the athletic trainer to examine strategic issues such as mission congruence and program goals and objectives, which shouldn't change often.

Program Self-Study

Part of the mission statement for the Memorial Hospital Sports Medicine Outreach Program specified that evaluation would occur on an ongoing basis to ensure quality care for the high school

SPORTS MEDICINE OUTREACH PROGRAM SELF-STUDY

INSTRUCTIONS

The self-study for the sports medicine program shall consist of four areas: general considerations, patients, staff, and program. The athletic trainer in charge of the program shall answer the questions below and prepare a report with supporting evidence to be submitted to the director of rehabilitation services and the vice president for patient services. In addition, the director of rehabilitation services, in consultation with the athletic trainer, shall select an appropriate external evaluator. The external evaluator's report shall be included in the self-study as an appendix.

GENERAL CONSIDERATIONS

1. What is the mission of the program? Is the mission statement consistent with the mission of Memorial Hospital? Is the mission statement consistent with national standards for the delivery of sports medicine services?

2. Does the program work well in the context of the Department of Rehabilitation Services? How does the program take advantage of available resources? Do the program's staff members work well together? Do they work well with the rest of the hospital staff?

3. Who provides leadership for the program? Are the program leaders effective?

4. What are the priorities of the program? Are they appropriate? Do they mesh well with the priorities of Memorial Hospital? Do the priorities of individual staff members mesh well with the priorities of the sports medicine program?

PATIENTS

1. Do patients achieve the short- and long-term goals established at the beginning of their treatment programs? Do patients have easy and quick access to evaluation and treatment services? Do the students of the Ashton County high schools use the program? If not, why not? Are the program's patient loads consistent with national averages?

2. Does the program help reduce the incidence of injury in the Ashton County high schools? If not, what factors account for this? In what ways can the program be improved in order to reduce the incidence of injury?

3. Are the students of the Ashton County high schools better educated about healthy lifestyles than students elsewhere? What efforts have been made to educate students regarding healthy lifestyles? What additional efforts should be and could be made in this area?

STAFF

1. How effective are staff members as providers of sports medicine services? Are some staff members ineffective? What can be done to resolve the problem?

2. Do staff members possess the standard credentials for delivery of sports medicine services? Do they engage in programs of continuing education?

3. Are staff members considered experts in their fields? Can they boast of professional accomplishments consistent with experts of regional or national reputation?

4. Are staff members performing in a manner consistent with their position descriptions and codes of professional conduct?

5. Is the size of the staff appropriate for the tasks it must accomplish? Could the same job be done with the same quality with fewer staff members?

(continued)

Figure 3.9 Self-study form for a hospital-based sports medicine clinic.

PROGRAM

1. Is each component of the sports medicine program effective? Which components are the strongest? Which are the weakest? How could the weak components be strengthened?

2. Is each component of the sports medicine program necessary? If not, should some components be eliminated? Should additional components be added to the program? Who would they serve? What is the desired effect of a new component?

3. Is the sports medicine program cost effective? Does the income it generates support its budget? Is it efficient? How could it become more efficient?

Figure 3.9 *(continued)*

student-athletes being served. One of the ways the hospital could evaluate the effectiveness of the program would be to design and implement a self-study process every three to five years (see figure 3.9). The self-study should critically examine all the major elements of the program and be shared with individuals involved with the sports medicine program. Reports from external evaluators and condensed transcripts of documentary evidence should be included as appendixes. It is also helpful to perform some form of a mini-assessment of a long-term plan approximately halfway on the established time line to determine what areas to focus on in order to reach the stated goals.

Outcomes

One of the major thrusts related to program evaluation that has developed since the late 1980s is objective measurement of patients' functional abilities using **outcomes assessment**. Outcomes assessment is a type of evaluation process that provides objective, measurable evidence that the care provided by the athletic trainer was effective in improving the patient's functional ability. Outcomes assessment is likely to play an increasingly important role in health care in general and for athletic trainers specifically. As Denegar and Hertel (2002) asked, "What do certified athletic trainers do that makes a difference in the health care of the physically active?" As the dollars available for health care continue to shrink at the same time that athletic trainers are seeking access to third-party reimbursement, quality assurance processes and utilization reviews will become critical factors in determining who will be paid and who will not. Health care professions that cannot demonstrate

that their interventions are effective and medically necessary will find themselves without access to third-party reimbursement in the increasingly competitive managed care market. In addition, organizations that cannot document that their interventions are cost effective will be bypassed in favor of those that can.

The focus on outcomes assessment is particularly important for athletic trainers employed in clinics and hospitals. These organizations remain financially sound only if they receive reimbursements for their services, either through government programs like Medicare and Medicaid or through private insurers. As the private insurance market continues to make the transition from a traditional fee-for-service model to a managed care model, it will be more important than ever for these organizations to be able to document that they improve their patients' function in an efficient and cost-effective manner. Hospitals and clinics that cannot produce documented evidence to demonstrate the effectiveness of their patients' functional outcomes will have difficulty getting the contracts from managed care organizations that will, to an increasing degree, be their lifelines.

Spending for medical research is reaching all-time high levels, yet challenges remain in translating basic science research into clinical applications (Moses et al. 2005). For the profession of athletic training to advance and subsequently justify the undisputed benefit of the certified athletic trainer, it will be necessary to avoid a glaring disconnect between the increasing body of knowledge produced by athletic training researchers and clinical practice (Hertel 2005). It is also vital that published data be compiled in such a way that the average athletic trainer in a clinical setting could locate and

Example of a CAT

Effects of combining OKC and CKC exercises on quad strength and knee laxity in athletes recovering from ACL reconstruction

Clinical bottom lines: 1. In athletes who have undergone anterior cruciate ligament (ACL) reconstruction, a combination of open kinetic chain and closed kinetic chain resulted in greater improvement of quadriceps strength than closed chain exercises alone. 2. A combination of open kinetic chain and closed kinetic chain exercises did not improve knee laxity statistically versus closed kinetic chain exercises alone in this population.

Citation: Mikkelsen, C., Werner, S., and Eriksson, E. Closed kinetic chain alone compared to combined open and closed kinetic chain exercises for quadriceps strengthening after anterior cruciate ligament reconstruction with respect to return to sports: A prospective matched follow-up study. *Knee Surgery, Sports Traumatology, Arthroscopy.* 2000; 8: 337-342.

Clinical question: In athletes who have undergone ACL reconstruction, is a combination of open kinetic chain (OKC) exercise and closed kinetic chain (CKC) exercise more effective than closed kinetic chain exercise alone in improving quadriceps strength and knee laxity?

The study: The purpose of the randomized controlled trial (RCT) was to look at the rehabilitation of ACL reconstruction using a combination of OKC and CKC exercises versus the same program using only closed kinetic chain exercises. Subjects received treatment from the same therapist that took the measurements. The study used both a pretest and a posttest. The RCT was not blinded. Reliability procedures were not established.

The study patients: The study consisted of 44 athletes, 34 males and 10 females, aged 18-40 years who were recovering from ACL reconstruction using a bone–patellar tendon–bone graft at the same hospital.

Experimental groups: All subjects were randomly assigned to one of two groups. One group performed a combination of open kinetic chain and closed kinetic chain exercises ($n = 22$). The other group performed closed kinetic chain exercises alone ($n = 22$). Therapy lasted six months. The participants were very similar to that in my clinical question.

The evidence: The outcome measures were quadriceps torque, measured by a Kin-Com dynamometer, and knee laxity, measured by KT 1000 arthrometer. The study showed statistical evidence that there was a measurable difference in quadriceps torque ($p < 0.01$) but no difference in knee laxity by those who performed a combination of open chain and closed chain compared to closed chain exercises.

Comments: 1. The study is limited as it only shows short-term effects of open kinetic chain exercises on the ACL reconstruction. Also, the researchers used equipment that not all therapists may have to measure outcomes. 2. Further studies should be done to show the long-term effects of ACL reconstruction on knee laxity. 3. The study provided statistical evidence that a combination of OKC and CKC exercises increased quadriceps torque compared to CKC exercises alone.

Appraised by: Riley Phelps
Date Appraised: August 7, 2008

Reprinted by permission from University of Nevada, Las Vegas. Available: http://pt.unlv.edu/ebpt/index.html.

comprehend the essentials of research findings. For example, it has been estimated that the average health care provider would need to read 19 journal articles per day every day of the year to remain abreast of the changes in health care (Hootman 2004). Others have stated that it takes an average of 17 years to translate research findings into clinical practice (Fineout-Overholt, Melnyk, and Schultz 2005). The use of critically appraised topics (CATs) has been helpful in condensing research information from peer-reviewed studies (Law 2002a). A CAT is a summary, in a couple of pages, of a focused clinical question. The information is divided into categories such as clinical question being addressed, date of completion of the CAT, treatment approaches, comparative interventions, and the outcomes obtained.

Outcomes assessment is important for athletic trainers who work in professional, collegiate, and high school settings. Although systematic assessment of outcomes has not traditionally occurred in these settings, the increasing pressure that most athletic trainers are under from cost-conscious administrators makes it important to be able to document that athletic trainers provide an excellent service in an economical fashion. Outcomes data could potentially serve a useful purpose in justifying new staff or in defending against an athletic director who wants to contract all sports medicine services to an outside agency. Streator and Buckley (2000) suggest that outcomes studies in these settings should help answer the following questions:

- Does the involvement of an athletic trainer in the athletic program result in decreased incidence of injury?
- Does the involvement of an athletic trainer in the athletic program result in reduced insurance claims?
- What are the cost savings associated with employing athletic trainers in the athletic program?

Additionally, results of outcomes assessments may assist with identifying the medical coverage required for each setting and support the need for full-time athletic trainers and an improved ratio of athletic trainers to athletes. Currently, in many high schools fortunate enough to have a full-time athletic trainer on staff, the athletic trainer is responsible for the supervision of hundreds of athletes. In these situations, the lone athletic trainer must prioritize work assignments in order to be where the risk of injury is greatest, thus neglecting coverage and care for many other student-athletes.

In the college and university setting, positive outcomes can be used for recruiting purposes; school officials, administrators, and coaches can provide parents of incoming student-athletes with information about the provision of care for their children.

Many methods are used to conduct outcomes assessments. The four most common models, however, are patient chart documentation, randomized clinical trials, patient satisfaction surveys, and patient-reported outcomes. Each has strengths and weaknesses (see table 3.1). All four are important sources of outcomes data. The usefulness of each of these methods, however, depends on the degree to which standard research protocols that reduce the likelihood of yielding inaccurate conclusions are employed. Outcomes studies that fail to employ control groups, to randomize patient selection and therapeutic methods, or to blind the researchers and the subjects may yield suspect results. Note also that many factors beyond the control of the athletic trainer can affect the outcome of a patient's care, including factors related to initial clinical findings

Table 3.1 Strengths and Weaknesses of Outcomes Assessment Models

Model	Strengths	Weaknesses
Patient chart documentation	1. Provides outcomes for specific patients 2. Required for Medicare reimbursement	1. Labor intensive 2. Dependent on charting skills of practitioner 3. Does not systematically control for situational variables
Randomized clinical trials	1. Uses rigid controls to reduce confounding factors 2. Controls variance 3. Useful for examining specific problems	1. Requires the use of a control group 2. Poor focus on broad or multiple issues 3. Time intensive
Patient surveys	1. Easy to administer 2. Useful for examining a broad range of issues 3. Useful for assessing patient satisfaction	1. Instruments must be subjected to a validation process 2. Lack of patient specificity 3. Self-reported data are often unreliable
Patient-reported outcomes	1. Easy to administer 2. Standardized scoring 3. Useful for assessing patient pain and function	1. Reliability and validity can vary between different instruments 2. Relies on patient honesty 3. Not all measures are applicable to athletes

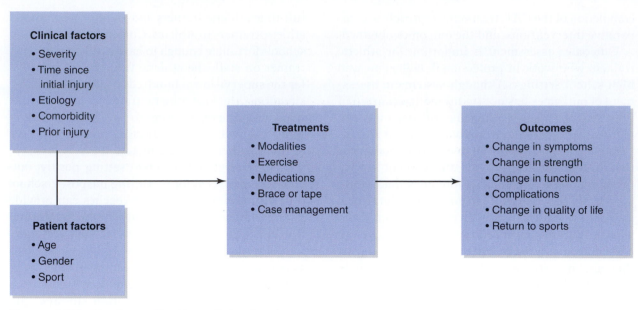

Figure 3.10 Factors affecting clinical outcomes.

Reprinted by permission from S. Streator and W.E. Buckley, "Clinical outcomes in sports medicine," *Athletic Therapy Today* 5, no. 5: 60 (2000).

and patient characteristics (Streator and Buckley 2000) (see figure 3.10).

One of the original athletic training outcomes assessment tools was completed by what was called at the time the NATA Reimbursement Advisory Group, which performed a three-year outcomes study. The study used an instrument called the Athletic Training Outcomes Assessment (ATOA) to link specific treatments with outcomes and to assess athletic training procedures for efficacy and efficiency (Keirns, Knudsen, and Webster 1997). The ATOA considered several factors, including type of injury, body part, type of treatment, affective variables, comorbidities, and patient outcome expectations (see figure 3.11). This outcomes study had many of the weaknesses of other outcomes studies that use self-reported patient surveys, including the lack of a control or comparison group (Albohm and Wilkerson 1999). Campbell (1999) reported that data from the three-year study yielded the following results:

- Athletic training methods produce excellent overall outcomes, with the best results in functional outcomes and physical outcomes.
- Athletic training techniques are effective in treating injuries at all body locations, especially in the lower extremities and spine.
- Industrial patients treated with work-hardening techniques by athletic trainers experienced excellent outcomes.

- The total number of treatments provided is a positive factor in determining positive outcomes.
- Patients have a high degree of satisfaction with athletic trainers and their services.
- Athletic training outcomes are consistent across site types, referring sources, and payer groups.
- As the number of days increased between an injury and the onset of treatment provided by a certified athletic trainer, the patients' favorable perceptions of their outcomes decreased.

Another outcomes study that has helped demonstrate the efficacy and efficiency of the care provided by athletic trainers was conducted by an independent outcomes research company, Focus on Therapeutic Outcomes, Inc. (FOTO). The FOTO study, conducted in 1999, compared patient responses to care provided by athletic trainers with that provided by physical therapists in the same clinical setting. The study showed that the outcomes associated with the care provided by athletic trainers, including various measures of value and patient satisfaction, were similar to those associated with care provided by physical therapists. Although the FOTO study provides a good starting point for the systematic study of athletic training outcomes, it has received criticism because it did not assess measurable patient function outcomes valued by the insurance

ATHLETIC TRAINING OUTCOMES ASSESSMENT

TO BE COMPLETED AT INITIAL ENCOUNTER

Site athletic trainer code: _____ Patient name:_____ Age:_____ Sex: _____

Site type: _____	Referring source: _____	Payer: _____
1. Sports medicine clinic 2. Clinic—High school or college 3. High school athletic training room 4. College or university athletic training room 5. Professional athletic training room 6. Industrial setting	1. Self 2. Coach or supervisor 3. Insurer 4. Primary care physician or generalist 5. Orthopedic physician or specialist	1. Medicaid 2. Medicare 3. Managed care 4. Workers' Compensation 5. CHAMPUS (government or military) 6. Private insurance 7. Institution 8. Patient

TO BE COMPLETED BY ATHLETIC TRAINER AT INITIAL EVALUATION

Duration between injury or surgery and beginning of athletic training treatments: _____ days

(Put 0 if treatments begin on the same day as the injury or surgery.)

Location of injury or surgery: _____

(Indicate the primary location only. If another injury exists, identify as a comorbid factor.)

1. Toe(s)	4. Lower leg	7. Hip	10. Abdomen	13. Cervical spine	16. Arm	19. Wrist
2. Foot	5. Knee	8. Pelvis	11. Lumbar spine	14. Head	17. Elbow	20. Hand
3. Ankle	6. Thigh	9. Groin	12. Thorax	15. Shoulder	18. Forearm	21. Finger(s)

Type of injury: _____

(Indicate the primary injury only. If another injury exists, identify as a comorbid factor.)

1. Joint dysfunction	4. Sprain: grade 1	7. Skin or wound infection	10. Fracture
2. Joint degeneration	5. Sprain; grade 2	8. Bursitis	11. Avulsion
3. Joint hypomobility	6. Sprain; grade 3	9. Musculotendinous injury	12. Neurologic disease

TO BE COMPLETED BY PATIENT AT INTAKE AND DISCHARGE

Patient—Your responses to this questionnaire will help your athletic trainer and this clinic determine rehabilitation outcomes for specific medical conditions in response to specific treatments. This will help us optimize our treatment services to you and other patients. Your responses will be kept confidential and will not affect your care in any way. Thanks for your assistance.

AT INTAKE						AT DISCHARGE				
Critical problem	Severe problem	Moderate problem	Minor problem	No problem	Instructions—Please rate your current capacities specific to the injury for which you will receive, or have received, treatments. Please answer all questions as best you can, even if some of the questions seem somewhat irrelevant to you. Circle the appropriate response according to the (0 1 2 3 4) scale; 0 – critical problem, 1 – severe problem, 2 – moderate problem, 3 – minor problem, 4 – no problem.	Critical problem	Severe problem	Moderate problem	Minor problem	No problem
0	1	2	3	4	**Work activities**—lifting and lowering, holding and handling, carrying, pushing and pulling, bending over, squatting and stooping, kneeling, crawling, reaching, turning and pivoting, gripping and pinching, fingering	0	1	2	3	4
0	1	2	3	4	**Sports, recreation, wellness activities**—running, jumping, throwing, catching, kicking, swinging, withstanding impacts, weightlifting, specific activities (sport, recreation, wellness)	0	1	2	3	4
0	1	2	3	4	**Movement**—getting into desired positions, range of motion, speed of motion, bilateral differences (e.g., limping), need for support device	0	1	2	3	4

Figure 3.11 Excerpt from Athletic Training Outcomes Assessment.

Adapted from JAMES A.F. STONER, MANAGEMENT, 2nd Edition, ©1982, pp. 268, 271. Prentice Hall, Englewood Cliffs, New Jersey.

industry. Future studies should be structured to analyze improvements in patient function, which will better enable the insurance industry and other important external markets to assess the cost-effectiveness of athletic training care.

Evidence-Based Practice

Over the last couple of decades, efforts have increased internationally to support assessment techniques and interventions as they relate to all aspects of medicine. The term **evidence-based medicine** has evolved as an approach to improving practice efficacy. Among other variations of this term are *evidence-based practice* and *evidence-based health care*. Sackett, considered one of the forefathers of evidence-based medicine, and his colleagues (1996) coined the phrase and defined it as "the conscientious, explicit, and judicious use of current best evidence in making decisions about the care of individual patients" (p. 71). When incorporating the evidence into clinical practice, one should use a systematic approach in reviewing peer research data so that unbiased clinical decision making can occur (Belanger 2002). Steves and Hootman (2004) noted the following reasons for the importance of evidence-based medicine for athletic training:

- Improvement of care for the patients
- Promotion of critical thinking
- Ongoing and continued evaluation of treatment methods
- Ability for athletic training to further contribute alongside health professions in peer-reviewed published evidence
- Improved potential for third-party reimbursement
- Overall enhanced reputation for the profession

The authors have furthermore identified five components of evidence-based medical practice for athletic trainers to adhere to:

1. Define a critically relevant question.
2. Search for the best evidence.
3. Appraise the quality of the evidence.
4. Apply the evidence to clinical practice.
5. Evaluate the outcomes of the applied evidence.

Watson described the **relative value** of a particular intervention as it relates to the overall cost of providing the service (Law 2002b). With reference to five types of economic value (cost–consequence analysis, cost-minimization analysis, cost-effectiveness analysis, cost–utility analysis, and cost–benefit analysis), part of the perceived success of an intervention relates to how the intervention compares in outcomes results to other comparable treatments when the cost per delivery of the intervention is factored in. For example, if two interventions yielded the same result for a patient but one was less costly than the other, the intervention with the lower cost would be better to use for the overall population because this could translate into a significantly larger savings of dollars spent for health care. Pharmaceuticals is an area in which this is clearly seen. Many brand-name drugs also have a generic equivalent that is approved to provide similar outcomes at a much lower cost to the consumer.

Because approaches to clinical care using evidence-based medicine remain a critical component to the delivery of organized health care services, practitioners must stay abreast of contemporary approaches based on sound evidential principles. There is growing support for teaching the concepts of evidence-based medicine as a standard part of today's medical and health care curriculum in an effort to promote this style of clinical practice as a learned normative method (Burns and Foley 2005; Cliska 2005). The BOC considers the application of evidence-based medicine in the practice of athletic training a professional responsibility and now requires evidence-based practice CEUs to maintain certification as an athletic trainer. Similarly, the curricular content as outlined by CAATE includes using evidence-based medicine as a foundation for the delivery of care for all entry-level athletic trainers.

One outcome that has been sparingly introduced into clinical practice as a result of evidence-based medicine is the use of **clinical practice guidelines**, or **CPGs**. "Clinical practice guidelines are systematically developed statements to assist practitioner and patient decisions about appropriate health care for specific clinical circumstances" (Field and Lohr 1990, p. 38). Perhaps one of the more well-known CPGs is the one related to the assessment process for an acute ankle injury:

OTTAWA ANKLE RULES (OAR)

X rays are only required if pain exists in the malleolar zone and any one of the following is present:

- *Bone tenderness along the distal 6 cm of the posterior edge of the tibia or tip of the medial malleolus*
- *Bone tenderness along the distal 6 cm of the posterior edge of the fibula or tip of the lateral malleolus*
- *An inability to bear weight for four steps, both immediately and in the emergency department*

Challenges With Implementing Evidence-Based Medicine

Despite the need for the profession of athletic training to join all other medical and allied health providers in the implementation of sound, evidence-based practice, not all athletic trainers have embraced the concept in its entirety. The two most common reasons are that (1) a large percentage of athletic trainers are not practicing in a setting that requires oversight of outcomes as they relate to using evidence-based techniques (e.g., reimbursement) and (2) the concept of evidence-based medicine has been formally taught in entry-level athletic training education programs for only the past decade. More specifically, the following barriers to successful integration of evidence-based practice in clinical settings have been identified (Haynes and Haynes 1998):

- Amount and complexity of available research
- Difficulties in developing evidence-based clinical policies
- Limited access to evidence for some clinicians
- Ineffective continuing education programs
- Challenges with patient compliance

KEY POINT

Information relating to the professionally described role of evidence-based medicine for athletic trainers can be found in the following documents:

- National Athletic Trainers' Association. 2011. *Athletic training educational competencies.* 5th ed. Dallas: Author.
- Board of Certification. 2010. *Role delineation study/Practice analysis.* 6th ed. Omaha: Author.

KEY POINT

The next update of the curricular content for athletic training programs will be embedded in the CAATE accreditation standards.

Maher and colleagues (2004) have also described barriers to evidence-based practice, specifically in the physical therapy profession, identifying the following reasons behind the barriers:

- Publication bias, with authors submitting for publication only those studies that have yielded positive outcomes
- Indexing of journals, because many practicing clinicians do not have access to subscriptions for databases, and lack of databases that include trials performed earlier
- Difficulty of obtaining access to the full text of some published articles
- Language barriers when some studies are not published in English
- Limited number of systematic reviews that assist with assessment of internal validity of the published research
- Difficulty in translating published studies into clinical practice
- Difficulty in drawing conclusions from the evidence when conflicting reports are available
- Difficulties of influencing the integration of the evidence into a patient's own health care decision-making process

It is clear that much more needs to be done for a complete cultural shift toward universal acceptance of evidence-based medicine to occur. Collaborative efforts toward removing the perceived and real barriers to implementing evidence-based medicine will allow for further advancement of quality health care services based on sound evidence. Furthermore, all scientists, educators, and clinicians will need to come closer to a consensus for rating systems that are used to both evaluate and report the evidence. One important concept that has plagued the profession of athletic training as well as medicine as a whole is the fact that in some cases, positive patient outcomes can be achieved despite the lack of peer-reviewed scientific studies that explain why. A lack of studies to support an assessment or intervention does not mean that the approach does not work.

Summary

Program management encompasses the summative process that athletic trainers must consider when overseeing an organization or activity. All programs and organizations should begin by establishing a vision statement that serves as a succinct description of what the program should eventually become. A mission statement is also an important planning tool that can convey the goals and philosophies of a program and further identify, for example, the particular services to be offered, the primary market for those services, and the technology to be used in delivery of the services. All developing programs should include a strategic planning process in an effort to foresee elements of implementation. Strategic planning processes should include some form of self-analysis, such as a SWOT analysis. Strengths, weaknesses, opportunities, and threats can be thoroughly assessed through internally and externally derived data collected from stakeholders to better align a program for success. These findings may also help formulate program policy and procedures that will assist in operational tasks.

Facility planning may be required for organizations envisioning any form of small- or large-scale type of business or event, and many considerations need to be taken into account to ascertain the necessities. When meetings are involved, a majority of the time is spent during the planning phases. Typically, the larger the meeting or conference, the more time is needed for planning. An established time line should be followed to ensure optimal success. Small departmental meetings also require planning, with agendas thought through in advance and disseminated to meeting attendees before discussion. Ongoing evaluations of conferences should be performed in an effort to assess the outcomes of the delivery of an event. Regular smaller meetings should also undergo a periodic review so that meetings can remain efficient, timely, and productive.

Program evaluation is an important component to assure the effectiveness of all programs that are delivered by athletic trainers. The goal is to ensure quality and continue to improve. Program evaluations should be done in a formal manner in a way that identifies strengths and weaknesses. An evidence-based approach should be undertaken in an effort to provide the most accurate and scientifically driven data to analyze.

Learning Aids

Case Study 1

The athletic director met Susan, the college's athletic trainer, in the hallway. After exchanging the news of the day, the AD said, "By the way, I've been working on the NCAA self-study, and one of the sections deals with drug education programs and policies. I know we are just a small college that doesn't have many problems with drugs, but I can't send this thing over to the president without addressing the issue, especially in light of the emphasis the NCAA places on it. Would you be willing to organize a program so that we can at least meet the NCAA guidelines?"

"What would you want such a program to include?" asked Susan. "This could potentially be a huge project."

"You're the expert," replied the AD. "Let me know what you come up with."

Susan had strong opinions on the use and abuse of alcohol and other drugs. Several of her family members had experienced the negative effects of drug and alcohol use. She had plenty of examples of how alcohol had affected her students. She decided that if she was going to take on this program, she wasn't going to allow half measures. She knew that for a problem as complex as drug and alcohol use among college students, she would have to develop a comprehensive program in order to be successful.

After checking with several other athletic trainers who had developed programs for their colleges, Susan began writing a proposal for the program. She decided to include the following elements:

- A standards-setting workshop led by a trained facilitator to help the coaches and team captains develop their own rules and sanctions for alcohol and other drug use
- A policy statement addressing the college's concern about the drug and alcohol issue with procedures to provide an action plan to deal with the problem
- A series of educational seminars and workshops for the student-athletes that would form the bulk of the drug and alcohol education program
- A research study to learn the extent of the problem on campus and determine the effectiveness of the program

The entire program would cost approximately $3,000 for the first 18 months. Because the athletic department wouldn't allocate funds for the project, Susan wrote a grant proposal to a local community foundation that covered the cost. Susan was pleased and confident. After six months of planning, the program was finally ready to go.

Questions for Analysis

1. Based on what you know of Susan's planning effort, how successful is the drug and alcohol education program likely to be? How would you have planned this program?
2. Who represents inside interests in this case? Who represents outside interests? How is this program likely to affect them? How should they be involved in planning it?
3. How much support do you think Susan will be able to develop for the program? What strategies should she use to gain support?
4. How should Susan evaluate the effectiveness of the program? What elements should she include in the evaluation plan?
5. How should Susan write the policy that she wants to see adopted? Develop an example of a process and a procedure that might support such a policy.
6. If you were in Susan's position, would you have handled anything differently? What alternative actions would you have taken?

Case Study 2

Fernando was halfway through his first year as the chairperson of the Department of Athletic Training at a midsized university. The department he led offered an accredited professional master's degree in athletic training. The department was housed in the College of Allied Health and had graduated an average of 10 students per year for the past eight years. Two full-time faculty members and three adjunct members who had release time from the athletic department staffed the department.

Fernando received a memo from the dean of the College of Allied Health informing him that it was his department's turn for a departmental review. In keeping with the new policy of allowing greater administrative freedom to department chairpersons, Fernando would be allowed to collect and present the evidence that he thought the provost and the dean's council should use to judge the effectiveness of the department. The dean told Fernando that he would have five months to submit his report.

A few days later, Fernando was having lunch in the faculty cafeteria when the dean walked over. "Fernando," the dean said, "you should know that the dean's council has been given instructions to reduce our budget by 10% next year. After discussing the problem, we all agreed that the only way to do it without weakening all the programs is to eliminate one of them. I wanted you to know that, unofficially, your department is one that is being considered in the cutback. No decision will be made until after the departmental reviews come in."

Questions for Analysis

1. What evidence should Fernando present when preparing the report for the departmental review? What plan for collecting the evidence would you develop if you were in Fernando's position?

2. Which aspects of the evidence should Fernando highlight, considering the uncertain future of his department? How could he best feature this evidence for maximum effect?

3. Would an external evaluator be useful in this situation? What qualities of the external evaluator would lend credibility to the report?

4. Besides the departmental self-study, what other steps could Fernando take to safeguard the future of the department? What are the likely effects of these actions? Could any of these actions have negative consequences?

Case Study 3

Marcus is beginning his second year as a graduate athletic training student at a small college. His class includes 16 students who want to attend the upcoming NATA Annual Meeting and Clinical Symposia in June. Although it is just a few hours away by car, they will need to raise money to offset the costs of conference registration, gas, hotel accommodations, and food.

The athletic training student club discussed the various methods of fund-raising, and most of the students expressed concerns over the amount of time they would need to spend on fund-raising efforts while they maintain an intense curricular load and clinical education requirements. They decided that the much-relied-on approaches of selling candy, holding car washes, having bake sales, and other similar events would not provide the level of funding they would need to reach their goal of sending everyone to the national meeting.

Marcus expressed his concerns to his club advisor during the first week of classes in September. His advisor mentioned that in recent conversations, some of the athletic training program's preceptors inquired about obtaining CEUs within the next few months because the end of the three-year reporting period was December 31 of this year, just four months away. Marcus' advisor told Marcus that he would help the club put together a CEU course. He also told Marcus that if the course were profitable, he would allow all of the proceeds to be used toward the students' trip.

Questions for Analysis

1. If Marcus were to encourage the club to participate in the planning of a fund-raising CEU program, what priorities would the students need to consider to determine whether or not the effort would be profitable?

2. With a little less than four months for planning, what challenges would the students face in determining the logistics of the course?

3. What criteria should the students use in identifying topics or a course content theme? How will they determine who will give the presentations?

4. How should the students assign responsibility among themselves to ensure that all aspects of course preparation are taken care of?

5. Could specific incentives be implemented to encourage participants to register early?

6. Given the current economic challenges that all businesses are facing, what steps could the students take to secure sponsorship for the program?

Key Concepts and Review

Understand and develop vision and mission statements for a sports medicine program.

Change is a pervasive aspect of organizational life that affects sports medicine programs. The development of vision and mission statements can help a sports medicine program create a philosophical infrastructure that will allow it to adapt appropriately to change. A vision statement should identify the service provider, the service to be provided, the recipients of the service, and the expected quality of the service. The mission statement is a broad, enduring statement of purpose that defines the scope of operations of the sports medicine program. The mission statement should direct the athletic trainer toward accomplishing specific tasks, motivate and inspire, and guide the development of goals and objectives.

Understand the principles underlying sports medicine strategic planning.

Planning is a set of activities that the athletic trainer should engage in to bring about a desired future state for the sports medicine program. Strategic plans are broadly written guides for developing specific program goals and objectives. The development of a strategic plan involves identifying the needs of both outside and inside interests; gathering information that identifies the historical and present status of the program; and analyzing the strengths and weaknesses of, the threats to, and the opportunities for the sports medicine program.

Develop and link sports medicine policies, processes, and procedures.

Operational plans are explicit steps that guide the actions of athletic trainers so that they can accomplish specific tasks. A policy is an operational plan for expressing the organization's intended behavior relative to a specific program subfunction. Policies require the approval of people in legal authority, such as boards of trustees or owners. Processes are a collection of incremental and mutually dependent steps designed to direct the most important tasks of the sports medicine program. Procedures provide athletic trainers with specific direction for various processes.

Communicate and develop ownership in a sports medicine program among inside and outside stakeholders.

Planning will be ineffective unless the athletic trainer can elicit support for the plan by identifying and influencing allies, opponents, bedfellows, and adversaries. The agreement–trust matrix can be a useful tool in this process. Athletic trainers should employ specific strategies with each of these groups to gain support for their programs and ideas.

Understand the principles of effective meeting and conference planning and management.

Most people view meetings as a necessary evil, but if properly organized they can be productive engines of decision making. Meetings are generally most effective if athletic trainers prepare in advance, divide the meeting into parts, control their own behavior, avoid new business and reports whenever possible, and have a future-oriented perspective. Conference planning is a specialized activity that some athletic trainer-administrators will undertake as part of their responsibilities. Planning an effective conference involves appointing a coordinator and a steering committee, establishing a theme and developing a program with the right speakers to accomplish the conference goals, establishing realistic time lines and budgets, selecting a site, developing a plan for registration, marketing the conference, planning for meals and entertainment, recruiting exhibitors and sponsors, preparing learning materials, and contracting for a variety of miscellaneous services.

Understand the principles of effective sports medicine program evaluation.

Athletic trainers should evaluate the effectiveness of their sports medicine programs to ensure that the programs will continue improving and to document program quality. Formative program evaluation identifies strengths and weaknesses and provides alternatives for improvement. Summative evaluation judges the quality of the program. Program evaluation is most valid when it uses the scientific method to compare program clients with people who do not have access to the program. This process is often difficult, expensive, and impractical. As much comparative data as possible should be used to evaluate the program. The use of an external auditor, along with chart auditing and outcomes studies, can facilitate unbiased assessments. A periodic self-study process that involves collecting evidence of program quality and answering questions crucial to program development is recommended.

Human Resource Management

After reading this chapter, you should be able to do the following:

- Identify the different forms of organizational culture that can exist in a sports medicine program.

- Formally define the relationships of the people working in a sports medicine program by developing an organizational chart.

- Learn the components of staff selection.

- Develop a position description and a position vacancy notice.

- Comprehend the recruitment and hiring process, especially as affected by discrimination and bias based on race, gender, disability, religion, and national origin.

- Define the differences between the three major supervisory models.

- Become familiar with the purposes, methods, and standards for evaluating athletic trainer performance.

- Recognize the key concepts associated with work–life balance as they relate to athletic training employment.

- Define the Fair Labor Standards Act and its effect on the employment of an athletic trainer.

Athletic trainers are professionals who are, in general, oriented toward providing clinical services. Most have never had training in how to manage human resources. Some athletic trainers excel at this aspect of administration without formal understanding of human resource systems, but they are the exceptions. The most complicated tools the athletic trainer will ever work with are people. Without a system for managing those assets, a sports medicine program is unlikely to accomplish its mission. If this sounds like a familiar occurrence, you may recall the Peter Principle from chapter 2. This chapter focuses on the human resource function of a sports medicine program and the skills athletic trainers need to be successful in this area.

Factors Related to the Sports Medicine Organization

The nature of the organization in which athletic trainers work has a powerful effect on many factors related to their employment. Three of the most important are the organization's culture, structure, and informal elements.

Organizational Culture

The first decision the athletic trainer in charge of a staff makes, consciously or unconsciously, is what kind of organizational culture the program will follow. **Organizational culture** includes the basic values, behavioral norms, assumptions, and beliefs present in an organization (Owens and Valesky

2014). The organizational culture of a sports medicine program largely defines what it means to be an athletic trainer in that setting. It influences the levels of commitment and loyalty of the athletic trainers working in the program.

Bennis and Nanus (2007) have described three general categories of organizational cultures (which they refer to as social architecture) that the athletic trainer should consider as part of sports medicine human resource management: collegial, personalistic, and formalistic.

- *Collegial culture.* The sports medicine program with a **collegial culture** is one in which the emphasis is on consensus, teamwork, and participation in most decisions by all members of the staff, who tend to view each other as peers. The head of the department allows and encourages everyone to offer input so that the decision-making process is consensual. Although this type of organizational culture appears ideal, it is inappropriate in some settings. For example, when quick decisions are required, the consensus-oriented style of the collegial culture is inappropriate because formal authority is spread among the members of the staff. If the staff is small, the collegial culture is probably both appropriate and useful. For a larger staff, this style may make it more challenging to reach a consensus of opinion.

- *Personalistic culture.* A **personalistic culture** in a sports medicine program places little emphasis on policy and procedure. Each member of the staff makes her own decisions. Teamwork and group consensus are not high priorities. Although program leaders might be available for advice and counsel, the staff athletic trainers' problems are perceived to be *their* problems, not the program's. The personalistic organizational culture is a form of controlled anarchy. This type of culture is seen with smaller staffs, or in some cases with somewhat larger staffs that operate independently out of multiple athletic training room facilities.

- *Formalistic culture.* The sports medicine program with a clear chain of command and well-defined lines of authority operates in a **formalistic culture**. The formalistic culture is typical of bureaucratic programs that heavily emphasize policy, procedure, and rules. This kind of organizational culture discourages risk taking and deviation from the established source of authority. Although this arrangement might seem undesirable for a sports medicine program, the formalistic style offers certain advantages. First, decisions can be made more

rapidly because various members of the staff have formal authority. Second, established policies and procedures can provide direction to staff athletic trainers and continuity in quality of service for clients. Finally, programs with large staffs might benefit from a formalistic culture because it divides and defines responsibilities and thereby enhances internal organization.

KEY POINT

Sports medicine programs typically exist in organizations that exhibit one of three kinds of organizational culture: collegial, personalistic, and formalistic. Each is typified by certain values, beliefs, assumptions, and behavior norms.

All work cultures that require individuals to work as a team to achieve overall success must rely on several common elements. While establishing cohesion among people in the work setting might involve numerous components, Lencioni (2002) has identified five areas of importance, or dysfunctions, that he feels must be addressed in order for a team to reach its goals.

- *Absence of trust.* Trust is lacking when members of a team are not willing to acknowledge to one another that they are imperfect. Mutual trust underlies team success. Lencioni suggests that teams with trusting members are more likely to be cognizant of and admit to their strengths and weaknesses, seek assistance when needed, and accept feedback and criticism about their areas and roles; they have learned how to be more focused on important issues.

- *Fear of conflict.* Teams that fear conflict will not make the best decisions. Teams that do not have a fear of conflict tend to have lively and interesting meetings, solve real problems quickly, minimize politics, and move forward by extracting and exploiting the ideas of all team members.

- *Lack of commitment.* Teams with members who lack commitment to the organization tend to create an environment characterized by ambiguity about directions and priorities and to breed a lack of confidence and fear of failure. They tend to revisit discussions again and again without coming up with meaningful solutions. In contrast, a committed team aligns itself around common objectives, develops an ability to learn from mistakes, takes advantage of opportunities before competitors do, and moves forward or changes direction when necessary without hesitation or guilt.

- *Avoidance of accountability.* Avoiding accountability creates resentment among team members who possess different performance standards, which likely leads to mediocrity. Key deliverables and deadlines are missed unless other team members pick up someone else's burden, likely leading to further team resentment. With accountability, all performers, especially those with a poor track record, will feel pressure to improve. Accountable members of a team will raise the standards for expectations and reduce the amount of time necessary for corrective action related to performance management.

- *Inattention to results.* The fifth dysfunction of a team is inattention to results. When team members do not pay attention to results, the result is failure to grow and stagnation. This is a common fault of many organizations in which leadership has been in existence for a relatively long time and is comfortable and set in the ways of operating. A person or operation that remains still while competitors and even colleagues improve has been "run over by the train." Attention to results leads to a greater likelihood of retaining achievement-oriented employees and minimizing individualist behaviors, as well as yielding unselfish employees who will at times put the team's goals and interests above their own.

Organizational Structures

Every sports medicine organization has a structure. The **organizational structure** of the sports medicine program plays an important role in how well staff members accomplish the program's mission. Each athletic trainer in the program has a different job to perform. Although duties may overlap and one athletic trainer may have duties similar to another's, each is responsible for distinct duties. The exception, of course, is the sports medicine program staffed by only one athletic trainer, a situation that is not uncommon at most high schools and some small colleges. Organizational structure need not be a concern for athletic trainers in these environments.

When designing the organizational structure of a sports medicine program, athletic trainers must consider the desired span of control. **Span of control** refers to the number of subordinates who report to a given supervisor. Although management researchers disagree on the precise formula for establishing a span of control, most agree that supervision of employees, including athletic trainers, is easier and more effective if supervisors are directly involved with three to six subordinates (Morash, Brintnell, and Rodger 2005). Organizational structures are typically depicted in organizational charts.

The **organizational chart** is a graphic illustration that shows the formal relationships between the various athletic trainers and other health care workers in a sports medicine program. Organizational charts are useful because they show staff members their roles in relation to the overall program. This task is especially important for newly hired athletic trainers because they lack a historical perspective of "how things are done around here."

KEY POINT

Organizational structure—the formal relationship that each person has to another within an organization—is best described by one of three types of organizational charts: function oriented, service oriented, or matrix.

Although a graphical depiction of the organizational structure of a sports medicine program can take many forms, most are charted according to function or service or in a matrix structure.

Function-Oriented Organizational Chart

"Function-Oriented Organizational Chart" is adapted from JAMES A.F. STONER, MANAGEMENT, 2nd Edition, © 1982, pp. 268, 271. Prentice Hall, Englewood Cliffs, New Jersey.

The organizational chart based on function is probably the most common in sports medicine settings. This type of approach seems to work best for smaller organizations that focus on a few areas of service. A functional organizational structure makes supervision easier because supervisors specialize along lines of expertise (see figure 4.1). Functional organizational structures can work well in sports medicine clinics or universities with large staffs, because they facilitate allocation of staff members to projects for which they have special skills and knowledge and can consolidate to more efficient and similarly aligned tasks. Typically, these tasks do not change quickly, and they meet the needs of a stable environment. For example, a policy for managing drug education and testing may not change frequently, although it will be reviewed as often as needed by the group charged with the overall function of the program.

Functional organizational structures also have several disadvantages. Making rapid decisions in these structures can be difficult because requests often have to make their way up the chain of command. Functional organizational structures can also make it difficult to establish accountability for particular areas of responsibility. Consider the structure depicted in figure 4.1. If athletic training students are consistently failing the Board of Certification (BOC) examination, who should be held accountable? Is the athletic trainer in charge of clinical education at fault, or is the recruiting and placement coordinator guilty of bringing poor students into the program? Finally, the functional approach to organizing a sports medicine program can isolate staff members because it places little emphasis on sharing ideas or on teamwork to accomplish program goals. From a team perspective, groups, committees, and especially departments within an organization that work in a function-oriented fashion tend to become possessive at times and to view compromise and collaboration as a weakness or as losing something. Groups that approach issues with this type of mentality are said to be functioning in a silo manner, without a positive interest toward interdisciplinary teamwork.

Service-Oriented Organizational Chart

"Service-Oriented Organizational Chart" is adapted from JAMES A.F. STONER, MANAGEMENT, 2nd Edition, © 1982, p. 274. Prentice Hall, Englewood Cliffs, New Jersey.

Another way to define the structure of a sports medicine program is to organize the staff according to the services they provide. Figure 4.2 provides an example from a large university that operates a sports medicine clinic in addition to the traditional sports medicine services provided by athletic department

athletic trainers. With the exception of the box for the coordinator's position, the boxes in this chart represent athletic trainers who are responsible for

Advantages and Disadvantages of a Functional Structure

Advantages

- Works best in a stable environment
- Promotes and uses expertise within staff members
- Enables specialization of staff skills
- Requires minimal internal coordination within a functionally assigned unit
- Requires fewer interpersonal skills

Disadvantages

- Can cause difficulty in decision making between functional areas
- Can lead to communication challenges between areas of function
- Slows response time between functional units in large programs
- Can lead to bottlenecks because tasks are performed sequentially
- Lessens innovation and narrows perspective
- Might create conflicts over program priorities and staff responsibilities between functional units
- Limits emphasis on sharing ideas and teamwork between functional units
- May lead to a silo effect

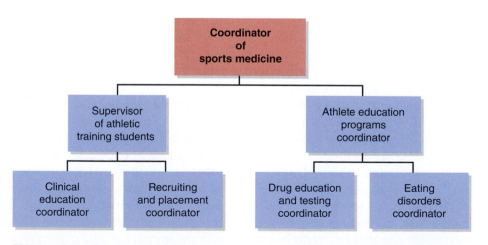

Figure 4.1 Sports medicine organizational chart: division by function.

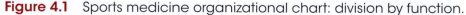

certain client groups. This type of organizational chart is especially appropriate for programs that serve a diverse clientele.

Like its function-oriented counterpart, the service-oriented organizational model provides both advantages and disadvantages. One of the advantages of this system is that it facilitates coordination of services to any one client group because of the relatively strict division of responsibility. Accountability is easier to obtain because athletic trainers work with well-defined client groups. Finally, the chief decision maker can usually act more quickly and easily because intermediate supervisors have more authority to make their own decisions.

Among the disadvantages of this system are problems balancing power and authority. When service groups are tightly defined, athletic trainers working with a particular client group might tend to place the interests of that unit over the mission of the total program. Power struggles between members of the various program units may result. Another disadvantage with the service-oriented organizational structure is that it sometimes inflates personnel costs. Strictly delimiting service groups means that the expertise of an athletic trainer working in one unit is often unavailable to an athletic trainer working in another. Consequently, additional athletic trainers are required to balance the expertise between units. Supervisory expenses go up proportionally.

Matrix Organization Chart

Many athletic trainers will be tempted to structure their sports medicine programs in terms of function or service. Unfortunately, most traditional sports medicine programs do not match these models. Athletic trainers should consider an alternative to

function or service paradigms: the matrix structure. The **matrix structure** combines the strongest features of the service and function models (Bazigos and Harter 2016).

In matrix structures, athletic trainers and other members of the sports medicine team report to two or more "bosses," depending on the project they are working on. The organizational chart for a matrix organization has both horizontal and vertical elements. An organizational chart for a university's

Advantages and Disadvantages of Service-Oriented Organizational Structures

Advantages

- Suited to fast change
- Allows for high visibility of athletic training programs
- Allows full-time concentration on tasks
- Clearly defines responsibilities
- Permits parallel processing of multiple tasks

Disadvantages

- Fosters politics in resource allocation
- Inhibits coordination of activities
- Limits what tasks can be addressed
- Permits in-depth competencies to decline
- Creates conflicts between tasks and priorities
- Can inflate personnel costs

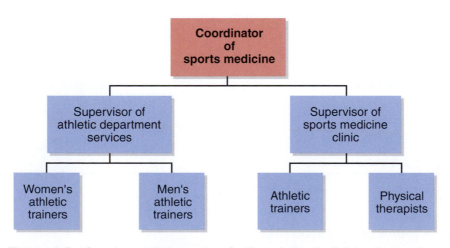

Figure 4.2 Sports medicine organizational chart: division by service.

sports medicine program might be structured similarly to the one in figure 4.3. The vertical elements show the chain of command in the program. The horizontal elements depict project teams that take advantage of the athletic trainers' specialization in certain areas. Not everyone has to be placed on a project team. Some athletic trainers will lack expertise in some areas. Others will be new to the organization and might need time to become acclimated. In educational settings, some of the athletic trainers might have release time to teach sports medicine courses, making it difficult to assign them to project teams.

The advantages of the matrix system as a model for deploying athletic trainers include the ability to efficiently use the staff's expertise. In addition, the matrix structure reduces coordination problems and enhances economic efficiency by assigning only the necessary number of athletic trainers to any given project.

The matrix model also has disadvantages. Athletic trainers need a high level of interpersonal communication skill to work effectively with var-

Advantages and Disadvantages of the Matrix Organizational Structure

Advantages

- Gives flexibility to the organization
- Stimulates interdisciplinary cooperation
- Involves, motivates, and challenges people
- Develops athletic trainers' skills
- Frees program coordinator for planning

Disadvantages

- Can create a feeling of anarchy
- Encourages power struggles
- Might lead to more discussion than action
- Requires high level of interpersonal skill
- Can be time consuming to implement

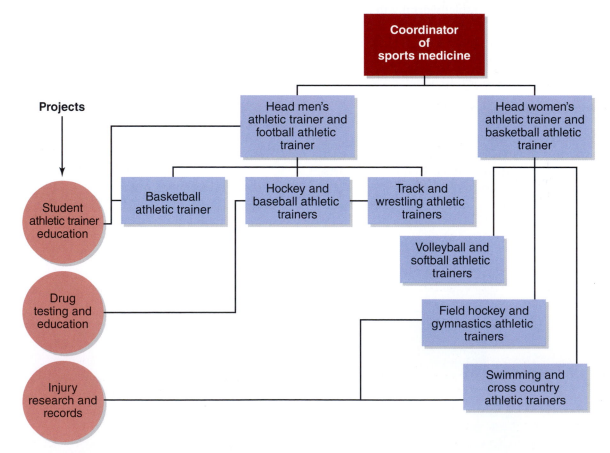

Figure 4.3 A matrix organization structure.

ious coworkers on different tasks. Without highly developed interpersonal skills, it may be difficult to get along with others. Another disadvantage of the matrix system is that athletic trainers can become frustrated and morale can suffer when people are switched between projects or when one project ends and another begins. Because many projects have a finite life span, this is a common problem.

Informal Organizations

Organizational structures, with their accompanying charts, are a useful starting point in helping athletic trainers and those with whom they work understand their roles in a sports medicine unit. Unfortunately, these devices rarely tell the whole story about how a sports medicine unit really functions. The formal organization, as defined by the officially approved organizational chart, is usually accompanied by the informal organization. Although the formal organization represents the theoretical relationships among the various members of the sports medicine unit, the informal organization represents the relationships as they exist and change from day to day. Whether athletic trainers are managers or employees, only those who understand both the formal and informal organizations will succeed in any given setting.

Why do athletic trainers and others join informal organization groups? They do so for many reasons, but Drafke (2002) believes that these are the most common:

1. *Social contact.* The informal organization allows people to join small groups and form relationships, thus filling an important human need. People develop friendships at work. The informal organization allows this to occur.

2. *Satisfaction of needs.* The relationships developed at work can provide for many of the psychological needs that most people have. The informal organization often bolsters self-esteem because it allows people to exercise power and assume leadership in a small group even when they have no formal authority to do so.

3. *Power.* Many people join groups in the informal organization because they sense that they will enhance their power by doing so. A group is often able to influence the outcome of a decision, whereas an individual might not be.

4. *Peer pressure.* Athletic trainers frequently join a group in the informal organization because of peer

KEY POINT

Relationships between people in an organization often have nothing to do with the formal organizational structure. People form relationships in organizations for at least 11 reasons: social contact, satisfaction of needs, power, peer pressure, problem solving, goal congruency, shared understanding, information and communication, knowledge and expertise, formal organizational support, and physical proximity.

pressure to do so. A person who doesn't ally himself with a group might be shunned.

5. *Problem solving.* Most people in the informal organization look to their peers as the first source in obtaining advice on how to solve work-related problems. This method is frequently less intimidating than seeking the advice of their superior on the formal organizational chart.

6. *Goal congruency.* Informal organization groups often form because of shared beliefs or goals. These goals might or might not be limited to work-related functions. Athletic trainers might choose to join a group based on common interests with other members of the group.

7. *Understanding.* Often an individual joins a group in the informal organization because the group members encounter similar kinds of problems at work. Athletic trainers are more likely to ally themselves with other groups of athletic trainers because of this shared experience and desire for understanding.

8. *Information and communication.* The informal organization is potentially a tremendous information source. Athletic trainers often choose which groups to join based on how much information the group is privy to. Athletic trainers who share information about organizational issues—whether officially sanctioned or not—will find others flocking to their group to hear the latest news. Knowing when to pass on unofficial information and when not to is an important survival skill.

9. *Knowledge.* The person who occupies the manager's role in the formal organization does not always have the most knowledge on a given subject. Athletic trainers will frequently seek out others in the informal organization for answers to their questions rather than going directly to their supervisors.

10. *Formal organization support.* The power structure of the informal organization commonly functions to keep the department or institution going when the formal organization is flawed or temporarily incomplete. The strategy of taking action now and apologizing later, as opposed to asking permission, is common in both health care and athletic organizations. This strategy often works because the informal organization influences day-to-day operations more than the formal organization does.

11. *Physical proximity.* Many people join groups in the informal organization because they work with the group members every day. Indeed, it is difficult to join a group when contact is infrequent.

Staff Selection

The basis for human resource management in sports medicine is **staff selection**. Although the term *staff selection* might imply only identifying and hiring new athletic trainers, it has a much broader meaning in law. The Equal Employment Opportunity Commission's *Uniform Guidelines on Employee Selection Procedures* (n.d.) defines *staff selection* as any procedure used as a basis for any employment decision. Athletic trainer hiring, promotion, demotion, retention, and performance evaluation are all considered selection activities by law (see figure 4.4). To comply with the *Uniform Guidelines,* athletic trainers must be sure their employment practices do not adversely affect any group protected under the law. The only exception to these rules occurs when an organization can prove that it discriminates because of "business necessity." The following sections provide practical suggestions for athletic trainers with staff selection responsibilities.

PEARLS OF MANAGEMENT

Staff selection is commonly assumed to include just that—selection of employees. Staff selection is actually a much broader construct and includes any procedure used to make employment decisions.

Position Description

A formal document that contains information about the required qualifications for, and the work content, accountability, and scope of, a job is known as a **position description**. The position description is an important communication link between the athletic

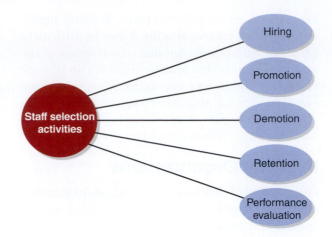

Figure 4.4 Staff-selection activities in sports medicine.

trainer and the supervisor that creates a common understanding of the role the athletic trainer should play in the program. Although many supervisors assume that their staffs agree with them about the duties for which they are responsible, Myers (1985) concluded that less than 50% of the employees he surveyed agreed with their supervisors on the standards and responsibilities of their jobs. When position descriptions are poorly written or are absent altogether, athletic trainers are unlikely to be able to meet the undefined expectations of their supervisors. Decades ago, Ray reported that many athletic trainers do not have position descriptions (1991). In addition, many athletic trainers' position descriptions are poorly written, couched in trait-oriented language, or lacking in weights for various job descriptors. Unfortunately, this may still hold true in many settings given the lack of athletic trainers in administrative positions with the knowledge to develop accurate and contemporary job descriptions.

The athletic trainer's position description should be divided into two sections: the job specification and the job description (see figure 4.5). The **job specification** describes the qualifications an athletic trainer should have to fill the role. An element that helps clarify the job specification is the **person specification**. The person specification translates the job specification into meaningful qualities that the person must have to be successful in the role. It also helps operationalize and define what those qualities must be for this particular job. A **job description should clearly** list the responsibilities for which the athletic trainer will be held accountable. It can be helpful if each responsibility is assigned a weight so that the athletic trainer understands which duties

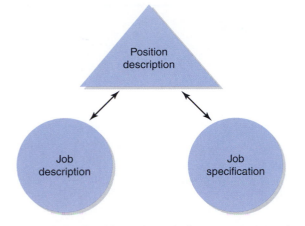

Figure 4.5 Position description components.

are considered the most important, therefore being able to prioritize and focus one's efforts in relevant areas.

The weights assigned to various responsibilities can be determined in a variety of ways. One method is to determine what percentage of the athletic trainer's time will be devoted to a particular responsibility. This method would place more weight on taping ankles or wound care than on performing CPR. An alternative would be to assign weights according to how critical the job responsibility is. Using this method, performing CPR would clearly be weighted more heavily than taping ankles or wound care. No matter which method is used, the weights must reflect the values of the organization. The casual observer should be able to see a clear representation of the organization's mission in the weighting of job responsibilities. Another important element in successful weighting of job responsibilities is a realistic assignment of weights. If every job responsibility is weighted as a 5 on a 1-to-5 scale of importance, the position description will not help the athletic trainer understand what is most important and what is less critical. It is also a good idea to clarify which qualifications are minimal and which are preferred for the position. This lets the potential applicants know what is minimally required while simultaneously suggesting that the organization might be looking for people with more educational background, clinical experience, or research skills depending on additional considerations related to the position being advertised.

Athletic trainers who write position descriptions struggle with several important questions. Should the responsibilities be specific or general? Should the document describe what ought to be or what is? Although no definitive answers meet the needs of every situation, general guidelines do exist. Being as specific as possible when delineating the duties and responsibilities of the athletic trainer is generally useful. Explicit descriptions are important because they provide clear direction for the athletic trainer. To avoid allowing employees to perform only minimal job responsibilities, a common tactic that human resource personnel use is to include a general phrase within the document to the effect of "and any other relevant duties required to perform the job as assigned by the coordinator of sports medicine." Additionally, it is recommended when describing the qualifications needed to perform the job that an employer lists both minimal qualifications and preferred qualifications. **Minimal qualifications** identify the essential skills needed to perform the job. This may include holding appropriate athletic training certification, a license in the state to practice, and possibly two years of clinical experience. **Preferred qualifications** assume that all minimal qualifications are met, and a candidate furthermore possesses additional skills and experience. Examples of preferred qualifications may include having five years of experience, possessing a manual therapy certificate, and prior history working with a specific subgroup of patients or athletes.

Careful consideration should be given to choosing who contributes to the writing of a job description. When staff members, or incumbents, write their own job descriptions, they tend to be narrowly focused and to ignore tasks they do not enjoy, no matter how important they are to accomplishing the mission of the sports medicine program. For this reason, the program head should perform a final check on all position descriptions. The combination of input from the supervisor and the subordinate into the position description will more likely result in a balance between the needs of the employee and those of the sports medicine program. Position descriptions for new athletic trainers should reflect the standard practices of the athletic training program so that the new employee can begin to adapt to the work setting and should reflect only the characteristics of the job, not ambiguous personal characteristics such as loyalty, initiative, and trust.

Finally, no matter which approach is used, everyone should review the position description and modify as needed to reflect changes in the athletic trainer's qualifications or the work environment. Potential changes to an existing position description should be clearly discussed and explained with the person currently in the role. For an example of what a position description might look like, see figure 4.6.

POSITION DESCRIPTION

Date: July 1, 2018

Job title: Assistant athletic trainer

Department: Intercollegiate Athletics

Status: Salaried nonfaculty

Incumbent: Judy Armstrong

Supervisor: Linda Black, head women's athletic trainer

Written by: DeMarcus Lewis, coordinator of Sports Medicine, and Judy Armstrong
Approved by: Jorge Garcia, director of Intercollegiate Athletics

JOB SPECIFICATION

Factor	Job specification	Person specification
Education	Requires minimum of master's degree	Must have a master's degree
Certification	Requires credentials consistent with Ohio law and recognized national standards	Must be BOC certified, hold a valid Ohio license, and be certified in CPR
Working conditions	Requires travel over weekends and holidays, and exposure to all kinds of weather	Must have flexible schedule and be in good physical condition
Physical demands	Requires lifting injured athletes, manual dexterity, and administration of CPR	Must be able to lift heavy weights and have functional use of all four extremities

JOB DESCRIPTION

Job responsibilities	Relative importance (1 = low, 5 = high)
Coordinates and delivers athletic training services to members of the field hockey and gymnastics teams including, but not limited to, coordination of physical exams, evaluation and treatment of injuries at practices and games, design and supervision of rehabilitation programs, counseling within the limits of expertise, and prepractice and game taping	5
Refers injured athletes to appropriate physicians according to guidelines in the Standard Operating Procedures	5
Submits injured athlete status reports to coaches by 11:00 a.m. of the day following the injury	4
Maintains computerized injury and treatment database according to guidelines in the Standard Operating Procedures	3
Coordinates NCAA Injury Surveillance program by conducting in-service training for student athletic trainers, collecting and checking the accuracy of individual and weekly injury report forms, and mailing completed forms to the NCAA by Monday of each week	3
Prepares annual injury and treatment report for all sports by June 1	3
Exhibits behaviors in strict compliance with the NATA Code of Ethics or BOC Standards of Professional Practice	5
Performs other duties not specifically stated herein but deemed essential to the operation of the sports medicine program as assigned by the coordinator of Sports Medicine or the head women's athletic trainer	Varies

Figure 4.6 Sample position description.

Recruitment and Hiring

Attracting and retaining qualified, competent staff members is crucial to the overall success of a sports medicine program. **Recruitment** of athletic trainers and other allied health care professionals should be viewed from two perspectives: the long-range need for human resources within the sports medicine program and the immediate staffing needs.

The long-term staffing plan depends, to a significant degree, on the strategic plan of the sports medicine program. How is our client base likely to change? How will the accomplishment of our goals and objectives affect our need for staffing? The long-range recruiting plan should consider several factors, including the likelihood of promotion or transfer of present staff members, upcoming retirement plans, and the projected availability of athletic trainers and other allied health care workers in the labor pool. All these factors are important. For example, if the program structure will support an additional athletic trainer but the pool of qualified applicants is inadequate, the human resources plan for the sports medicine unit might need to be revised. Each of these factors should be evaluated annually so that future staffing needs can be met.

The other perspective in the recruitment process is the immediate need for staffing the sports medicine program. Immediate staffing needs typically arise because of five changes in the makeup of the present staff: radical program changes, termination (for either personal or professional reasons), retirement, noncompliance, and death. Each of these can result in the immediate need to fill a vacant position (see figure 4.7).

Neither long-term nor immediate staffing needs of the sports medicine unit can be fulfilled unless those needs are successfully integrated into the overall institutional or departmental staffing plan. Athletic trainers are often frustrated when their staffing requests are denied or put on hold. Too often, the athletic trainer-manager responds to this negative outcome by saying, "Athletic training always gets shortchanged around here. Our needs are always considered last priority." Frequently, the reason for these decisions is not that athletic training and its needs are low priorities, but that athletic trainer-managers have not carefully cultivated relationships with institutional decision makers, who face pressure from many competing interests. The athletic trainer-manager must communicate

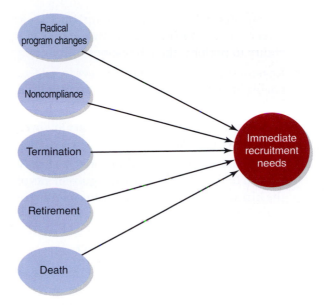

Figure 4.7 Factors influencing immediate recruitment needs.

the staffing needs of the sports medicine program to institutional decision makers so that they will receive frequent reminders about how important those needs are to the operation of the program.

Many institutions that employ athletic trainers have developed specific procedures for recruiting and hiring all personnel. In these institutions, the athletic trainer in charge of staffing the sports medicine program has little choice but to become well informed about the policies and procedures and to adhere to them scrupulously. Most institutional recruitment and hiring policies and procedures are designed to prevent blatant forms of discrimination based on race and gender. In many cases, the athletic trainer is required to document every step of the recruitment and hiring process to ensure that all qualified applicants have equal opportunity in the process. Human resource departments are required to implement a standard set of procedures for their recruitment and hiring practices to prevent discriminatory practices. Such standards should include the following practices:

- Hiring restrictions are not based on one's gender, national origin, age, or religion (or other protected classes), but rather one's qualifications to perform the job.
- The essential functions listed in the job specifications are valid indicators of the ability of an athletic trainer to perform the job.

- Questions asked in the hiring interview directly relate to the prospective employee's ability to perform the job responsibilities.
- Reasonable accommodations are made to enable people with disabilities or people of various religious beliefs to perform the job.
- Standard and equitable procedures are followed for reviewing each applicant.
- Search committee members are formally trained in the ethical and legal requirements of the hiring process in order to be in compliance with federal law.

Validity and Reliability in Hiring

Besides ensuring that racial, gender, and other biases are systematically purged from the hiring process, the athletic trainer in charge of staffing must consistently use hiring criteria that are predictive of success in the position. Validity in staff selection criteria is important for several reasons. First, the use of valid hiring criteria is more likely to produce an athletic training staff that functions well in its role. Second, using valid hiring criteria enhances efficiency in the staff selection process because productive employees are less likely to leave the organization, which would create gaps that would have to be filled. Finally, valid hiring criteria can help demonstrate that the hiring process was fair and free from bias.

Establishing validity in hiring criteria is a difficult process that often takes years to accomplish. A significant amount of trial and error might be involved in validating the process. In general, athletic training managers ought to scrutinize every established criterion for a particular position and ask themselves two questions:

- Could a person who did not meet this criterion be reasonably expected to succeed in this position?
- How likely is it that a person who meets this criterion will succeed in this position?

If the answer to the first question is yes, the criterion is not valid and should be discarded. The answer to the second question is a bit trickier. The athletic trainer-manager must predict a probability value based on her knowledge of the position and her experience. If the answer to the second question is "quite likely," then the criterion is probably valid. If, on the other hand, the athletic trainer-manager

cannot predict how successful candidates would be even if they met the criterion, the criterion is probably not valid. We use the modifier *probably* because the only way a manager can definitively assess the validity of employment criteria is by collecting data over time and determining the relationship between various employment criteria and success or failure in the position.

Reliability in staff selection is the degree to which employment standards and practices are applied with consistency to all candidates. As with validity, reliable procedures are important for ensuring that bias is reduced to a minimum. Reliable procedures also help produce the same information when applied to different candidates. For example, suppose that all candidates for an athletic training position with a large urban police or fire department were required to submit to a drug-screening procedure. If the procedure resulted in an unacceptably high rate of false positive or false negative results, it would be an unreliable staff selection criterion because its use provides different information for candidates with similar characteristics. Ensuring that all candidates go through an identical screening process, including the questions asked during the interview, will enhance reliability.

Hiring practices vary greatly from organization to organization. Some sports medicine programs employ an informal process, whereas others adhere to rigid procedures. Most will use a system that resembles the following 10-step process.

Step 1: Request for Position

Athletic administrators, general managers, principals, and clinic administrators will not consider filling a vacancy or adding a new position unless the athletic trainer makes a specific request. Some organizations require that the athletic trainer complete a specific form as part of the request process. Others require a position description. Administrators will generally screen requests for additional personnel more cautiously than they will requests for position replacements. Such requests should be detailed enough to document need, based on both current and forecasted program conditions. The athletic trainer-manager could use many potential sources of information to justify the position. Outcomes data, patient load, revenue statements, and student–faculty ratios are just a few examples of the kinds of justification most administrators will require before they approve a position.

Common Steps for Recruiting and Hiring Sports Medicine Personnel

1. Request for position
2. Position request approval
3. Position vacancy notice
4. Application collection
5. Telephone and web-based interviews
6. Reference checks
7. On-site interview
8. Recommendation and approval for hiring
9. Offer of contract
10. Hiring

Step 2: Position Request Approval

After the athletic trainer in charge has submitted the request to the appropriate administrative officer, the request will probably be approved, denied, or held up pending further study. Athletic trainers should try to anticipate the data that administrators will need to make a decision.

Step 3: Position Vacancy Notice

Once the request for position is approved, the athletic trainer might be required to advertise the position vacancy to satisfy collective bargaining agreements and state and federal guidelines. Position vacancies should be posted both internally, so that current sports medicine staff who want to apply for a position may do so, and externally. Position vacancy notices may be posted externally in the following locations:

- National Athletic Trainers' Association online placement vacancy notice service
- NCAA: The Market
- The Chronicle of Higher Education
- HigherEdJobs.com
- LinkedIn.com
- Publications of SHAPE America (Society of Health and Physical Educators)
- Publications of the American Physical Therapy Association
- Publications of the American College of Sports Medicine
- Local newspapers

Finally, many athletic trainers find it useful to send a copy of the position vacancy notice to program directors of accredited athletic training programs, alumni mailing lists, or other forms of e-mail distribution lists composed of athletic trainers.

The position vacancy notice should not be a carbon copy of the position description but should include a summary of the major responsibilities, a list of required and preferred qualifications, and a brief description of the major attributes of the institution or organization. In addition, the position vacancy notice should include the name, address, e-mail address, and telephone number of the person responsible for coordinating the hiring effort for the sports medicine program along with a list of required application documents. Typical application documents include a resume or **curriculum vitae (CV)**, letter of application, letters of reference, and transcripts. Many institutions require notice of nondiscrimination as part of all position vacancy notices (see figure 4.8).

Although creating the position vacancy notice is an important step in the hiring process, athletic trainers who want to attract the best candidates to their programs must rely on their networking skills to do so. Athletic trainer-managers responsible for staff selection should maintain a file on people they think would be excellent candidates for future positions in their organization. When openings occur, they should contact these people directly and encourage them to apply. A word of caution regarding this technique is appropriate. Athletic trainers who actively recruit from the ranks of other sports medicine programs run the risk of being accused of stealing another organization's employees. This situation can lead to bad feelings and damaged institutional relationships. Although avoiding this unpleasant side effect of network-based employee recruiting can be difficult, the best approach is generally to work with the candidate to develop a strategy to minimize the consequences and preserve the relationship. For example, clear goals related to professional development will allow employers to be cognizant of one's career growth plans. In most cases candidates will not want their employers to know that they are considering another position until they are reasonably certain that they will in fact be hired by the new organization.

Nowhere is network-based recruiting more important than in the effort to identify, recruit, screen, and hire members of minority or other underrepresented groups. Athletic trainers who

---

OHIO TECHNOLOGICAL UNIVERSITY

ASSISTANT ATHLETIC TRAINER

OTU is seeking applications for the position of assistant athletic trainer in the Department of Intercollegiate Athletics. Primary responsibilities include the delivery of athletic training services for the field hockey and gymnastics teams, although occasional work with other teams will be required. This position also includes responsibility for coordinating the sports medicine program's injury research and records program, including maintenance of the computer database and coordination of athletic training students involved in NCAA injury surveillance data collection.

Minimum qualifications include a master's degree, BOC certification, an Ohio athletic training license, and current American Red Cross CPR certification.

Salary is negotiable and will be commensurate with experience. This position is a 10-month, renewable term, salaried nonfaculty contract.

Ohio Technological University has an enrollment of 25,000 students and is located in an urban center of more than 250,000. OTU offers 41 undergraduate majors and 15 graduate degree programs. The university is a member of the NCAA Division I and offers eight sports for men and eight for women. OTU is an equal opportunity, affirmative action employer. Women and members of minority groups are encouraged to apply.

Candidates should send a letter of application, resume, three letters of reference, and undergraduate transcript by June 1 to the following:

DeMarcus Lewis
Coordinator of Sports Medicine
Ohio Technological University
Urban Center, OH 40000
(217) 555-5555

Figure 4.8 Sample position vacancy notice.

want to enhance the racial and cultural diversity in their programs face a challenge because the number of certified athletic trainers who are members of an ethnic minority is relatively small. To encourage members of minority groups to apply for their positions, athletic trainers can employ these strategies:

1. Send the position vacancy notice to the athletic trainers at all historically black colleges and universities (HBCUs).

2. Send the position vacancy notice to the program directors at universities that offer accredited athletic training programs.

3. Send the position vacancy notice, along with a personal letter, to certified athletic trainers who identify themselves as members of a minority or other underrepresented group.

4. Make direct contact with minority athletic trainers they are familiar with and personally invite them to apply for the position.

Even with the use of all four strategies, recruiting minorities to a program may take a long time. At all times, employees involved with recruitment should consult with their human resources department to ensure appropriate steps are taken and to seek their expert advice with position searches.

Step 4: Application Collection

The next step in the process is to receive and screen applications for the position. A common practice is to appoint a committee of interested people with a legitimate stake in hiring the athletic trainer to screen applications. The operation of search committees varies widely. Some operate on consensus, whereas others follow strict parliamentary procedure and vote on the suitability of various candidates for the position. In some cases, the committee suggests a name (or the top two or three candidates) to a director, dean, or other high-ranking administrator who is charged with making the final decision.

In any case, incoming applications should be sorted into three groups:

1. Unqualified applicants
2. Qualified applicants with complete application files
3. Apparently qualified applicants with incomplete application files

As the application deadline approaches, the committee should send a letter to apparently qualified applicants with incomplete files requesting an immediate response if they wish to remain under consideration for the position. The committee should keep on file a copy of all correspondence with applicants as evidence of good-faith hiring practices on the part of the institution or organization.

What process should the committee use to assess a candidate's credentials? No foolproof method exists, but athletic trainers should be aware of certain "red flags" as they evaluate the materials submitted as part of the application package.

Application Letter   Athletic trainers should ask themselves the following questions as they read an application letter (see figure 4.9 for a sample letter).

- Is the letter personalized? An application letter addressed "To Whom It May Concern" indicates a gross lack of preparation on the part of the candidate.

- Is the letter well written? The application letter demonstrates the writing skills of the potential employee. A candidate whose application letter is poorly written and full of grammatical errors is likely to write poorly after he or she is hired.

- Has the letter been proofread? One common error is not changing the name of the school, the employer, or a person in the letter when a candidate is preparing multiple letters that contain somewhat similar information.

- Does the letter briefly describe the candidate's experiences and qualities without duplicating the contents of the resume?

- Does the letter describe why the candidate thinks he or she is qualified for the particular position? Letters that do not contain this

information are often form letters that candidates routinely include with all job application packets.

Resume   Athletic trainers should ask themselves the following questions as they read an applicant's resume (see figure 4.10 for a sample resume).

- Is the resume professionally prepared? A poorly formatted resume often shows that the applicant has poor organizational skills.

- Does the resume contain all the usual categories of information? Common categories include personal information, educational background, professional experience, honors and awards, and references. Other categories that might be appropriate include publications, presentations, grants, and volunteer and community service.

- Does the resume reflect a continuous time line from the date the candidate entered school until the present? Gaps in the record are not necessarily bad, but they should be investigated if the candidate is chosen for a telephone interview.

- Does the candidate's experience reflect the kind of position for which she is applying? If the candidate has never worked in a setting similar to the one for the job she is applying for, it will be difficult to predict how well she is likely to perform based on experience.

- Do the previous professional experiences listed on the resume reflect stability? A resume filled with many jobs of short duration raises questions about the employability of the candidate.

- Are the references listed on the resume well-known, reputable members of the profession? References with whom the athletic trainer is personally acquainted are more likely to provide an honest appraisal of the candidate's qualities—both good and bad. Do the references include people who served in supervisory roles for the candidate? How long has a reference known the candidate and in what capacity?

- Does the resume reflect the candidate's experiences without exaggeration? Many candidates attempt to make their experiences sound more glamorous than they really were. For example, if a candidate indicates that he was an assistant athletic trainer at a Division I university and you deduce that this took place while he was a

February 5, 2018

DeMarcus Lewis, ATC
Coordinator of Sports Medicine
Ohio Technological University
Urban Center, OH 40000

Dear Mr. Lewis:

The purpose of this letter is to request that I be considered as a candidate for the assistant athletic trainer position at Ohio Technological University. I have been a high school athletic trainer for the past five years and am very interested in furthering my career at the university level. I am particularly interested in the position at OTU because it would allow me to build on the skills I have developed since finishing my master's degree. On a personal note, I am also interested in this position because it would allow me to move back to a region of the country where my parents and most of my family reside.

As you can see from my resume, two of the sports with which I have experience are gymnastics and field hockey. I have enjoyed working with these sports at the high school level, and I am excited to have the chance to work with college-level gymnasts and field hockey players. I have asked the coaches of the teams I have worked with in my present position to write to you in support of my application. I am confident that they will be able to help you gain a better sense of my athletic training skills in these two sports. I believe that my experiences as a college-level gymnast also help qualify me for your position.

Thank you very much for considering my application. Enclosed you will find a resume and a list of references. I would be grateful for the opportunity to interview with you and your staff at any time you think would be appropriate. If you have questions regarding my background or application, please do not hesitate to contact me.

Sincerely yours,

LaTasha Hays, MS, ATC

Figure 4.9 Sample application letter.

junior in college, he has probably inflated his experience as an athletic training student at that university.

- For an entry-level athletic trainer, does the resume reflect skills beyond the basic expectations for all entry-level athletic trainers?

Letters of Reference An athletic trainer should ask herself the following questions when reading the letters of reference:

- How long has the reference known the candidate and in what capacity? A person who has known the candidate for a longer period of time in a capacity related to the position being sought is able to provide more substantive information. Having known the candidate for a short period of time can make it difficult to provide information. Also, someone who is a classmate, acquaintance, family member, government official, or religious or spiritual leader may not be able to provide an accurate assessment of a candidate's ability to perform athletic training–related tasks.

- Does the writer recommend the candidate for the position? Some people are honest enough to indicate that in their opinion a candidate is not well suited for a particular position, although this type of comment is rare.

- Does the writer balance the candidate's strengths and weaknesses? Every candidate has both, and the useful letter of reference will mention them.

- Does the information in the letter confirm what appears on the resume? Inconsistencies should be verified through a telephone call to the person who wrote the letter of reference.

- Is the letter of reference excessively short or vague in its assertions? People who don't really want to recommend a candidate will often write a very short letter confirming the candidate's employment or educational status and little else. Another common technique is to use language that is so bland and nondescriptive that it becomes difficult to determine whether the writer actually recommends the candidate or not.

- Does the letter include references to actual job performance? A strong letter of reference will focus on the quality of the candidate's performance. Weak letters often focus on personality traits that, while valuable and desirable, might not reflect the quality of the candidate's work.

- Does the letter address the referring individual's perception that the candidate will be successful in the position being sought? Candidates may be better suited for certain positions than for others. Candidates should choose people as references based on the position they are applying for and should select people who can provide the most accurate assessment in relation to the particular job.

Step 5: Telephone and Web-Based Interviews

After the qualified applicants have been identified, members of the search committee should interview especially promising candidates by telephone or through a Web-based program such as Skype or Google hangout. Telephone and Web-based interviews in advance of on-site interviews are useful for weeding out unsuitable applicants and providing additional information not readily communicated in application letters or resumes. The interviewers should be friendly and informative, but they should avoid making statements that the candidate might interpret as promises or oral contracts that might be binding on the institution. Questions asked in the telephone or Web-based interview should elicit additional information unavailable in the application documents. Interviewers should ask each candidate the same questions in the same order to ensure reliability. Questions should always focus on candidates' job-related behavior, not on personal characteristics. Examples of legal and illegal questions that athletic trainers should be aware of when conducting interviews are presented in the following sidebar (Falcone 2008; Fry 2016).

Step 6: Reference Checks

After further narrowing the applicant pool through telephone and Web-based interviewing, the search committee should begin checking references. This aspect of the recruitment and hiring process is important because it allows the potential employer to validate the information supplied by the candidate. Some application materials need not be checked. Notarized transcripts, diplomas, and certificates are usually, but not always, valid. Expiration dates and signatures should be checked.

Examples of Legal and Illegal Interview Questions

Illegal questions

- Are you a United States citizen?
- Do your religious beliefs allow you to work on Sundays?
- Are you married? Do you have children?
- Do you have illnesses or disabilities?
- Did you serve in the military? What kind of discharge did you receive?
- Where did you learn to speak Spanish?

Legal Questions

- Could you, after employment, submit verification of your legal right to work in the United States?
- Weekend and holiday work is a condition of this position. Is that acceptable to you?
- Can you perform the essential job functions of this position with or without accommodation?
- Did you serve in the military? Were any of the jobs you performed similar to those in this position?
- Do you speak languages other than English that would be useful in this position?

Amy Hays, MS, ATC

1234 South Armstrong St.
Way-Out-West, CA 90000
999-555-2000
amyhays@network.com

Professional Goals

I would like to use the experience I have gained as a certified athletic trainer in the high school setting in a more competitive and athletically challenging environment. I would especially like to secure a position in a Division I university.

Educational Background

2011	Master of Science in Athletic Training, Big State University
2009	Bachelor of Science, Regional University (Major—Athletic Training Minor—Biology)
2007	Associate of Arts, Wiley County Junior College

Professional Experience

2009–Present   **Way-Out-West High School** I serve as the head athletic trainer in a high school comprising 2000 students and 20 sports, including

Boys' Sports		Girls' Sports	
Football	Gymnastics	Field hockey	Gymnastics
Cross country	Volleyball	Cross country	Volleyball
Soccer	Track	Soccer	Track
Basketball	Baseball	Basketball	Softball
Swimming	Tennis	Swimming	Tennis

In addition, I coordinate the school's drug and alcohol prevention program. My responsibilities also include maintenance of injury and treatment records.

2007–Present   **Western County Triathlon** I serve as the medical director for this event, which draws over 1,000 participants from all over the state.

2007–Present   **Summertown Gymnastics Club** I teach gymnastics at this club during the summer.

Certifications

2009–Present	Certified Athletic Trainer, Board of Certification
2008–Present	Certified Basic Life Support Instructor, American Red Cross

Memberships

2007–Present	National Athletic Trainers' Association
2009–Present	Far West Athletic Trainers' Association
2009–Present	California Athletic Trainers' Association

Honors and Awards

2009	Athletic Training Scholarship, Big State University
2006	Most Valuable Gymnast, Regional University

(continued)

Figure 4.10   Sample resume.

Publications

Hays, A. (2007). Scaphoid non-union in a gymnast: A case study. *California Sports Medicine,* 2(3):14–16.

References

These people have given their permission to be contacted for additional background on my experiences and qualifications:

Ms. Renee Bigelow
Athletic Director and Gymnastics Coach
Way-Out-West High School
1245 Western Dr.
Way-Out-West, CA 90000
999-555-8903
Rbigelow@wayoutwest.edu

Dr. Martin Dykstra, ATC
Program Director
Graduate Athletic Training Program
Big State University
Bigville, OH 40001
444-555-1111
Martindykstra233@bsu.edu

Ms. Lillie Thompson
Field Hockey Coach
Way-Out-West High School
1245 Western Dr.
Way-Out-West, CA 90000
999-555-8903
lthompson@wayoutwest.edu

Figure 4.10 *(continued)*

The most valuable information source is usually the applicant's previous employers or, for entry-level applicants, internship supervisors or former preceptors. An applicant's performance in similar employment settings is the best predictor of how the person will perform the new job. Notes from all conversations should be kept in the applicant's file for future reference by other members of the search committee.

Step 7: On-Site Interview

On-site interviews are costly and time consuming. Only those applicants who are obviously well qualified for the job should be interviewed on-site. Candidates about whom the search committee has serious reservations should not be interviewed. The on-site interview is important for both the candidate and the organization. The interview allows the candidate to become familiar with the work setting, and it allows the search committee to see the candidate in the work setting.

The on-site visit can be organized in many ways. Most visits should include interviews with institutional stakeholders such as coaches, athletes and other physically active patients, athletic administrators, owners, team physicians, athletic training faculty, and other athletic trainers. Time should be set aside for the candidate to ask questions about the job. Candidates should have an opportunity to tour the facilities and inspect their potential worksites. The visit should typically be one or two days long, depending on the level of responsibility of the position and the number of people who need to be involved in the interview process. If an employer is conducting an on-site interview for a candidate, the visit might be structured like the one in figure 4.11.

The people with whom the candidate will work closely should have the largest amount of interview time with him or her. Interviews with people the candidate will have limited contact with or those with only a tangential interest can be more limited in time and scope. One option to save time is to invite a group to lunch so that the candidate can meet several people at once, rather than reserving time in the schedule for each one. Candidates interviewing for faculty positions should have time allocated for meeting with students enrolled in the program. This interaction can be beneficial for both the candidate and the students.

Bringing a candidate to campus for an on-site interview means it is believed that the person

---

ITINERARY FOR THE VISIT OF JOHN OLMSTEAD

Candidate for the position of head men's athletic trainer

MONDAY, JUNE 11

10:00 a.m.	Arrive at Urban Center Airport, met by DeMarcus Lewis
10:30 a.m.	Meet with Linda Black, head women's athletic trainer, Fieldhouse athletic training room
11:45 a.m.	Lunch with Athletic Training Students Club representatives Jim Gleason and Elaine Williams
1:30 p.m.	Meet with Jorge Garcia, director of intercollegiate athletics, central administration building
2:45 p.m.	Meet with Dr. Reid Chesterfield, team physician, Student Health Service
3:30 p.m.	Meet with Greg Campbell, head football coach, Memorial Stadium
4:15 p.m.	Meet with Lucy Sneller, director of human resources, central administration building
5:00 p.m.	Check into Campus Inn
6:30 p.m.	Dinner with DeMarcus Lewis, coordinator of sports medicine, and Rick Ellis, assistant athletic trainer, Campus Inn Grill

TUESDAY, JUNE 12

7:30 a.m.	Breakfast with Tom Hernandez, head men's basketball coach, University Club
8:30 a.m.	Meet with members of the search committee, Fieldhouse conference room
11:00 a.m.	Fly home; Jim Gleason will accompany you to the airport
11:00 a.m.	Search committee meeting, Fieldhouse conference room

Figure 4.11 Sample on-site interview itinerary.

possesses the minimal qualifications for the position based on the documents reviewed to date and the preliminary interview process. During the on-site visit, a part of the process should be used to confirm the candidate's ability to fill the role based on further inquiry and discussion. In addition, and perhaps most important at this point, the idea is to determine the fit of the candidate. As with any team, simply having the best players at every position does not necessarily guarantee a winning season unless the chemistry is right and the teamwork is effective. Determining whether or not a candidate is a good fit for an organization may be difficult to do objectively. Feedback from all of the stakeholders that have taken part in the interview process is helpful; feelings, perceptions, and other indicators may be relied on to make such a decision.

An important aspect of the on-site interview that many managers fail to recognize is the need to sell the job to the candidate. Too often, we assume that the mere offer of a job will be enough to induce a candidate to accept. This is frequently not the case. A significant part of the interview process should be devoted to highlighting the benefits of the job, the organization, and the community.

Reliability in the on-site interview is just as important as in the telephone and Web-based interviews. Regardless of how the interview is organized, a structured process will enhance the reliability of the selection procedure. In a structured interview, the interviewers, preferably the same people, ask each candidate the same questions in the same order. This process helps improve the chances that the search committee members will have the information they need to make distinctions between the candidates.

It is also helpful to schedule time for rest periods or breaks for the candidate, as well as social time when the employers and candidate can interact in a less formal environment. This can occur during casual dinners after a formal interview has taken place. If candidates are asked to give a presentation of any kind as part of the interview process, providing time for setup can be helpful to the candidate, especially if audiovisual or other technological aids do not always operate as expected.

Step 8: Recommendation and Approval for Hiring

After the candidates have been interviewed on-site, the search committee must make a recommendation for hiring to the person in the organization with formal authority to approve it. Supporting documentation, including the candidate's resume, transcripts, letters of recommendation, and interview notes, should accompany the recommendation for hiring so that the decision maker has the necessary information to make a final choice. Search committee members should be sure they make a final recommendation for hiring based solely on the qualifications of the candidate and not on personal characteristics unrelated to the job, such as race, marital status, national origin, or creed.

Step 9: Offer of Contract

After the search committee has selected the most outstanding candidate, whoever is authorized to negotiate a contract with the candidate should call and orally extend an offer of employment. If the parties can agree on terms of employment over the telephone, the authorized institutional representative should prepare a formal employment contract consistent with institutional rules, collective bargaining agreements, and state and federal laws. The contract should include the starting date for the job, length of employment, salary and benefits, position title, and job responsibilities as specified in the position description. In addition, the contract should include a clause stating that the athletic trainer agrees to abide by the terms and conditions delineated in the institution's employee handbook. Two copies of the signed contract should be sent to the athletic trainer with instructions to sign and return one of the copies by a given date, usually within 10 to 14 days. Oftentimes employers would like a decision, or at the very least a response with questions or negotiable items, sooner. The reason for this is if the position is not accepted, the employer will need to make a decision as to whether or not to offer the job to another candidate in a timely manner or to reopen the search process. Less formal ways of handling the offer of contract are certainly available, but the less formal the process, the greater the chances for misunderstanding and trouble later.

Step 10: Hiring

After a candidate has signed a written employment contract, the institution should send a letter to the other applicants thanking them for their interest in the position and informing them that the position has been filled. In some cases, it is considered gracious to personally call candidates who were interviewed on-site and not offered the job to inform them of the hiring. Too many institutions, however, ignore this important courtesy. Another step that some institutions take at the end of the hiring process is to distribute a press release to the media announcing the addition of the new athletic trainer to the sports medicine staff. This valuable public relations tool for the sports medicine program makes the new athletic trainer's induction into a relatively unfamiliar work setting more comfortable. Providing the newly hired athletic trainer with an orientation manual can be helpful during the preparation and transition process. Information on topics such as training that needs to be completed, policies and procedures for computer access and usage, and other daily functions necessary to perform the job should be included.

Finding Your Job

Everything up to this point in this section has been written from the perspective of the athletic trainer-administrator who is looking for just the right person to join her staff. Because many of you reading this text are either undergraduate or graduate athletic training students who aren't yet in a position to be doing the hiring, it seems fitting to include a few tips for helping you find your first job. Although the preceding material will help you understand the recruiting and hiring process from an employer's point of view, you should consider many additional facets of employment when looking for a job.

Identifying Job Openings

If you are a student just getting ready to graduate and enter the workforce, one of the questions you have undoubtedly asked is, "Where can I find a job as an athletic trainer?" Athletic training positions are advertised in many places. The career center at your university may have a database of recently posted positions. Similarly, your professors probably receive many e-mails each month advertising athletic training positions in a variety of settings. Once the place many people started their job search, today the classified help wanted section of your local newspaper is usually not a rich source of athletic training positions, but you may find local schools, hospitals, or companies advertising there from time to time. Other ways to identify potential athletic training jobs include the following:

- *Networking.* Your ability to develop and stay in touch with the many contacts you have made while in school might be the best job search strategy you can employ. The supervisors and teachers you have had in various classes, clinical experiences, internships, and health-related summer jobs will know about positions as they become available. Make sure that all these people have a current copy of your resume, and keep in touch with them so that they will know that you are looking for a job. Dunne (2002) recommends that you let everyone in your life—including family, friends, advisors, and mentors—know that you are job hunting. You might be surprised by the way you find out about your first job! Professional networking begins in the classroom: Someday your classmates will be practicing certified athletic trainers whom you will have built relationships with. It is beneficial to maintain friendships throughout school and beyond, despite minor episodes or incidents that might irritate you during a brief point in time. Burning bridges can serve no benefit for future networking purposes.

- *Cold calling.* This technique can be especially effective if your job search is restricted to a limited geographic area. For example, if you have to find a job in a certain city, you should compile a list of all the agencies, clinics, hospitals, schools, universities, and professional sports organizations that are likely to employ athletic trainers in that city. Send all these a letter indicating your interest in working for them as an athletic trainer (even if you aren't sure whether they have openings—they may save your letter for a future opening). Include a resume with your letter. Follow up with a phone call to see whether the organization received your materials and inquire about openings. This task is time consuming. If the geographic area that you are searching is large, this method can take a long time, but it is a valuable tool because you will be saturating a particular market with your name. While cold calling can be effective in identifying position openings that otherwise would not be easy to find, it is important to avoid overdoing contact with any single employer, which may be perceived as nagging.

- *Web-based databases.* Athletic trainers can take advantage of many Web-based job search services. Some are specific to athletic trainers, whereas others are broadly structured for all kinds of health care professionals. NATA provides one of the most important Web-based services, but there are many others. Besides searching specific athletic training–related databases such as district and state pages, you can simply use Internet search engines like Google or Yahoo and search terms such as *athletic trainer* and *job* or *position* to develop a long list of potential positions in nearly every employment setting. Web-based search engines that are more specific to health care jobs, and especially athletic training jobs, will yield results on positions more suitable for an athletic trainer. In addition, universities, colleges, and school districts have human resource pages where they post position vacancies. Note that jobs in other countries may be advertised under a different heading such as athletic therapist (Canada) or physiotherapist (United Kingdom, Australia).

- *Conventions, conferences, and job fairs.* National and regional conventions, conferences, and job fairs are a common and convenient place for employers to recruit athletic trainers. The annual conventions of NATA, SHAPE America, and the American College of Sports Medicine all host job fairs that provide employers and job seekers a venue to meet, interact, and interview. If you plan to look for a job at one of these conventions, bring plenty of copies of your resume and show up prepared to interview. Athletic training state and district meetings often serve as good opportunities for job seekers.

Choosing Where to Apply

Once potential opportunities have caught your interest, you will need to decide which ones are worth pursuing. This can be a time-consuming process that involves learning about each position. Whether it is an athletic training job or a graduate assistantship you are seeking, the process of inquiry will be similar. To objectively evaluate each opportunity, you can use a matrix such as the one in figure 4.12 to assess the individual components of each position and also perform a comparative summary analysis. Items for consideration in the vertical column of the matrix can be added or deleted based on criteria you feel are important to evaluate. Some things to consider when weighing the relative merits of an employment offer include the potential for job growth, benefits, salary, environment for communication and collegiality, job security, and job flexibility (Konin 1997).

Using the chart, rate the categories for each employment setting. Use a scale of 0 to 10, with 10 representing the best situation for you.

	EMPLOYMENT CONSIDERATION					
	Job 1	Job 2	Job 3	Job 4	Job 5	Job 6
Salary						
Other benefits (e.g., CEUs, licensure dues, cell phone)						
Job flexibility						
Location of job						
Distance from home						
Safety of area						
Reputation of employer						
Health benefits						
Professional development opportunities						
Staff morale						
Facilities						
Cost of living in the area						
Job security						
Supervisor						
Policies and procedures in place						
Average commute						
Typical working hours						
Potential for advancement						
Contract length (9, 10, 11, or 12 months)						
Volume of travel required						
Reporting line						
Total rating						

Figure 4.12 Guide to choosing a job.

Making Contact

After you have compiled a list of potential employers, the next step is to make sure that they become aware of your interest, background, credentials, and skills. A well-prepared resume and cover letter are the most common ways to accomplish this, but you can and should use other methods to help you stand out from the crowd. Depending on how your cover letter and resume were delivered, it is usually a good idea to follow up with either an e-mail message or a phone call to make sure that the potential employer received them, unless the job posting specifically requests that you not contact them. For some jobs this will be your first conversation with the employer, and making a good impression is important. Yate (2002) suggests that this contact experience should have four goals:

- Get the employer's attention
- Generate interest in your application
- Create a desire in the employer to know more about you
- Encourage the employer to take action on your application

Here are a few ways to help you accomplish those goals:

- Express your enthusiasm for the opportunity to work in the organization.

- Fill in the employer on additional experiences you may have had since sending in your materials. Keep in mind that if you are an entry-level athletic trainer, you possess all of the same skills every recently certified entry-level athletic trainer has based on learned competencies and proficiencies. Thus, additional experiences can help separate you from others.

- Remind the employer of the special skills or experiences that help you stand out from the crowd, but do this in a manner that doesn't exaggerate your experiences.

- Ask the employer whether he has preliminary questions that he would like to ask you.

- Identify your time line for availability as it relates to a start date and your overall flexibility for work scheduling.

- Thank the employer for his time.

- Stay in touch with all potential employers in this way until the position is filled or you have accepted another job.

Resume Writing

In many cases, one's first chance to make an impression on a potential employer takes the form of a resume. It is helpful to seek advice from others regarding the development, formatting, and updating of a resume so that it is attractive to an employer. However, be prepared to receive as many opinions on how to prepare a resume as the number of people you seek advice from. While there is no one perfect method or style of resume writing, you can follow general guidelines on how to present an appealing document.

All resumes follow a format that is designed to subdivide the background information for a person and present it in reverse chronological (most recent first) order. The following subcategories are suggested for inclusion for an athletic training graduate or relatively new certified athletic trainer:

- *Personal contact information.* This should include formal and preferred name, current mailing address, e-mail, and phone numbers.

- *Goals and objective.* It is helpful to list a single focused professional goal. This may be a relatively short-term goal, such as the type of setting you want to work in, or it may be slightly more long term, for example what you want to accomplish within the next three to five years as an athletic trainer.

- *Educational experience.* List all of the educational programs you have attended or graduated from. Include the name of the school, geographical location of the school (city, state), year of attendance or graduation, and major and minor areas of study.

- *Certifications and licenses.* List all certifications and licenses held, including the date that it was awarded. For example, "2016 to present" shows that it is still valid. Include your license number for any state you're licensed in and your National Provider Identifier (NPI). Be specific about each certification, and include who granted it, such as American Red Cross CPR/AED for the Professional Rescuer. If you are not yet certified by the BOC, state when you anticipate your certification.

- *Employment experience.* List all places of employment. Be sure to include the name of the employer, your position and title, primary responsibilities, dates of employment, and location of employment setting (city, state).

- *Honors and awards.* Identify relevant honors, awards, and achievements that you have earned relative to your professional career, academic endeavors, or social contributions. If the name of an award is not self-explanatory, include a brief sentence that describes the achievement. Academic and professional awards should always be highlighted on a resume. Examples of other honors and awards that you may or may not want to list include Boy Scouts recognition or captain of a high school athletic team. It may be a good idea to list such honors if in total they represent a pattern of leadership or accomplishment. As one's professional career advances, honors like these may become less relevant to athletic training skills.

- *Presentations and publications.* Include professional presentations you have given (exclusive of formal classroom assignments) or work you have published; examples are a poster at a regional district athletic training meeting, a community sports safety presentation to coaches or parents, or an abstract published in a proceedings manual.

- *Memberships.* List the organizations or associations that you are a member of. This may include student athletic training associations, NATA, academic honor societies, and community groups.

List the years of your affiliation, and if the name of the organization is not self-explanatory, include a sentence that explains its purpose. Be sure to list leadership or official positions you have held in these organizations.

- *Additional information.* There may be items you think are important to list on your resume that do not seem to fit into a specific category. You may also not want to have one item under a subheading as it may look like a lesser accomplishment. If this is the case, you can create subcategory headings of your own or simply use the subheading Miscellaneous. An example might include a nonpaid shadowing experience you completed that was beneficial to your career. This might also be a place where you can list additional languages you speak or computer or other related skills you possess.

- *References.* List the names and current contact information of people who have agreed to provide a recommendation for you. Include their name, title and affiliations, employer, mailing address, e-mail address, and phone number. In an initial interview, employers may ask for your permission to contact anyone related to your school or work history. If you grant this, they may call people you've worked with, even if you don't include them on your reference list.

As previously mentioned, opinions vary regarding what to include or not include on a resume. The following are considerations that should be left up to you:

- *Personal information.* Some people list their age, health status, hobbies, family members, and even religious affiliation. Depending on the employment setting that you are seeking, this information may or may not be relevant.

- *High school.* Where someone attended high school becomes less relevant the longer her career. In some cases, a high school attended is listed on a resume because it has some connection to the potential employer or employment setting.

- *Nonathletic training work experience.* Because athletic training is a health care profession, work experiences as a waitress, clerk, retail manager, or other jobs may not be relevant in demonstrating capability as an athletic trainer. However, in some cases, listing these experiences may demonstrate work ethic or skills such as leadership, supervision, accounting, interpersonal skills, or software management that are similar to those required of a successful athletic trainer. Most would agree, however, that listing these experiences is more helpful to a newly certified athletic trainer than to one who has been removed from entry-level education for years.

- *Grade point average.* Students who have obtained an above-average grade point are encouraged to list this on the resume as part of their academic experience. Be sure to list not only the earned grade point average, but also the potential maximum, for example, 3.7/4.0. If you have earned honors or high honors, this should be listed. However, if you earned honors for just one or two semesters out of a possible eight, you might want to consider whether or not to include this information.

- *Employment departure.* All employment experiences should be listed, regardless of their duration. With noticeably short stints of employment, it may be wise to list the reason for departure in an effort to proactively explain what might otherwise be viewed as a red flag. Acceptable reasons for departures may include family or home relocations, a return to school for further education, illness, or other life-changing circumstances.

- *Order of events.* The decision about what order to list items is a simple one. If you have held three jobs, you can list them in reverse chronological order, with the most recent one first (recommended), or in chronological order beginning with the first job. Regardless of which method you choose, the order should be the same for all subcategories of the resume.

- *References available on request.* Some professionals recommend not including references with contact information on a resume but instead the statement "References available on request." Although the issue is open to debate, it would appear that including information on references makes for a more thorough resume, allowing potential employers who choose to contact your references to do so without having to track you down. Furthermore, from a networking perspective, listing the names of your references may trigger a connection of some kind with the employer. This could prompt a quicker phone call to discuss your candidacy based on name recognition alone.

Cover Letter

A cover letter should always accompany a resume. The cover letter should be succinct, presenting an overview of your interest in and qualifications for the job. The cover letter typically includes the following:

- Introductory paragraph stating formal intent to apply for the position
- Body of letter highlighting your experiences in a single paragraph
- Careful meshing of your abilities with the employer's needs in a single paragraph
- Summary paragraph informing the recipient of how you can be contacted

Figure 4.13 shows an example of a cover letter.

Common Mistakes to Avoid

While there are numerous ways to write a resume and cover letter, there are also common mistakes that employers see, and these errors can create a negative impression of the applicant. Careful proof-reading and attention to detail will help you avoid these mistakes.

- *Inappropriate e-mail address.* Contact e-mail addresses that do not look professional, such as partydude@email.net, make a bad impression.
- *Nonapplicable career goal or objective.* Applicants sometimes forget that the career goal or objective listed on the resume should be specific to each position they are applying for and should be modified accordingly. For example, the career goal "To serve as head athletic trainer in a secondary school setting" should be changed or deleted if the applicant has decided to send the resume with an application for a university position.
- *Incorrect names.* Candidates applying for multiple positions often use the same basic cover letter, and failing to change the name and affiliation of the addressee is not uncommon. This is simply a matter of careless proofreading and makes an unfavorable

---

January 14, 2018

Mr. Marty Stamkos
Athletic Director
Light High School
Tampa, FL 33533

Dear Mr. Stamkos,

In response to your recent posting for an athletic trainer position at your high school, I would like to formally submit my application for consideration.

After carefully assessing the position description, I believe that my past experiences and current leadership capabilities would serve as a complementary fit at Light High School. As my resume reflects, my career experience as a certified athletic trainer has included four years in a secondary school setting, the past two as the head athletic trainer. In addition, I am CPR certified and will soon become a certified strength and conditioning specialist.

My leadership experience and interpersonal skills are strengths that will enable me to provide quality care and services to the student-athletes. I am dependable and organized and also show a dedication to my work that others have commended me for regularly. I believe that all these characteristics would enable me to perform in an exemplary manner at your school. It is my continued career goal to be an athletic trainer in a secondary school setting, and your program appears to be exactly the type of setting I would like to work in.

Thank you for consideration of my application. I can be reached at any time on my cell phone or by e-mail if you feel that I am a qualified candidate and are interested in setting up an interview.

Sincerely,

Wes Oates, ATC

Figure 4.13 Sample cover letter.

impression, even though employers know that candidates do apply for multiple positions simultaneously in an effort to find the right job.

- *Misspellings.* Misspelling addressees' names or listing their credentials incorrectly is a common error that can be avoided with careful proofreading. Similarly, applicants misspell names of individuals listed as references and provide inaccurate or outdated contact information, which causes difficulties for potential employers who want to contact references.

- *Name dropping.* It may be appropriate to inform a potential employer that you learned of the opening through a particular person. However, listing people's names can give the impression that you hope their professional reputation or stature will increase your chances of obtaining a position and is not often seen in a favorable light.

- *Redundancy.* The cover letter should emphasize and highlight key components of a resume. More important, it complements and should serve as an opportunity to expand on the resume. Using the cover letter to merely repeat what is on the resume is not the best way to sell yourself to a potential employer.

- *Exaggeration.* The cover letter serves to explain why you feel you are a good fit for a job. Even though the cover letter is crafted to portray your background and your interest in the job, you should be careful not to exaggerate your skills or accomplishments. Guard against overstating your merits, especially if you are a recent graduate, because it will be assumed that you possess entry-level skills. If there is a job qualification that you do not meet, explain your plan to meet it in the near future. For example, if they are looking for a CPR instructor and you are not one, explain that you have found a class in the area where you could become a certified instructor in a timely manner.

- *Listing basic accomplishments.* In listing responsibilities and accomplishments in a job or clinical experience, do not include basic tasks that every athletic trainer performs. Employers will expect that you can carry out responsibilities such as taping ankles, cleaning the athletic training room, and evaluating and treating injuries, and these should not be listed as skills or accomplishments.

- *Aggressiveness.* It is helpful to note your availability for interviews. However, many consider it inappropriate to state that you will contact the employer soon after sending a resume. It is acceptable in some cases to follow up to ask about the status of a job inquiry. However, it is not necessarily as appropriate to state, for example, "If I do not hear from you within one week I will contact you to set up an interview."

Interviewing

Interviewing for a job can take several forms. Employers sometimes conduct preliminary interviews by telephone before arranging face-to-face interviews with the most promising candidates. As suggested earlier, some employers conduct interviews at conferences and job fairs, whereas others prefer to bring the applicant to the employment site. Whatever the interview technique or location, your first task as the interviewee is to prepare. Although you'll certainly need to be able to answer the employer's questions during the interview, you should also be able to summarize your experiences, qualifications, and skills in approximately 30 seconds. You should be able to articulate your professional philosophy. Be prepared to explain how you deal with difficult problems, using examples from your past. Find out as much as you can about the organization before the interview—the organization's website is a great place to start this part of your preparation. All this takes planning and practice. You should arrange for a videotaped mock interview so that you can practice and receive feedback. Many career counseling centers on college campuses offer this service.

The list of questions that one can be asked during an interview is endless. There are standard, expected questions such as "What are your strengths and weaknesses?" Other questions tend to be people's personal favorites and are unlikely to be anticipated during preparation for an interview. The following are examples of questions that a candidate for an athletic training position might be asked:

- What would others say are your strengths and weakness?
- Explain how you would be a team player. Perhaps provide an example of a previous athletic training–related experience.
- How can you specifically make our organization better?
- Why should we hire you?
- What unique skills do you possess, and how will that make you a good AT?
- Are you willing to work nights or weekends or both and travel when necessary?

- What are your professional goals for five years from now? Ten years from now?

- What are your thoughts on the current state of health care as it relates to athletic training services?

- Currently, we are struggling with reimbursement issues. What suggestions might you have to assist us with efforts to obtain fair remuneration for the services that we provide?

- Recently, we had an athletic training student who was asked to perform a manual technique on a patient that the student was not comfortable performing. Normally, the AT performs the treatment, and the results provide the patient with two to three days of pain relief. On this particular day, the AT had a family illness and could not make it to work. It also happened to be the last treatment session for the patient, given the fact that she was going to leave for a three-day drive to California where she lives in the winter. If you were the athletic training student in this situation, what would you do?

- What type of salary are you looking for?

- With respect to this position, what are the most important issues that will determine whether or not you would accept should we decide to offer a position to you?

- Are you familiar with CPTs? If you answer no: How would you plan to learn about them before beginning employment with us? If you answer yes: What code would you choose to use for a patient who has ABC health care as an insurance provider and participates in a hydrotherapy session for 45 minutes under your supervision?

- Why do you want to work with us?

- How do you handle stress? Please elaborate.

- How do your goals tie into the mission of our program and institution?

- What is the first thing you would like to do if hired here?

- How could we help you here with your professional goals and interests?

In addition to these professional and work-related questions, it is not uncommon for employers to ask a candidate what might be considered a unique type of question unrelated to athletic training simply in an effort to judge the candidate's innovativeness and creativity. These are also questions intended to elicit spontaneous answers:

- If you could be a piece of furniture, what would you be and why?

- Who is your favorite cartoon character and why?

- If you could be any animal, what would you be and why?

- What city in the United States has the best pizza?

- Tell me about the last good movie that you saw.

Lastly, employers try to hire positive-minded people who will be motivated to work and who do not thrive on negativity or pessimism. Be prepared to respond to questions that may be traps. The intent of this type of question is to provoke a candidate to speak in a negative manner about a previous employer, colleague, or situation. Here are some examples:

- What did you dislike about your last job? Why did you leave?

- Did you ever have professors you didn't like? What didn't you like about them?

- Tell me something that you do not like about yourself.

- Please describe your idea of a bad job.

First impressions are critical. Although the employer has seen your cover letter and resume, the interview is probably the first time he or she will meet you in person. Although employers should certainly be concerned about your knowledge, skills, and experience as important predictors of job performance, they will also be developing an impression of how well you are likely to fit into the culture of the organization. They will determine in a relatively short time whether they like you—and whether the other employees with whom they work will like you. The following tips will help you develop a good first impression with prospective employers:

- *Dress professionally for the interview.* Any externals (clothes, grooming, excessive jewelry) that distract the employer from your conversation will create a poor impression. You want them to remember your experience and personality, rather than tattoos, piercings, colorful socks, or cologne that may have been distractive. (See figure 4.14.)

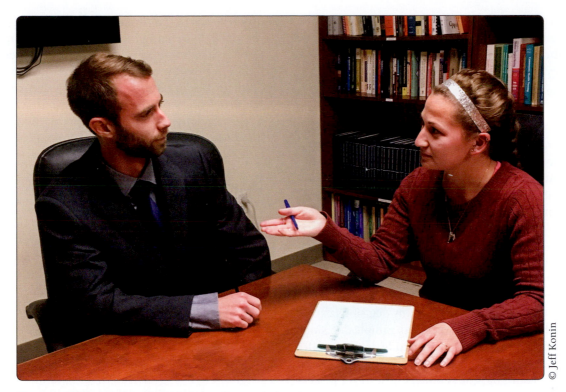

© Jeff Konin

Figure 4.14 Professional dress for an interview.

- *Learn as much about the organization as you can before the interview.* Besides trying to learn the names of the people in the organization, attempt to discern in advance the culture of the place so that you can frame your answers in a way that will have as much effect as possible. Ideally, talk to people who work in the organization or know it well enough to give you advice. Review their website and search the Internet to see whether they've been in the news lately.

- *Be enthusiastic.* Express interest in the things the employer tells you about the organization. If you think that this is a place where you could be happy working, be sure to say so. Employers want happy, motivated employees. You'll have to demonstrate that you can be both.

- *Be courteous.* Although it may seem obvious that an applicant should show courtesy, failing to say simple things like "please" and "thank you" has derailed the job prospects of many talented people. As someone being interviewed for a position in an organization, you are a guest in that place for a day. Your interviewers will remember your behavior long after they have forgotten your answers to specific interview questions.

Closing the Deal

An interview will create a first impression in the mind of the employer. You should take steps to build on that first impression after the interview ends by repeating in modified form the steps you took to contact the employer before the interview. Here are a few things you can do to help the employer remember you after you have left:

- *Send thank-you notes.* Send notes to every person with whom you spoke during your interview. The notes should be specific to the conversation you had with that person (for example, "I enjoyed learning about your facilities at Big Time University. My experiences there as an undergraduate were outstanding."). Be sure to thank the employer for taking time to interview you for the position. Encourage the employer to contact you if additional questions or concerns arise. You can send these notes by either mail or e-mail, but it is best to send them immediately after the interview.

- *Postinterview references.* Although you probably had several people write to the employer on your behalf before the interview, you may want to have one of your most trusted and enthusiastic sponsors contact the employer after the interview ends—especially if the sponsor is personally acquainted with the employer.

- *Keep in touch.* Stay in touch with the employer after the interview so that you can both keep current with the search and to demonstrate enthusiasm and eagerness for the position.

- *Prepare for a job offer.* Soon after your interview, you may be called and offered a job. An offer frequently includes all of the terms for employment, including the salary. To be prepared, you should have some idea of the terms of employment that would be acceptable to you. NATA surveys athletic trainers annually and posts their reported salaries; the information is categorized by the type of employment setting, gender, years of experience, amount of education, geographical location, and other categories of relevance. Many decisions can be made when a job offer is received. Simple decisions include accepting the offer or turning down the offer on the spot. If you know immediately based on the offer and your goals, it is always best to act professionally and provide your certain decision. However, if you are undecided and need time to process the offer, it is acceptable to request this. Be prepared to state how much time you will need to decide, and be sure that it is reasonable in the eyes of the employer. The employer really wants to know that you are excited and ready to accept the offer. If you need additional time to decide, use the time wisely. Consult with mentors, family members, and others you trust. If you opt to counteroffer in any way, be sure it is a reasonable offer, and one that shows you put serious thought into your request. While some employers may accept your counteroffer, others may meet you some place between their offer and yours, and yet other employers may simply state that the offer was nonnegotiable. If the latter is the case, be prepared to walk away from the original offer if it is not what you want. Keep in mind that salary is not the only point of negotiation. Benefits such as professional development funding support, membership and licensure fees, and opportunities for growth are just a few examples of negotiable terms. Always keep negotiations on a professional level because the end result is to secure employment through the process. Starting a new job with a positive relationship is always the best approach.

- *Don't burn bridges.* Be sure to maintain amicable relations with the employer even in the face of rejection. You never know when another opportunity to work in that organization might arise. Your response to *not* being hired can be just as important to your reputation as an offer of employment. You might not be the right person for the job at this point in the organization's history, but that does not mean you won't be in the future. If you receive a rejection letter, write back to thank the employer for considering you for the position and send your best wishes.

Personnel Deployment

The cost of employing people makes up the largest portion of the budget for most service-oriented enterprises, including those in which athletic trainers typically work. If an educational institution, health care facility, or business that employs athletic trainers is to operate effectively and efficiently, it must deploy the right number of staff at the right times and in the right places. Too often, employers hire athletic trainers and, without doing adequate planning for reasonable workloads that yield effective patient outcomes, expect them to manage every aspect of athlete or employee health care needs.

Factors Affecting Personnel Deployment Decisions

Nelson, Altman, and Mayo (2000) recommend that institutions consider the following five elements when planning staff deployment:

1. *Activities to be performed.* What jobs are critical to the successful operation of the sports medicine operation? When and where are these tasks performed? The answers to these questions should flow from the goals and objectives of the sports medicine program as outlined in chapter 3. Activities not related to the program's mission, goals, and objectives draw needed staff resources away from the things that matter most.

2. *Required abilities.* What level of professional competence is required for each of the identified tasks? Which professional credentials, licenses, or certifications are required by law or commonly accepted standards? When considering the kinds of abilities required for the activities performed in the program, organizations should think about more than technical athletic training skills. Equally important are things like communication skills, interpersonal skills, and organizational and management skills.

3. *Number of required staff.* How will the number, timing, and location of tasks, along with rules governing reasonable workloads, affect the number of personnel required to accomplish the mission? (See the discussion of the Fair Labor Standards Act later in this chapter.) Standards that help establish the necessary number of athletic trainers cover some employment settings in which athletic trainers work. NATA has established recommendations and guidelines for the number of athletic trainers needed to staff college and university sports medicine programs adequately (see the later section on appropriate medical coverage).

4. *The way in which the staff currently uses its time.* Are the athletic trainers currently in place using their time efficiently? Effectively? Are they working on the right kinds of tasks given their level of training and expertise? Several methods exist for analyzing staff activities. Using a combination of existing records, supervisor observations, and employee self-reports, it is possible to determine the kinds of activities that athletic trainers are involved with. Mayo and Goodrich (2002) recommend conducting both numeric and process analyses from time to time as a way to determine the appropriateness of staff activities (see the next section on workload analysis).

5. *Finding staff to accomplish the goals of the program.* Are resources available to hire additional athletic trainers if they are needed? Can athletic trainers be reassigned to achieve greater efficiency? Can other personnel assume some of the duties now assigned to athletic trainers? Too often the first impulse—especially in athletic training, in which understaffing has been a chronic problem for many years—is simply to hire more staff to accomplish the mission of the sports medicine program. The athletic trainer-administrator has the responsibility, however, to accomplish the mission at the least possible cost. Given that staff salaries and benefits make up most of the costs, additional hiring is not always the best action. The athletic trainer-administrator should consider other options such as task reallocation, task elimination, outsourcing for certain tasks, and use of part-time personnel for some aspects of the program. One activity that consumes a great deal of athletic trainers' time is having an open clinic. ATs often wait around in the athletic training room for several hours per day in case an athlete needs to come in for treatment. ATs could be more efficient with their time if athletes were

required to schedule appointments, similar to other health care providers.

Workload Analysis

The athletic trainer-administrator can use many methods to monitor the work being performed by his staff for the purpose of determining appropriate staffing levels. Mayo and Goodrich (2002) recommend two that seem appropriate for sports medicine settings: numeric analysis and process analysis.

- **Numeric analysis** is the process of determining a staff member's workload by calculating and comparing the amount of time a person spends on certain tasks with the outputs—the measurable results. An example of numeric analysis commonly employed in sports medicine clinics is the number of patients treated by each staff member per day, per week, per month, or per year. A similar example from athletic training education would be the number of credit hours taught by a faculty member per semester or per year. Calculations of this type are most useful if they are tracked over time so that increases or decreases in workloads can be observed. Where national standards exist, numeric analyses can also serve as helpful indicators for determining whether a particular staff member or a group of athletic trainers is working below, at, or above the standard.

- **Process analysis** is a technique for streamlining the number and complexity of steps needed to provide a service to a customer. Tasks that require the fewest number of steps—and whose steps are the simplest to perform—typically require fewer people to perform. Athletic trainer-administrators who want to staff their programs at the lowest reasonable level should brainstorm with their staffs to identify all the steps required to complete any given task. Two or more athletic trainers may be performing the same task using different steps. Analyzing those steps may produce a consensus on the most efficient way to perform the task.

A word of caution regarding process analysis is appropriate. Although this technique can be useful in sports medicine and other health care settings, risks are associated with its rigid implementation. Health care professionals may understand that a certain degree of conformity to organizational processes is necessary for efficiency, but they are likely to complain if they must sacrifice their professional autonomy and judgment. For example, if a school's head athletic trainer advocates a taping method that uses 6 fewer inches (15 cm) of tape per procedure and imposes this method on the other members of the staff, she should not be surprised if her staff meets the directive with limited enthusiasm. Although the procedure is technically more efficient, the cost savings are likely to be minimal. Athletic trainer-administrators must balance gains in efficiency with the staff's need for professional autonomy.

Appropriate Medical Coverage

Although the staff deployment concepts outlined in the previous section apply to almost any business or industry, NATA provides recommendations for appropriate coverage for different settings. These guidelines provide colleges, universities, and secondary schools with a system for determining the number of certified athletic trainers required to render adequate health care services to their student-athletes. The model on which the guidelines were established was developed from published injury data, national surveys of collegiate medical coverage, guidelines from a variety of sports medicine organizations, and other sources. Similar documents now exist that offer guidelines and suggestions for appropriate medical coverage in other settings. The most current version of the formula used to establish appropriate staffing can be found on NATA's Web page.

Staff Supervision

The concept of management as defined in chapter 2 includes the notion that managers coordinate the activities of a group of people toward a common goal. They accomplish this partly through supervision. **Supervision** is a process whereby authority holders observe the work activities of an employee to improve the outcomes of the employee's work or the professional development of the employee. Supervision is different from summative evaluation. The purpose of summative evaluation is to place a value on the quality of an employee to determine appropriate employment actions, including retention, promotion, demotion, transfer, discharge, and compensation level.

Supervision is one of the most difficult managerial functions for an athletic trainer to master for several reasons. First, unless the employees whom the athletic trainer supervises are perfect in every way, supervision requires some degree of confrontation. Second, almost every supervisory problem is unique in some way. Responding to the employment-related problems of athletic trainers requires creativity and emotional investment in the staff and their development. Finally, effective supervision requires the athletic trainer to consider the opinions and perspectives of others. Athletic trainer-supervisors should develop strategies to reduce the level of bias they bring to situations so that the needs of both the sports medicine program and its employees can be met. Athletic trainers can use many supervisory models. Tanner and Tanner (1987) have described four: inspection, production, clinical, and developmental. This discussion combines the inspection and production models because their differences are minor.

It is not uncommon for athletic trainers in supervisory roles to find themselves in a position of supervisory neglect. Directors of athletic training clinical services and directors of athletic training education programs are not often directly supervised by other athletic trainers. Clinical athletic training directors may be supervised by an athletic director or a principal at a school, whereas those in academia may report to a department chair or dean with a nonathletic training background. It is imperative for athletic trainers in these circumstances to educate their supervisors on their role and function so that their supervision and summative evaluations are performed fairly and are reflective of their duties. In 2006, it was reported that while 46% of NATA membership was composed of women, only 37% of women held supervisory positions and leadership roles (Perez et al. 2006). In June 2016, NATA membership statistics reported that nearly 55% of the members were women, although no information was available to determine what percentage of those are in supervisory or leadership roles (NATA 2016).

Motivation

Before we look at the various supervisory models, it will be helpful to consider the role that supervisors play in motivating employees. Motivation of workers is generally considered an important supervisory function, yet it remains a poorly understood and applied management concept in most work settings. The supervisory models described in this section differ in many ways from each other, in part because of the different assumptions they make about the nature of motivation in the workplace.

PEARLS OF MANAGEMENT

Athletic trainers may be required to supervise other employees to improve their work outcomes or professional development. The three kinds of supervisory models are inspection–production, clinical, and developmental.

The inspection–production model, for example, has its roots in the scientific management movement of the early 1900s. One of the most important assumptions underlying that theory is that financial reward is the sole motivation for people to work. We now know that motivation in the workplace is a complex phenomenon influenced by many factors besides the promise of financial gain.

Motivation is a complex concept. Answers to three basic questions are necessary to understand the part played by motivation in the supervisory roles that athletic training managers must assume (Porter, Bigley, and Steers 2002).

1. What energizes human behavior?
2. What directs or channels human behavior?
3. How can human behavior be maintained or sustained?

Each of these questions lies at the heart of the broader question, "How do I motivate the athletic trainers under my supervision to do the best job possible?" None of these questions has easy answers, and that is the primary reason this book does not have a table titled How to Motivate Athletic Trainers. We have learned quite a bit about motivation, however, and it seems that the concept can be broken into four basic components:

1. Needs or expectations of the employee
2. Employee behavior
3. Employee goals
4. Feedback from the supervisor or other sources

Although this model does a good job of explaining workplace motivation at its simplest level, it is a poor predictor of employee behavior in actual job settings. At least four confounding factors complicate this model:

1. *Motives can only be inferred, not seen.* Knowing why employees act the way they do at work is often difficult. Although their behavior might be observable, the motivation for that behavior is often not. For example, if an athletic trainer puts in extra time in the athletic training room by volunteering to cover special events and other similar functions, we would know only that she is a hard worker. We wouldn't know what her motivation is for consistently volunteering. Perhaps she wants the extra money. Maybe she has a limited social life and meets her affiliation needs only through her work. Maybe she wants someone else's job and sees this as a way to demonstrate that she is capable and worthy of promotion or other leadership opportunity.

2. *Motives conflict with each other and are subject to change.* Most of us deal with conflicting motivations in many segments of our lives. These motives are usually not static; they change, as do the other situational variables in our lives. For example, an athletic trainer's behavior might be the result of conflicting motivations. If she has young children at home, the motivation to get ahead at work might conflict with her desire to fulfill her role as a parent. If she is the primary breadwinner, she might see the extra work as an opportunity to supplement the family income. As her children grow older, their needs (and hers) will change, resulting in a different set of motivating factors.

3. *Individual differences exist with regard to motives.* If everyone responded to the presence of motivators in the same way, supervision would be easy. However, what motivates one person is often insufficient to motivate another. One athletic trainer might be motivated (by something) to work extra hours in the athletic training room. Another athletic trainer might not be. This athletic trainer might be the last to arrive and the first to leave every day. He could receive extra pay by covering special events, but he chooses not to. The two athletic trainers have the same motivator (extra pay) but exhibit different behavior.

4. *Goal attainment modifies behavior in different ways.* Besides the fact that people are motivated by different things, they often respond differently to achievement of the same goals. Consider an athletic trainer recently appointed to the head athletic trainer position, who then coasted, rarely volunteering for extra work even if it meant extra pay. Assume that another athletic trainer would like to be head of the program one day. Will she also coast after she achieves that goal? Will she continue to volunteer for extra duties? Or will she work even harder in the hope that she might be promoted to a position on the athletic director's staff?

As you can see, although motivation seems to be a straightforward concept, its application is complex and difficult to predict. As you read the following sections, keep in mind the assumptions that each supervisory model makes about the nature of human behavior at work.

When you eventually attain a position in which you must supervise athletic trainers and other health care professionals, you will have to choose a supervisory style that meshes with your basic assumptions about what motivates people.

Inspection–Production Supervision

The primary characteristic of the **inspection–production** model of supervision is an emphasis on authoritative managerial efficiency. Athletic trainers who prefer this approach to supervision insist on strict observance of program policies and procedures. This model views the services provided by the sports medicine program as products and the athletic training employees as the raw materials used to develop those products. In the inspection–production model, supervising athletic trainers requires all employees of a sports medicine program to develop a comprehensive list of goals for the year. Then they carefully check progress toward accomplishing those goals during the course of the year. The overriding emphasis of this model is on accomplishment of program goals and objectives and on attainment of the program mission.

The following are advantages of the inspection–production model:

- It can be effective in helping a sports medicine program accomplish its goals.
- It sets well-defined limits on job-related behavior for all employees and consequently enhances common understanding of the athletic trainers' roles.
- It is usually associated with formalistic bureaucratic organizations that have many levels of supervisory management.

Using the inspection–production system of supervision in service-oriented enterprises, including sports medicine programs, has several disadvantages:

- This model was originally developed and implemented in industrial settings where

inputs and outputs could be easily measured. Measurement of inputs and outputs in most sports medicine settings is difficult. Although some measures of program success or failure should be developed, interpretation of them will vary widely depending on the audience.

- Another problem with this model is the nature of the work that athletic trainers do. Most athletic trainers perform a variety of jobs, and not all of them are easily observed or quantified. For example, if a supervising athletic trainer wanted to be sure that a staff athletic trainer was meeting the program standard for taping effectiveness and efficiency, he could simply observe her as she prepared a team for a practice or game. But how would he inspect the effectiveness and efficiency of her counseling skills? Her rehabilitation skills?

- The inspection–production method of supervision can cause professional employees such as athletic trainers to feel unappreciated and unfulfilled. Because the dominant ethos is program goal accomplishment and not professional development, athletic trainers will rarely appreciate what little developmental feedback they receive. They will tend to view such feedback in negative terms.

Clinical Supervision

In the athletic training setting, supervised clinical education is directed by a **preceptor**. A preceptor is defined by CAATE as a certified or licensed professional who teaches or evaluates students or both in a clinical setting using an actual patient base (Commission on Accreditation of Athletic Training Education 2012). Furthermore, **clinical education** is defined as the application of athletic training knowledge, skills, and clinical abilities on an actual patient base that is evaluated and feedback provided by a preceptor. As the profession of athletic training continues to develop and respond to the role delineation of the practicing athletic trainer, the standards and definitions will continue to evolve.

Among the many supervisory techniques that can be applied within the clinical supervision model, one of the most promising for athletic trainers is work sampling (Harris 2009). Work sampling identifies the type of work that athletic trainers do and the amount of time they spend doing it. Hence, it can be an effective tool for both clinical supervision and job analysis. Work sampling consists of logging the activities of athletic trainers at randomly selected times and analyzing the data to judge the nature and quality of the work that they are performing. Appropriate activities facilitate the goals and objectives of the sports medicine program. Inappropriate activities duplicate effort, lack a connection to the purposes of the program, fulfill purely personal or social wants, or allocate too much time to tasks that are not suited to the athletic trainer's qualifications.

The following are advantages of clinical supervision:

- Emphasizes collegial working relationships and cooperative planning
- Promotes the professional status of the athletic trainer and involves the athletic trainer in as much of the supervisory process as possible
- Focuses on a consultative rather than authoritative role for the supervising athletic trainer

The primary disadvantages of the clinical system of supervision are the following:

- The supervising athletic trainer must devote large blocks of time to supervising individual employees. Because clinical supervision requires direct observation of an athletic trainer's performance and most supervising athletic trainers have significant responsibilities in the treatment of injured clients, finding the time to implement a truly clinical system of supervision is difficult.
- Accurate interpretation of observed supervision data requires training.

Developmental Supervision

Developmental supervision involves collaboration between a supervising athletic trainer and employees. The emphasis is on helping employees develop professionally while meeting the needs of the sports medicine program. The overriding philosophy of developmental supervision is participative management—employees discuss common problems and suggest and implement creative solutions. The system is intended to improve both the sports medicine program and its employees by increasing employee involvement in problem solving. It acknowledges the interdependence of the goals of the program and those of the athletic trainers.

The primary advantage of the developmental model is its emphasis on personal growth and its integration of athletic trainer and sports medicine program goals. The developmental system tends to build an organizational culture that emphasizes meeting the needs of athletic trainers to improve program quality. Athletic trainers working in organizations with this focus are generally happy and content with their professional development.

However, well-developed, happy employees do not guarantee overall program success. Collegiality and collaboration are desirable only when they bring different perspectives and new ways of thinking to difficult problems. Heavy emphasis on collaboration can delay problem solving because of the need to preserve the collegial organizational climate.

Best Supervisory Model

Which supervisory model is best? Is one model more appropriate for a university setting? For a sports medicine clinic setting? These questions are difficult to answer because the three supervisory models have not been empirically investigated in sports medicine settings. But we can intuitively draw a few tentative conclusions. First, most sports medicine programs should probably integrate elements of each model into their supervisory plans. When possible, programs should use collaborative problem solving because athletic trainers will have a greater sense of ownership in the resulting solutions. When questions arise about the effectiveness of an athletic trainer, direct observation of his work and suggestions for improvement by the supervising athletic trainer would probably be useful. At times, however, the supervisor will have to take other actions. If an employee has not responded well to attempts at collaborative problem solving or suggestions from the supervisor, the supervising athletic trainer may have no alternative but to impose a solution to correct the actions of the employee.

Performance Evaluation

Performance evaluation is the process of placing a value on the quality of an athletic trainer's work (Raab et al. 2011). Performance evaluation is important for at least two reasons:

1. It can help a supervising athletic trainer make valid and reliable distinctions between athletic

trainers who are performing at or above program expectations and those whose work is unsatisfactory.

2. A properly implemented system of performance evaluation helps the athletic trainers being evaluated identify areas of weakness and eliminate or reduce them.

PEARLS OF MANAGEMENT

Performance evaluation is an underused and generally poorly performed human resource tool in athletic training. Performance evaluation systems and methods should meet established standards so that they are legal and fair, useful, accurate, and practical.

Figures 4.15 and 4.16 provide examples of performance evaluation instruments. Remember, however, that a performance evaluation instrument that is not based on a specific athletic trainer's weighted job description and not designed for a particular purpose is useless. Performance evaluation is *not* the annual completion of a form. Performance evaluation is a process that takes place throughout the year that involves mutually establishing goals, creating performance standards for accomplishing those goals, measuring the level of accomplishment, mutually understanding how well the athletic trainer met her goals, and mutually developing plans to remediate performance deficiencies and continue professional development. Measuring performance often requires the input of the athletic trainer being evaluated, the athletic trainer's peers, the supervisor, the clients, and the consulting physicians. A performance evaluation instrument not built on these principles would be so riddled with caveats, it would be meaningless. In some circumstances, coaches are also asked to provide input regarding the performance of the athletic trainer. While their feedback is viewed by some as relevant, it is important to take into account that coaches are biased in their expectations of an athletic trainer and not always objective in their judgment of how appropriately the athletic trainer is performing his role. At times, a coach's opinion on how well an athletic trainer performs may simply be an opinion about how compliant the athletic trainer is with the coach's requests.

Status of Performance Evaluation in Athletic Training

Printed resources for athletic trainers on performance evaluation are few, and most are outdated and advocate a trait-oriented approach (Parks 1977; Penman and Adams 1980). Trait-oriented evaluation systems place a value on athletic trainers' performance by assessing human qualities. For example, if a supervisor were to evaluate a staff member's performance using a trait-oriented approach, he would likely label her aggressive, unfriendly, and difficult to get along with. Unfortunately, none of these terms refer to the quality of her work. Although trait-oriented systems are the easiest to implement, they usually lack validity and reliability.

In many settings, formal evaluation of the performance of athletic trainers does not occur annually. For example, many years ago Ray reported on the performance evaluation in all athletic training settings, and found that only 35 percent of athletic trainers employed in the professional athletics setting reported being evaluated annually (1991). Of those who were evaluated regularly, most perceived their performance evaluations differently from their supervisors. For example, athletic trainers and their supervisors had different perceptions about whether *Competencies in Athletic Training* and *Standards of Practice for Athletic Training* were used as a basis for evaluating athletic trainer job performance. One of the most likely reasons for this discrepancy was that nonmedical supervisors, such as athletic directors and school principals, who were unfamiliar with the athletic trainer's job responsibilities conducted a significant number of the evaluations. In addition, only about half of those supervisors had formal training in how to conduct a performance evaluation or interpret the data derived from the evaluation. The Athletic Trainers' Society of New Jersey has developed a summative performance report tool designed to serve as a model for athletic trainers employed in a secondary school setting (Athletic Trainers' Society of New Jersey 2014).

Another reason athletic trainers and their supervisors have different opinions on the nature of performance evaluation is that many athletic trainers, even if they are formally evaluated, never receive feedback regarding their performance from their supervisors. This lack of communication is an important reason for the lack of understanding between athletic trainers and their supervisors.

Ohio Technological University
Department of Intercollegiate Athletics
Annual Performance Evaluation Instrument

Employee being evaluated: Judy Armstrong

Evaluation: July 1, 2017–June 30, 2018

Supervisor conducting evaluation: DeMarcus Lewis

Date of feedback conference: July 10, 2018

This information may be shared only with the following: Judy Armstrong, Linda Black, DeMarcus Lewis, Jorge Garcia

Data sources used in the performance evaluation: Supervisor's direct observations and feedback from team physicians and athletic trainer coworkers as provided on the Ancillary Data Source form.

PURPOSE

The purposes of the annual performance evaluation include (1) helping employees to identify strengths and weaknesses of their performance in job-related responsibilities so they can work with their supervisors to improve performance, and (2) collecting job-related performance information that may be used for the following staff selection activities: promotion, demotion, retention, dismissal, and compensation. Only job-related performance may be used as the basis for this evaluation.

ROLE-SPECIFIC RATINGS

Instructions to evaluator: Assess the performance of the employee for each specific job responsibility. Rate only those responsibilities included on this employee's position description. Provide performance quality ratings using a 1-to-5 scale. Provide performance frequency ratings using a 1-to-5 scale.
Multiply performance quality ratings by performance frequency ratings by relative importance points (from position description) for overall performance ratings. Provide rationale for each rating.

PERFORMANCE QUALITY RATINGS

1–Job responsibility is performed at an unacceptable level of quality (significant improvement is expected).
2–Job responsibility is performed at a below-average level of quality (significant improvement is expected).
3–Job responsibility is performed at an average level of quality (most other employees perform at this level).
4–Job responsibility is performed at an above-average level of quality (some improvement is possible).
5–Job responsibility is performed at an outstanding level of quality (no improvement is possible).

PERFORMANCE FREQUENCY RATINGS

1–Job responsibility is performed 0%–20% of the time.
2–Job responsibility is performed 21%–40% of the time.
3–Job responsibility is performed 41%–60% of the time.
4–Job responsibility is performed 61%–80% of the time.
5–Job responsibility is performed 81%–100% of the time.

(continued)

Figure 4.15 Performance evaluation instrument.

JOB RESPONSIBILITIES FOR JUDY ARMSTRONG

Responsibility	Performance quality rating	Performance frequency rating	Relative importance points	Total possible	Total achieved
	Rationale:	Rationale:	5	125	
Coordinates and delivers athletic training services to members of the field hockey and gymnastics teams including, but not limited to, coordination of physical exams, evaluation and treatment of injuries at practices and games, design and supervision of rehabilitation programs, counseling within the limits of expertise, and prepractice and game taping.					
Refers injured athletes to appropriate physicians according to the guidelines in the Standard Operating Procedures.	Rationale:	Rationale:	5	125	
Submits injured athlete status reports to coaches by 11:00 a.m. of the day following the injury.	Rationale:	Rationale:	4	100	
Maintains computerized injury and treatment database according to the guidelines in the Standard Operating Procedures.	Rationale:	Rationale:	3	75	
Coordinates NCAA Injury Surveillance Program by conducting in-service training for athletic training students, collecting and checking the accuracy of individual and weekly injury report forms, and mailing completed forms to the NCAA by Monday of each week.	Rationale:	Rationale:	3	75	
Prepares annual injury and treatment report for all sports by June 1.	Rationale:	Rationale:	3	75	
Exhibits behaviors in strict compliance with the NATA Code of Ethics.	Rationale:	Rationale:	5	125	
				700	

WORKING CONDITIONS

Instructions: Describe unusual working conditions beyond the control of the employee that may have affected his or her ability to perform the assigned duties.

CRITICAL INCIDENTS

Instructions: Describe critical incidents that occurred during the evaluation period that are consistent with the strengths and weaknesses of the employee's job-related performance.

PERFORMANCE IMPROVEMENT PLAN

Instructions: List the steps the employee should take in order to improve his or her job-related performance.

EMPLOYEE RESPONSE

Instructions: Describe points of agreement or disagreement with your supervisor's evaluation of your job-related performance.

Figure 4.15 *(continued)*

Ohio Technological University
Department of Intercollegiate Athletics
Annual Performance Evaluation
Ancillary Data Source Instrument

Employee being evaluated: Judy Armstrong

Evaluation: July 1, 2017–June 30, 2018

Supervisor conducting evaluation: DeMarcus Lewis

This information may be shared only with the following: Judy Armstrong, Linda Black, DeMarcus Lewis, Jorge Garcia

PURPOSE

The purpose of this instrument is to help supervisors provide employees with valid and reliable feedback regarding their performance by allowing them to collect information from peers and coworkers. The information may also be used to make employee selection decisions regarding promotion, demotion, retention, dismissal, and compensation.

Instructions: Use the specific job responsibilities below from the employee's position description to guide your assessments. *Assess only the employee's performance on these responsibilities.*
Assess only those responsibilities that you directly observed.

JOB RESPONSIBILITIES OF JUDY ARMSTRONG

Responsibility	Comments
Coordinates and delivers athletic training services to members of the field hockey and gymnastics teams including, but not limited to, coordination of physical exams, evaluation and treatment of injuries at practices and games, design and supervision of rehabilitation programs, counseling within the limits of expertise, and prepractice and game taping.	
Refers injured athletes to appropriate physicians according to the guidelines in the Standard Operating Procedures.	
Submits injured athlete status reports to coaches by 11:00 a.m. of the day following the injury.	
Maintains computerized injury and treatment database according to guidelines in the Standardized Operating Procedures.	
Coordinates NCAA Injury Surveillance program by conducting in-service training for student athletic trainers, collecting and checking the accuracy of individual and weekly injury report forms, and mailing completed forms to the NCAA by Monday of each week.	
Prepares annual injury and treatment report for all sports by June 1.	
Exhibits behaviors in strict compliance with NATA Code of Ethics.	

_____   _____   _____
Signature   Position   Date

Figure 4.16   Performance evaluation ancillary data source form.

Performance Evaluation Methods

Practitioners of performance evaluation have long disagreed about which methods are most effective for rating employee job performance (Reinhardt 1985). To date, no formal agreed on or established tool or process has been reported in the athletic training literature. No single method of performance evaluation matches every setting or meets the needs of every organization. Table 4.1 summarizes the strengths and weaknesses of the seven most common performance evaluation methods.

Performance Evaluation Standards

In a hallmark work completed by the Joint Committee on Standards for Educational Evaluation (JCSEE), *The Personnel Evaluation Standards* significantly influenced the practice of performance evaluation in a variety of settings. These widely accepted evaluation principles remain helpful to educational professionals in improving their personnel evaluation systems. Many policy boards have adopted them as the official standards for judging performance evaluation systems. Although *The Personnel Evaluation Standards* were written for educational settings, they are rooted in valid and reliable evaluation principles and can be applied in noneducational settings. Athletic trainers employed in professional athletics, sports medicine clinics, and industry can benefit from the application of these standards because validity and reliability of performance evaluation are important in their job settings as well.

KEY POINT

Performance evaluation systems for athletic trainers should be legal and fair, useful, practical, and accurate.

There are 27 personnel evaluation standards in four broad categories: propriety, utility, feasibility, and accuracy. A description of each standard follows. Although the list seems long, keep in mind that performance evaluation is an important part of the athletic trainer-manager's responsibilities. Even small deviations from the ideal can result in damaging consequences for the employee, the supervisor, and the institution.

The following 27 standards are reprinted by permission from Joint Committee on Standards for Educational Evaluation, *Personnel evaluation standards*, 2017, ©Joint Committee on Standards for Education Evaluation.

Table 4.1 Strengths and Weaknesses of the Most Commonly Used Performance Evaluation Methods

Method	Weaknesses	Strengths
Management by objectives	Tends to emphasize job characteristics that can be measured over those that cannot.	Employee is able to give input into the standards by which he or she is evaluated.
Written essay	Is dependent on subjective data and validity is dependent on writer's skill and judgment.	Evaluator can write a detailed profile of the employee's work.
Critical incident report	Can be subject to writer bias; often based on subjective data; negative incidents usually receive more notice than positive.	Provides more detail regarding the employee's work.
Graphic rating scale	Scale elements often are not valid or job related.	It is simple to administer and low cost.
Forced-choice rating	Fails to provide specific feedback; not useful in human resource planning; does not relate job performance to selection criteria.	It is simple to administer and low cost.
Ranking	Difficult to discriminate performance levels on multitask jobs; discourages cooperation among work group members.	Simplifies the task of allocating rewards.
Behaviorally anchored rating scales	Most useful for employees with identical job responsibilities; expensive and time-consuming to develop; difficult to update as job responsibilities change.	Evaluates behaviors rather than traits and is specific to single job category.

Propriety Standards

The following seven **propriety standards** help ensure that performance evaluation is legal and fair.

- *P1 Service Orientation.* Personnel evaluations should promote sound education, fulfillment of institutional missions, and effective performance of job responsibilities, so that the educational needs of students, community, and society are met.

- *P2 Appropriate Policies and Procedures.* Guidelines for personnel evaluations should be recorded and provided to the evaluatee in policy statements, negotiated agreements, and/or personnel evaluation manuals, so that evaluations are consistent, equitable, and fair.

- *P3 Access to Evaluation Information.* Access to evaluation information should be limited to the persons with established legitimate permission to review and use the information, so that confidentiality is maintained and privacy is protected.

- *P4 Interactions with Evaluatees.* The evaluator should respect human dignity and act in a professional, considerate, and courteous manner, so that the evaluatee's self-esteem, motivation, professional reputations, performance, and attitude toward personnel evaluation are enhanced or, at least, not needlessly damaged.

- *P5 Balanced Evaluation.* Personnel evaluations should provide information that identifies both strengths and weaknesses, so that strengths can be built upon and weaknesses addressed.

- *P6 Conflict of Interest.* Existing and potential conflicts of interest should be identified and dealt with openly and honestly, so that they do not compromise the evaluation process and results.

- *P7 Legal Viability.* Personnel evaluations should meet the requirements of all federal, state, and local laws, as well as case law, contracts, collective bargaining agreements, affirmative action policies, and local board policies and regulations or institutional statutes or bylaws, so that evaluators can successfully conduct fair, efficient, and responsible personnel evaluations.

Utility Standards

The following six **utility standards** ensure that an athletic trainer's performance evaluation is useful (Joint Committee on Standards for Educational Evaluation 2017).

- *U1 Constructive Orientation.* Personnel evaluations should be constructive, so that they not only help institutions develop human resources but encourage and assist those evaluated to provide excellent services in accordance with the institution's mission statements and goals.

- *U2 Defined Uses.* Both the users and intended uses of a personnel evaluation should be identified at the beginning of the evaluation so that the evaluation can address appropriate questions and issues.

- *U3 Evaluator Qualifications.* The evaluation system should be developed, implemented, and managed by persons with the necessary qualifications, skills, training, and authority, so that evaluation reports are properly conducted, respected, and used.

- *U4 Explicit Criteria.* Evaluators should identify and justify the criteria used to interpret and judge evaluatee performance, so that the basis for interpretation and judgment provides a clear and defensible rationale for results.

- *U5 Functional Reporting.* Reports should be clear, timely, accurate, and germane, so that they are of practical value to the evaluatee and other appropriate audiences.

- *U6 Professional Development.* Personnel evaluations should inform users and evaluatees of areas in need of professional development, so that all educational personnel can better address the institution's missions and goals, fulfill their roles and responsibilities, and meet the needs of students.

Feasibility Standards

The following three **feasibility standards** foster practicality in performance evaluation (Joint Committee on Standards for Educational Evaluation 2017).

- *F1 Practical Procedures.* Personnel evaluation procedures should be practical, so that they produce the needed information in efficient, nondisruptive ways.

- *F2 Political Viability.* Personnel evaluations should be planned and conducted with the anticipation of questions from evaluatees and others with a legitimate right to know, so that their questions can be addressed and their cooperation obtained.

- *F3 Fiscal Viability.* Adequate time and resources should be provided for personnel evaluation activities, so that evaluation can be effectively implemented, the results fully communicated, and appropriate follow-up activities identified.

Accuracy Standards

The following 11 **accuracy standards** are intended to improve the validity and reliability of a performance evaluation and thereby lend accuracy to the system (Joint Committee on Standards for Educational Evaluation 2017).

- *A1 Validity Orientation.* The selection, development, and implementation of personnel evaluations should ensure that the interpretations made about the performance of the evaluatee are valid and not open to misinterpretation.

- *A2 Defined Expectations.* The qualifications, role, and performance expectations of the evaluatee should be clearly defined, so that the evaluator can determine the evaluation data and information needed to ensure validity.

- *A3 Analysis of Context.* Contextual variables that influence performance should be identified, described, and recorded, so that they can be considered when interpreting an evaluatee's performance.

- *A4 Documented Purposes and Procedures.* The evaluation purposes and procedures, both planned and actual, should be documented, so that they can be clearly explained and justified.

- *A5 Defensible Information.* The information collected for personnel evaluations should be defensible, so that the information can be reliably and validly interpreted.

- *A6 Reliable Information.* Personnel evaluation procedures should be chosen or developed and implemented to ensure reliability, so that the information obtained will provide consistent indications of the evaluatee's performance.

- *A7 Systematic Data Control.* The information collected, processed, and reported about evaluatees should be systematically reviewed, corrected as appropriate, and kept secure, so that accurate judgments about the evaluatee's performance can be made and appropriate levels of confidentiality maintained.

- *A8 Bias Identification and Management.* Personnel evaluations should be free of bias, so that interpretations of the evaluatee's qualifications or performance are valid.

- *A9 Analysis of Information.* The information collected for personnel evaluations should be sys-tematically and accurately analyzed, so that the purposes of the evaluation are effectively achieved.

- *A10 Justified Conclusions.* The evaluative conclusions about the evaluatee's performance should be explicitly justified, so that evaluatees and others with a legitimate right to know can have confidence in them.

- *A11 Metaevaluation.* Personnel evaluation systems should be examined periodically using these and other appropriate standards, so that mistakes are prevented or detected and promptly corrected, and sound personnel evaluation practices are developed and maintained over time.

Fair Labor Standards Act and Athletic Training

Traditionally, the culture of athletic training has prescribed long hours at modest pay to meet the needs of injured athletes whose schedules rarely conform to the typical 40-hour workweek. Coaches, athletic directors, and athletes have come to expect that athletic trainers will stay in the athletic training room until they have attended to the last person, even if doing so requires 60 or 70 hours per week. Many in the profession who desire a higher quality of life are now challenging this culture, both in terms of a more reasonable workweek and a compensation package befitting the level of education required for practice in athletic training. One of the primary issues of concern to athletic trainers is whether they are exempt under the Fair Labor Standards Act (FLSA) (U.S. Department of Labor 2011). Congress originally passed the **Fair Labor Standards Act** in 1938 and has since amended it several times. This is an issue that has been proactively addressed by NATA over the past few years and currently sits in the decision-making hands of the federal administration. The FLSA is responsible for establishing minimum wage and overtime pay guidelines. In 2014, a Presidential Memorandum was signed directing the U.S. Department of Labor (DOL) to update the regulations defining which white-collar workers are exempt from the FLSA minimum-wage and overtime requirements. NATA first provided official comments to the Office of Management and Budget (OMB) on the proposed revisions to the Standard Occupational Classification (SOC) in 2014. The goal was to have athletic trainers reclassified under a category that better reflects their education, licensure and credentialing, training, and practice setting. In 2016, a reclassification was completed by the DOL with a proposed implementation date of December 2016. Just before its implementation, a U.S. district judge suspended the Department of Labor's overtime rule indefinitely based on concerns of whether the DOL had authority to make such rules.

The overtime final rule served to (1) increase the standard salary threshold under which white collar workers are eligible for overtime pay, and (2) increase the annual salary threshold above which "highly compensated employees" are exempt from overtime pay. A category of the final rule that applies most specifically to athletic trainers is referred to as the professional employees category. This category sets forth guidelines that determine whether or not an athletic trainer is eligible for overtime pay. If an athletic trainer's salary and job duties do not meet all of the guidelines, then he or she is eligible for overtime pay under the new rule. By contrast, if the AT's salary and job duties satisfy all of the guidelines, then he or she is not eligible for overtime pay.

Under the professional employees category, three subcategories exist: creative professional, learned professional, and teaching professional. An athletic trainer would most likely fall under the learned professional category, and if so, is exempt from overtime and minimum wage standards.

The following guidelines are used to determine whether or not one qualifies:

- The employee must be compensated on a salary or fee basis at a rate not less than $913 weekly (with adjustments made every three years).
- The employee's primary duty must be the performance of work requiring advanced knowledge, defined as work that is predominantly intellectual in character and that includes work requiring the consistent exercise of discretion and judgment.
- The advanced knowledge must be in a field of science or learning.
- The advanced knowledge must be customarily acquired by a prolonged course of specialized intellectual instruction.

The two important elements in these guidelines are "learned profession" and "exercise of discretion and judgment." A learned profession is one that requires advanced knowledge (usually beyond the high school level) in the field of science or education that the person obtained by prolonged and specialized instruction. Specific academic training as a prerequisite for entering a profession is usually required.

The "exercise of discretion and judgment" element is much less well defined and can be confusing when the issue of whether or not athletic trainers should be classified as professionals (and therefore be exempt from the FLSA) is addressed.

For example, in some states, the provisions of a credentialing act require that physicians supervise athletic trainers. Some athletic trainers have argued that because they do their work under the direction of a physician, they are not exercising discretion and judgment. In institutions without team physicians, athletic trainers might in fact exercise discretion and judgment, even though the work they perform is the same as that performed by nonexempt athletic trainers at a similar institution. Athletic trainers who teach at least 50% of the time are generally exempt and not entitled to overtime because teachers are considered professionals under the FLSA. Athletic trainers who spend more than 50% of their time in management or administrative roles might also be exempt.

KEY POINT

The Fair Labor Standards Act (FLSA) is a law intended to ensure that employees are justly compensated for work they do that exceeds the boundaries of the normal workweek. Athletic trainers might or might not be exempt from the provisions of the FLSA depending on how their jobs are structured.

Work–Life Balance

Work–life balance is a theory that focuses on blending and prioritizing a person's work responsibilities and lifestyle (e.g., leisure, health, family, social needs). The concept focuses on the recognition that people assume multiple roles within these two areas, and thus the demands of one may affect the others (Kalliath and Brough 2008). Work–life balance is a multilevel construct, and because the athletic training work environment makes many demands on a person's time and energy, concerns have emerged within the profession (Kossek, Baltes, and Matthews 2011; Kossek et al. 2014). These demands associated with working as an athletic trainer can make it difficult to find balance, creating a work–life conflict, and have led to concerns about professional commitment and a career that is viewed as transitory rather than steadfast.

Defining Balance

Two perspectives exist regarding a person's ability to achieve balance. Work–life conflict takes the view that work and life are incompatible, and conflict results. Conversely, the idea of work–life enrichment assumes that harmony can exist despite engaging in multiple roles. The first perspective centers on the idea that conflict is inventible because the requirements of multiple roles create competition for time, energy, and resources. These demands lead to the inability to meet all expectations (Goode 1960). Conflict, therefore, has an adverse effect on overall work performance and a person's health because it spills over into each role. Although conflict is suggested to affect work and lifestyle roles equally (Greenhaus and Beutell 1985), often family and personal time is most affected or even sacrificed because it is viewed as less flexible. The emphasis of work–life conflict is on the negative effects that filling multiple roles can have on work, home, and personal life. The second mindset, work–life enrichment, offers a more positive outlook: When engaging in multiple roles, people gain strength from each role they participate in, enhancing rather than depleting resources (Greenhaus and Powell 2006). Proponents of the idea of work–life enrichment believe that work and family roles are interdependent, and that they work together to promote positive relationships. When one experiences work–life enrichment, development of skills and knowledge in one role can increase performance and success in the other roles.

Barriers to Balance

Specific variables create conflict between work life and family and home life for athletic trainers, and these variables can be classified into three broad areas: individual (i.e., personality), organizational (i.e., the nature of the job), and sociocultural (i.e., gender stereotypes) (Dixon and Bruening 2007). Organizational variables have been the primary focus of research, and factors leading to conflict include long working hours, travel, and limited control over one's work schedule (Mazerolle, Bruening, and Casa 2008; Mazerolle et al. 2011). For people working in sport settings and health care systems, including athletic trainers, the concept of facetime is important (Dixon and Bruening 2007). The need to be present to complete all work-related tasks is a requirement and job expectation that can limit time for other activities as well as create an emotional and physical strain on the individual. Although the employment setting can influence the structure and length of the workday, most athletic trainers work more than 40 hours per week (Mazerolle, Bruening, and Casa 2008; Mazerolle et al. 2011), and that is the most frequently cited source of conflict. Concerns with salary, supervisor support, and lack of adequate staffing also impose barriers to work–life balance. Figure 4.17 illustrates the factors described as inhibitors to finding balance in athletic training.

Facilitators to Finding Balance

Concerns about work–life balance are not isolated to athletic trainers; considerable attention has been given by researchers, professional organizations, and government agencies to developing and finding

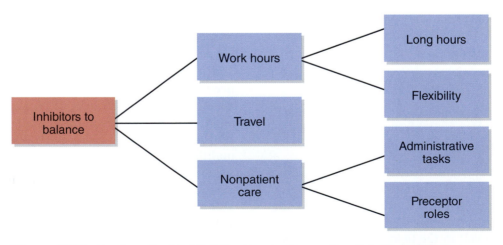

Figure 4.17 Factors that inhibit finding balance in athletic training.

work–life balance strategies and policies. Much like the barriers to balance, facilitators are viewed from an organizational, sociocultural, and individualized level (figure 4.18).

Workplace Initiatives

Workplace initiatives to establish work–life balance can be formal or informal (Kossek, Lewis, and Hammer 2010). The human resources department of an organization establishes formal workplace initiatives. Formal policies are often referred to as organizational or structural support for work–life balance and are designed to provide employees some control over their work schedule as well as enable them to combine employment with caregiving. Common examples include flexible work arrangements, dependent care initiatives, vacation time, sick and personal leave, and childcare and eldercare benefits. Informal initiatives can be defined as cultural work–life support. They are socially based within the organization and help create a climate that supports work–life balance. Cultural support takes place during interactions between the AT and her supervisor and between the AT and her coworkers. Despite the informality, cultural support is as critical as formal workplace initiatives to supporting work–life balance and creating a climate that promotes a positive view of this balance (Kossek and Hammer 2008; Hammer et al. 2009).

- **Flexible work arrangements** (Kossek and Lautsch 2008) allow employees to establish their own work schedules (e.g., work from 10 a.m. to 6 p.m. instead of 8 a.m. to 4 p.m.); these flexible work schedules can be classified as compressed (i.e., 10-hour days, over four days), split shifts, or part-time (through job sharing). The flexible work arrangements allow employees more freedom to organize their work so it fits with other aspects of their life. Flexible work arrangements increase employees' control over their work time and their ability to make decisions about their workday.

- **Mobile workplace** is an arrangement in which an employee works remotely, often from home, but it can be anyplace outside the office. This arrangement allows employees flexibility in how they perform their job. Tasks such as documentation and preparing bids for ordering supplies can often be done from any location with a secure Internet connection.

- **Dependent care initiatives** provide employees support to help them manage their family responsibilities more easily. Common initiatives are on-site dependent care, financial assistance toward dependent care, and allowing an employee the flexibility to take personal days instead of vacation days to deal with appointments and unexpected dependent care issues.

- **Leave of absence** refers to time allowed away from work because of an unusual circumstance, such as jury duty, a death, or the birth or adoption of a child. During this time away, employees receive their normal compensation for a predetermined

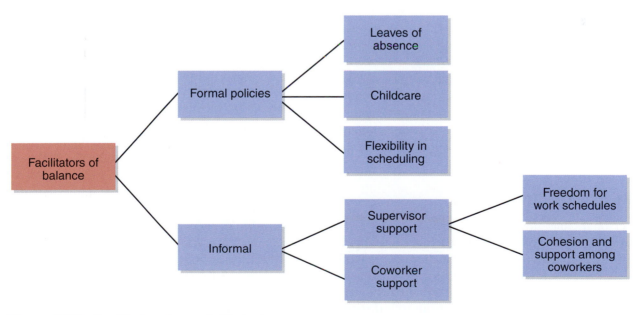

Figure 4.18 Facilitators to work–life balance.

period of time. Common leaves of absence include maternity and paternity leave and bereavement leave.

- **Employee assistance programs (EAPs)** are on-site workplace programs that assist and support an employee who may need short-term counseling. The programs are confidential and voluntary, and provide employees an outlet for services related to personal and work problems that may be influencing their lives. EAPs address a broad spectrum of issues, and consultants provide the service.

- **Health care initiatives**, or wellness programs, aim to improve an employee's quality of life through initiatives such as fitness programs, healthy lunch options, stress relief workshops, and discounts on prescriptions. By encouraging employees to invest in their health through measures such as annual checkups, these initiatives can lower employees' medical costs.

Informal Initiatives

Supportive supervisors are a key factor in an employee's ability to achieve work–life balance (Kossek and Hammer 2008). Supervisors can support work–life balance by allowing work-scheduling autonomy, planning schedules ahead of time, sharing a family-first mindset, and creating a cohesive work environment by communicating clearly and frequently. Supportive supervisors can also welcome workplace integration, a strategy that focuses on creating permeability between work and family roles when appropriate and necessary for balance (Rapoport et al. 2002). Supervisors can provide emotional and general work support as a means to facilitate balance for their employees.

Collegiality within the workplace is essential for work–life balance. Collegiality is the overall enjoyment employees feel around those with whom they work, and it is also the willingness of those employees to share the workload as a means to manage the demands of the workplace.

Individual Initiatives

Personal time, in which an employee steps away from his or her role of an athletic trainer, is important and provides time for rejuvenation. During this time the athletic trainer satisfies the personal need to engage in activities that are meaningful as well as rejuvenating. Engaging in a healthy lifestyle through

habits such as working out, eating right, and sleeping well is an important aspect of personal time.

Another strategy for achieving work–life balance is using effective time management skills. This allows an athletic trainer to prioritize each responsibility and task during the day, including patient care and personal obligations. To-do lists are necessary for meeting these obligations. Learning to say no can also be an effective time management tactic.

Work–life separation and integration are strategies that help reduce the negative spillover from work and home and vice versa. Separation creates distinct boundaries between work and home, allowing athletic trainers to focus their time and energy on one role at a time (e.g., no work e-mails after 6:00 p.m., no telephone calls from home between 9:00 a.m. and 1:00 pm). Integration, however, permits more flexibility between work and personal roles, allowing for spillover to occur when necessary (e.g., having lunch with a spouse during the workday, bringing a child to the office when school is not in session).

Summary

Athletic trainers in supervisory roles will find themselves involved with human resource management. The proper management of human resources and personnel begins with establishing an organizational culture. No one culture fits all circumstances. However, setting a tone for how the operation will manage people is critical in order for personnel to understand working expectations. An organizational chart that reflects the hierarchy of positions, reporting structure, and roles and responsibilities helps to clarify the personnel structure. Having in place an organizational culture and chart can lead to development of accurate position descriptions, which in turn facilitates the process of recruitment and hiring of employees that best fit the organization. Both the employer and the employee have much to consider when it comes to hiring. Both parties should take ample time to consider all aspects of each employment opportunity, and particular attention should be paid to the legal aspects of the hiring process and work environment to avoid discriminatory procedures. Appropriate supervision contributes to more accurate employer performance assessment, a process that should include both formal and informal feedback in a timely and honest manner. Supervisory approaches can vary, taking into consideration both how one best manages as an individual and how one should accommodate to meet the needs of subordinates. Work–life balance is important in all careers, and it can be particularly challenging in athletic training. Both formal and informal initiatives should be established to improve work–life balance, which should improve job satisfaction and employee retention.

Learning Aids

Case Study 1

The new manager of the Wellness Center, a physician-owned sports medicine and rehabilitation clinic, instituted a policy requiring all supervisors to evaluate their employees and recommend salary increases. This new program was an attempt to implement a merit pay system at the center. In the past, all employees received an across-the-board increase without regard to how they had performed during the past year.

Sandra supervised the center's six certified athletic trainers. Upon receiving the memo mandating the new policy, Sandra decided that she would simply write a narrative describing each of the athletic trainers. She thought that such a narrative would be a useful guide for the new manager in awarding pay increases because it would provide in-depth analysis of the strengths and weaknesses of each athletic trainer. The following are examples of the evaluations she submitted.

- *Brian Robinson:* Brian Robinson is one of the best athletic trainers employed by the center. He is thoughtful, works well with the patients, has a cheerful personality, and gets along great with the staff. Brian has received positive feedback from the athletic director at South High School, where he is assigned during the fall and spring. The athletes and parents seem to like him and there have been no problems that I am aware of, although I have only been out there a couple of times. My recommendation is that Brian be given a 3% salary increase.

- *Juan Diaz:* Although I think Juan is basically a pretty good athletic trainer, he has had several problems over the past year. Juan seemed to be in the middle of a couple of controversies at Martin Luther King High. I know King is an inner-city school and Juan has a lot of tough problems to overcome down there, but I just wish he could deal more effectively with them so we wouldn't have to spend time on them at the center. Juan hasn't been very effective in getting referrals to the center from his high school. As I mentioned earlier, although I think Juan does a good job as an athletic trainer, I can't recommend anything higher than a 1% increase for him this year.

Sandra was surprised when three weeks later, on the day after the salary increases were announced, Juan stormed into her office and informed her that he was going to sue both her and the Wellness Center for discrimination based on negligent evaluation.

Questions for Analysis

1. What were the strengths and weaknesses of the performance evaluation system that Sandra initiated?

2. How could the center's new manager have approached the problem more constructively and effectively? How would this have affected Sandra? How would it have affected Brian, Juan, and the other athletic trainers?

3. Describe the performance evaluation system you would implement if you were in Sandra's position. What concerns, if any, would you express to the new manager regarding the new policy?

Case Study 2

John had just bought the local professional football franchise. He had made his fortune in the fast-food restaurant business, starting with one small fried-chicken restaurant and building it into a multimillion-dollar chain with restaurants all over the world. At his first meeting with the club's staff, John announced that he was bringing in a consultant to do a management audit of every department. He explained that sound management was the cornerstone of his success in business and in life. He expected each member of the staff to adopt that philosophy. Sound management, in his opinion, was the key to success in any business, and professional football was a business.

A few weeks later, Jerome and the rest of the sports medicine staff spent the better part of two days answering questions and explaining the club's sports medicine operation to the management consultant. The consultant asked about policies and procedures. He examined the record-keeping system. He investigated the supply and equipment purchasing routines. He became familiar with how Jerome selected student athletic trainers for summer training camp. As far as Jerome could tell, the consultant left no stone unturned.

About a month later, the management consultant and John, the new owner, walked into the athletic training room and told Jerome that they wanted to discuss the results of the recent management audit with him. "Jerome," the consultant began, "for the most part, you are managing this part of the club's operations fairly effectively. You buy only what you need and you don't pay more than you have to. The procedures you have implemented are consistent with club policy, and they seem to be efficient and effective. But in talking with your assistants, the assistant coaches, and some of the players, I have determined that you don't do a very good job of using your staff to its fullest potential. The information they provided leads me to believe that you don't delegate authority enough. You try to do too much by yourself. Take a look at the organizational chart I developed of your operation as it currently exists." (See figure 4.19.)

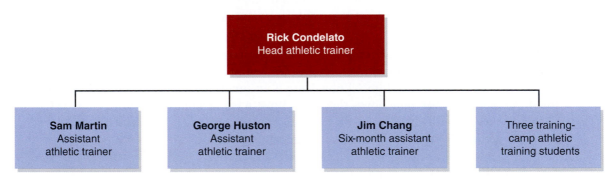

Figure 4.19 Organizational chart for Jerome's sports medicine program.

"Jerome," said John, "I want you to reorganize your staff so you can work more efficiently. From what everybody tells me, you're a good man and although I expect maximum effort, I don't want you to get burned out simply because you haven't organized your staff well enough. I expect to see your reorganization report on my desk by Monday of next week."

Questions for Analysis

1. What is wrong with the current organizational structure in Jerome's program? What problems are likely to arise based on the present structure?

2. How could Jerome reorganize to reduce the amount of work he is responsible for and still accomplish everything that needs to be done?

3. If you were in Jerome's position, what organizational structure would you devise to meet the mandate of the new club owner?

4. What strategies should Jerome employ to make sure that his assistants develop ownership in the new organizational structure?

Case Study 3

Alicia is a senior athletic training student at a midsized university in New England. She is looking forward to taking her athletic training certification exam in April and getting a job as a certified athletic trainer in a secondary school setting. One of her clinical instructors informed her that a high school in the same district is planning to employ its first full-time certified athletic trainer for the upcoming school year. Alicia is excited because the high school is located just 10 miles (16 km) from where she currently lives.

Alicia was encouraged to send a resume to the school's athletic director now so that he can be made aware of her interest in the position. This is the first time Alicia has put together a resume for an athletic training position. She wants to be sure that her cover letter and resume are perfect, with no errors. She also wants to make sure that her resume is reflective of her experience to demonstrate that she is the best person for the job.

Questions for Analysis

1. What challenges will Alicia have in preparing a cover letter and resume for a secondary school athletic training position before she achieves her certification?

2. Given that Alicia possesses many of the same skills as other entry-level athletic trainers, and arguably less experience than other athletic trainers who might apply for the same job at the secondary school, how can she promote herself as the best candidate for the position?

3. What are methods of networking that could benefit Alicia during the next few months before the formal posting of the position? Are there behaviors or approaches Alicia should avoid so she doesn't come across as too persistent in her interest for the job?

4. What type of information can Alicia gather to prepare for an on-site interview to demonstrate her interest, qualifications, and fit for the job?

Key Concepts and Review

Identify the different forms of organizational culture that can exist in a sports medicine program.

Organizational culture includes the basic values, behavioral norms, assumptions, and beliefs of a sports medicine program. The type of organizational culture will have an effect on human resource management. The three major types of organizational cultures are collegial, personalistic, and formalistic.

Formally define the relationships of the people working in a sports medicine program by developing an organizational chart.

An organizational chart best illustrates the relationships between the various members of a sports medicine program. Athletic trainers can describe these relationships in one of three ways: by function, by service, or in a matrix format.

Learn the components of staff selection.

Staff selection is a commonly misunderstood term. The Equal Employment Opportunity Commission's *Uniform Guidelines on Employee Selection Procedures* describes staff selection as any procedure used as the basis for an employment decision. Hiring, promotion, demotion, performance evaluation, retention, and discharge are all examples of selection activities as defined by federal law.

Develop a position description and a position vacancy notice.

A position description is a formal document that describes the qualification requirements, work content, accountability, and scope of a person's job. The weighted position description is an important first step in helping athletic trainers understand the expectations of their employers. The position description generally comprises two sections: the job specification and the job description.

Comprehend the recruitment and hiring process, especially as affected by discrimination and bias based on race, gender, disability, religion, and national origin.

Recruitment and hiring are two of the most visible, expensive, and time-consuming aspects of the human resources function in sports medicine. Recruitment activities should be viewed in terms of long- and short-term needs. The prime directive in recruiting and hiring is that all qualified applicants should receive equal consideration. Athletic trainers and other sports medicine personnel must be hired based on their qualifications, not on race, gender, religion, or national origin. The recruitment and hiring process usually follows these 10 steps: request for position, position request approval, position vacancy notice, application collection, telephone and Web-based interviews, reference checks, on-site interview, recommendation and approval for hiring, offer of contract, and hiring.

Define the differences between the three major supervisory models.

The three major types of supervisory models are inspection–production, clinical, and developmental. The inspection–production model emphasizes authoritative managerial efficiency. Clinical supervision is the process, borrowed from education, of direct observation of an athletic trainer at work and the subsequent development of plans to remediate deficiencies in performance. The overriding theme of developmental supervision is participative management.

Become familiar with the purposes, methods, and standards for evaluating athletic trainer performance.

Performance evaluation is the process of placing a value on the quality of an athletic trainer's work. In some settings, athletic trainers are not formally evaluated and lack position descriptions. Much of the performance evaluation literature intended for athletic trainers is based on a trait-oriented approach. Trait-oriented evaluation is usually biased and is rarely useful for improving performance. Athletic trainers should acquaint themselves with the 21 performance evaluation standards developed by the Joint Committee on Standards for Educational Evaluation. They are intended to guide the development of performance evaluation systems and to offer improvements in four major areas: propriety, accuracy, utility, and feasibility.

Recognize the key concepts associated with work–life balance as they relate to athletic training employment.

Work–life balance is a theory that focuses on blending and prioritizing a person's work responsibilities and lifestyle. The high demands associated with working as an athletic trainer can stimulate issues with finding a balanced lifestyle (work–life conflict), and have led to concerns related to professional commitment and a career that is viewed as transitory rather than steadfast.

Define the Fair Labor Standards Act and its effect on the employment of an athletic trainer.

The Fair Labor Standards Act is a federal law that establishes regulations for various aspects of employment, including minimum wage and overtime pay. It is intended to protect employees against unfair work practices. This law determines whether athletic trainers qualify for overtime or not, or if they are considered salaried employees.

5

Financial Resource Management

The common denominator in almost every management problem is money or the lack of it. Money is the engine that drives athletic enterprises, regardless of the level of competition. Sports medicine programs associated with athletic programs are subject to all the economic pressures that those programs experience, whether the setting is a high school, college, university, professional team, or hospital. For athletic trainers working in independent sports medicine clinics, the need for sound financial management practices is even more acute because economic downturns usually affect those operations more rapidly. The shallow resource pool typical of independent clinics compounds the effects of poor financial management. The amount of money an athletic trainer will have to operate a sports medicine program in an educational setting varies greatly depending on the level of competition engaged in by the institution's teams (National Collegiate Athletic Association n.d.). The economics of the health care industry at any given time also affects how athletic trainers manage financial resources. Around the turn of the century, there was a movement away from traditional third-party reimbursement toward managed care models, resulting in a drastically altered financial landscape for most sports medicine clinics. Highly profitable publicly traded health care corporations were gobbling up small, independent clinics at a phenomenal rate. Most sports medicine clinics have had to expand their services to include nontraditional activities such as performance enhancement, gym memberships, and nutritional counseling. Traditional rehabilitation is being transformed so that athletic trainers might see a patient only a few times, with the bulk of the rehabilitation consisting of liberal doses of advice and a program of home exercise. These changes have a significant effect on health care professionals—including athletic trainers—who operate, own, manage, and work in these environments.

The purpose of this chapter is to help athletic trainers become more astute stewards of their institution's financial resources by presenting the theory and application of various techniques for budgeting, purchasing, and inventory control. The chapter presents these three topics as distinct and separate processes, but in reality they are closely related to each other in a financial planning network (see figure 5.1). Although the ideas discussed in this chapter are applicable to almost any setting, athletic trainers should realize that certain types of sports medicine clinics, as small businesses, require more financial planning than this book can suggest. At a minimum, athletic trainers should consider six components of a financial analysis when operating a sports medicine clinic (Barnes 1997):

1. Sales
2. Costs
3. Profits
4. Revenue
5. Return on investment (ROI)
6. Growth earnings

Athletic trainers who manage independently owned and operated sports medicine clinics should

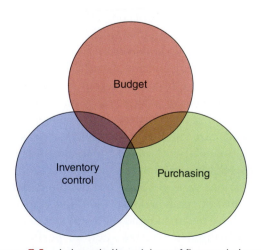

Figure 5.1 Interrelationships of financial activities of the sports medicine program.

seek the counsel of experienced management consultants, attorneys, and accountants. In addition, the U.S. Small Business Administration publishes a management series that can help these athletic trainers become more familiar with the variety of issues facing owners of all types of small businesses. Beyond learning this introductory information about fiscal management as part of the educational process, if and when a practicing athletic trainer is required to manage a budget can vary immensely. Those who take their first job in a secondary school setting or small college may be handed budgetary responsibilities immediately and can refer back to the basic principles introduced in this textbook. Others may practice athletic training for years before taking on a director role without any real-world budgetary experience.

Budgeting

Budgeting financial resources is a process that organizational leaders ask program heads to undertake. Athletic trainers and others responsible for planning and delivering sports medicine services must develop skills in planning and implementing budgets so that needed services are delivered in an effective, timely manner and allocation of financial resources is consistent with the strategic plans of both the institution and the sports medicine program.

A **budget** is an organized plan for coordinating resources, revenues, and expenditures. A budget also serves as a tool for estimating receipts and disbursements over a period of time. Beyond its practical uses as a restraint on resource waste and as a predictive tool for the financial health of a sports medicine program, a budget is a quantitative expression of the athletic trainer's management plan. As such, it is both a strategic plan for how the sports medicine unit will function over a given period and an operational plan for how it will accomplish its goals.

Although many practitioners think of budgeting as a task that begins and ends in a narrow time frame during a particular part of the year, the wise athletic trainer views budgeting as a continuous process of prioritizing, planning, documenting, and evaluating the goals of the sports medicine unit and translating those goals into concrete plans for how to expend available resources. Because athletic seasons stretch across all 12 months and new programs of all types are added to the athletic trainer's responsibilities, the budgeting process requires constant attention to funding status and ongoing evaluation for the next budget cycle.

Budgeting is different from forecasting. Forecasting is the process of predicting future conditions based on various statistics and indicators that describe the past and present situations. Typically, only a few people near the top of the organizational chart perform forecasting. Because budgeting is a type of planning, however, it requires input from the grass roots of the sports medicine program. An effective budget will consider the input of all employees on using the financial resources to meet documented program needs as opposed to simply allocating funds according to past traditions.

KEY POINT

Budgeting is the method that athletic trainers use to put a sports medicine program's mission into financial terms. Although several budgeting methods are feasible, none will be effective unless the athletic trainer properly plans for the budget process by developing a well-conceived needs assessment and by periodically evaluating the budget.

Types of Budgets

Most sports medicine budget planning is based on one of six budgeting models (Ray 1990):

1. Zero based
2. Fixed
3. Variable
4. Lump sum
5. Line item
6. Performance

Each of these methods can be an effective way to help athletic trainers plan the financial activity of their programs, depending on the particular circumstances and nature of the programs they direct. Depending on the financial health of the program and its parent institution, each budgeting method will normally be coupled with either permission to increase spending or a mandate to reduce spending.

The **spending-ceiling model**, also known as the *incremental model,* is the budgeting circumstance most often desired by sports medicine program directors (Bass n.d.). This method requires justifica-

tion only for expenditures that exceed those of the previous budget cycle. Budget increases are most often linked to the inflation rate, which presents problems for sports medicine programs because prices for medical goods and services typically rise faster than inflation does. Athletic trainers who use this method are usually able to balance financial resources and expenditures for two or three years, but often fall behind after that because of the difference between the inflation rate and the increasing cost of medical goods and services.

Sports medicine programs in financial crisis are often forced to combine their primary budgeting method with the **spending-reduction model**. Under the spending-reduction model, department heads, including directors of sports medicine programs, are required to reduce their budgets to preserve institutional funds. For obvious reasons, this method requires the most imagination and creativity of all the budget models. Because financial resources tend to be reduced periodically in most sports medicine settings, the wise athletic trainer would identify those goods and services that could be cut without seriously affecting the program. If a financial crisis does arise, the athletic trainer will be prepared.

Any of the following budgeting methods can be used in either a spending-ceiling or spending-reduction mode.

Zero-Based Budgeting

Zero-based budgeting is an administrative method that requires unit directors to justify every expense without reference to previous spending patterns. This method requires close attention to documentation of actual program needs. Although it requires more effort on the part of the athletic trainer, zero-based budgeting can be an excellent tool for developing priorities in a sports medicine program. Zero-based budgeting requires athletic trainers to evaluate each subfunction of the program and rank it according to how important it is to the accomplishment of the overall mission. The director should include a rationale for each item in the budget request, explaining why the expense is necessary and what alternatives there are to funding it.

Fixed Budgeting

Fixed budgeting is an appropriate process for sports medicine programs in financially stable environments. This method requires an athletic trainer to project both expenditures and program income, if any, on a month-by-month basis to determine total program costs and revenues for the fiscal year. This exercise is useful because it can help the athletic trainer determine the likely cash flow of the operation at various points in the year. This type of budgeting is probably most appropriate for large, well-established sports medicine clinics during periods of relative economic certainty. School sports medicine programs rarely use fixed budgeting because most of these programs are not income oriented.

Variable Budgeting

Variable budgeting requires that expenditures for any given time period be adjusted according to revenues for the same period. Unfortunately, the athletic trainer who coordinates the activities of a sports medicine clinic will rarely be able to predict the monthly balance of expenditures to revenues with perfect accuracy. Assume that the clinic director budgeted $25,000 for expenses in June, anticipating that revenues would be approximately $50,000. Under the variable budgeting system, if actual revenues were only $40,000, the clinic director would be required to reduce expenditures by 20% for that month. Like fixed budgeting, this method is rarely used in school-based programs.

Lump-Sum Budgeting

In lump-sum budgeting, a parent organization provides an athletic trainer with a fixed sum of money and the authority to spend that money any way he or she sees fit. Most athletic trainers who use lump-sum budgeting like it because it gives them the freedom to spend money where they think it is needed the most. Lump-sum budgeting requires an administrator to hold athletic trainers accountable after the fact. Many administrators like this type of budgeting as well because it allows the athletic trainer to best determine the needs and avoids a micromanaging approach to supervising.

Line-Item Budgeting

Line-item budgeting requires that athletic trainers list anticipated expenditures for specific categories of program subfunctions. Typical line items for a sports medicine program include expendable supplies, equipment repair, team physician services, and insurance (see figure 5.2). Line-item budgeting allows a parent organization to retain greater control over the sports medicine program because money budgeted for one line usually cannot be spent on another line without permission. The advantage of a line-item budget is that it is easy to understand and prepare. The disadvantage is that the athletic trainer has limited flexibility in responding to midyear financial crises because funds dedicated to one use cannot be easily transferred to another use.

Performance Budgeting

Performance budgeting breaks the functions of a sports medicine program into discrete activities

BUDGET COMPARISON REPORT

Acct. No.: 213702   **Dept.:** Sports Medicine   **Responsible person:** Stan Curtis

Object code	Account description	2017-2018 Expense	2017-2018 Budget	2018-2019 Request	Percent change
3110	Travel	229.25	300.00	300.0	0
3205	Supplies	7,632.32	9,000.00	9,475.75	5.3
3305	Printing	89.29	100.00	100.00	0
3315	Speakers	0	1,500.00	1,500.00	0
3320	Stipends	5,997.96	6,300.00	6,300.00	0
3360	Postage	257.65	300.00	300.00	0
3530	Repairs	313.15	500.00	500.00	0
3650	Phone	428.89	475.00	500.00	5.3
3720	Uniforms	430.00	500.00	500.00	0
3850	Periodicals	150.00	150.00	150.00	0
4035	Insurance	200.00	250.00	300.00	20.0
4100	Dues	90.00	100.00	100.00	0
Department total		**$15,818.51**	**$19,475.00**	**$20,025.75**	**2.8**

Figure 5.2 Sample line-item budget for a school-based sports medicine program.

and appropriates the funds necessary to accomplish these activities. Examples of activities typically associated with a school sports medicine program include prepractice and pregame team preparation, rehabilitation, injury treatment, administration, patient education, and emergency first aid (see figure 5.3). Expenses for each of these activities can be calculated and used to determine the overall budget. This method is similar to line-item budgeting in that minibudgets are developed for separate categories of expenditures. Sports medicine programs do not commonly use performance budgeting because of the expense and difficulty of analyzing specific activity costs.

Planning the Budget

The process for budget planning varies depending on institutional budgeting cycles and rules and the type of budgeting system being used.

Needs Assessment

The first step in any budget cycle involves a careful assessment of program needs. Witkin and Altschuld (1995, p. 4) define **needs assessment** as "A systematic set of procedures undertaken for the purpose of setting priorities and making decisions about program or organizational improvement and allocation of resources. The priorities are based on identified needs."

A **need** is generally considered to be something essential or important. A need may be something

that an organization already retains, or it may be something it aspires to acquire. People commonly confuse needs with solutions. A need should not be confused with the many possible solutions for meeting the need. Some of the solutions will have budgetary consequences, and some won't. The important thing to recognize for the purpose of the needs assessment, however, is that none of these options is a need. Each is a potential solution that might help eliminate the need in this case.

Needs assessment as it relates to budget planning should generally include the following three phases:

PHASE 1: EXPLORATION

During this phase, an athletic trainer should

- identify the needs of the sports medicine program,
- decide what information to collect for each of the identified needs, and
- decide where and how to collect the information.

PHASE 2: INFORMATION GATHERING

During this phase, an athletic trainer should

- collect as much information as possible for each of the identified needs,
- prioritize needs, and
- determine causes for each of the needs.

PHASE 3: DECISION MAKING

During this phase, an athletic trainer should

- develop alternative solutions for each need,
- determine budgetary implications for each solution,
- prioritize solutions, and
- integrate solutions into the program budget.

Funding-Source Decisions

The next step in planning a budget for a sports medicine program is for the athletic trainer and the division head (for example, athletic director, chair of the academic department, general manager, or principal) to agree on which fund will provide the various items that the athletic trainer needs. This discussion should cover all of the program's projected expenses. Too often, athletic trainers focus only on the costs associated with supplies and equipment during the budget-planning process, to

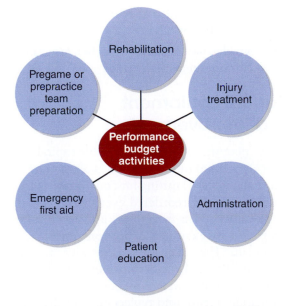

Figure 5.3 Performance budget activities.

the exclusion of other items important for running the program, including services, telephone, photocopying, and so on. After the athletic trainer and the division head have identified all program costs, they should allocate each to a particular budget. Protective pads, for instance, might fall into the sports medicine budget or the equipment budget. The health services budget might cover costs associated with physical examinations. Expenditures for travel to professional meetings might be part of the parent department's travel budget instead of the sports medicine budget. These decisions will depend on both the working relationship and the financial philosophies of the individuals involved.

Which fund these expenditures fall under will affect who controls the funds. For example, if an athletic trainer's travel to professional conferences is covered under the director of cocurricular activities' overall travel budget, the athletic trainer will probably be required to justify each meeting she wants to attend. In addition, she will likely be subject to all the restrictions on travel that apply to other district employees who report to the same director.

Another important decision involves whether the purchase of certain injury-protection equipment should be covered by the sports medicine budget or the budget of the team that will use the equipment. If only one team will use an item, it makes sense to include that item in the team's budget rather than the budget of the sports medicine program. If such items are placed in the budget of the sports medicine program, other teams might develop false expectations of the sports medicine staff.

For example, if an athletic trainer purchases knee braces to be used specifically by football players, then other coaches might expect him to purchase knee braces or similar devices for their athletes. The sports medicine program will probably be unable to continue to support this expense. A more rational approach would be for the football coaches to include the expense of the knee braces in their own budgets. Only in this way will the athletic trainer be able to avoid setting a precedent that he won't be able to afford for long.

Improved Budget Planning

The first year a budget is planned for the sports medicine unit is often the most difficult because no precedent exists on which to base financial plans. The process of budgeting for the first year of operation most closely approximates the zero-based budgeting model, because a rationale for each purchase must be developed without reference to established spending patterns. The presence of such spending patterns facilitates subsequent budget planning, which then approximates the spending-ceiling, or incremental, model. Athletic trainers can enhance their budget planning for sports medicine goods and services by following these guidelines:

- Keep a running inventory of all consumable and nonconsumable supplies.

- When budget submission time comes, calculate the amount of each type of consumable supply that has been used. Project and estimate how much more of the supply will be needed to complete the fiscal year, taking into account the different needs of the sport seasons yet to come.

- On the basis of estimates of how much of each type of supply will be needed to complete the fiscal year, and taking into account any changes that will take place during the next fiscal year (for example, new varsity sports, longer seasons), estimate the amount of each type of supply that will be needed for the next fiscal year.

- Consult with several vendors to obtain estimates of how much prices are expected to rise for the next fiscal year. With this information, develop anticipated prices for all the consumable supplies that will be needed for the next fiscal year.

- Establish long-term relationships with vendors and negotiate bulk rate purchasing opportunities.

- Be knowledgeable regarding the guidelines for bidding and purchasing.

- Consider partnering with other programs for greater purchasing leverage.

Capital Equipment and Improvements

Budget planning for nonconsumable capital equipment and capital improvements is often more difficult than budget planning for consumable supplies that are typically reordered every year. Therapeutic modalities, ice machines, and rehabilitation equipment are examples of nonconsumable capital equipment. These items are expensive, and many sports medicine directors are not able to include them in their annual supply budgets. Planning for acquisition, repair, and replacement of these items requires careful coordination between directors of sports medicine units and higher-level decision makers. Renovations, additions, and modifications to existing facilities are known as capital improvements. Maintenance of durable medical equipment can become a necessary task. Planning to cover the costs of maintaining equipment can range from in-house services to outsourced contractual agreements (Cashmore 2006). The following suggestions will help budget planners meet the needs of the sports medicine program in this area:

- Treat equipment repair as a consumable supply and include it as a line item in the annual operating budget. If the institution will agree to roll over the unused balance of this account from year to year, it can serve as a fund for capital equipment purchases.

- Develop priority lists for capital equipment and improvement requests complete with documentation of need. Suggest possible funding alternatives to decision makers.

- Make institutional fund-raisers aware of the priority list and the documentation of need so that they can keep those needs in mind when soliciting funds from contributors.

- Consider answering grant requests from funding agencies or engaging in research projects funded by industry. For example, Hope College became a testing site for a new analgesic cream, which brought the sports medicine unit more than $25,000. The college now uses the money to fund capital equipment purchases for the sports medicine program.

Budget Evaluation

Most directors of sports medicine units either ignore budget evaluation completely or perform it reluctantly. Evaluation of the budget, however, is important in the overall budgeting process, because it allows administrators to reach informed judgments on how well the institution is spending its financial resources. The following three relatively simple steps can help athletic trainers evaluate how well the budget process is working.

1. *Maintain dual accounting systems.* Besides monitoring the accounting done in the sports medicine unit, request computer printouts from the institution's business office to make sure that expenditures are charged to the proper funds.

2. *Evaluate service contracts.* During the annual evaluation of contracts for services such ambulance, insurance, team physicians, and athletic training

students, make sure that pay rates are competitive for the work being done. Keep a running log of all activities of each contractor, including the number of hours worked and the type of work performed.

3. *Compile statistical information.* Periodic statistical reports of how consumable and nonconsumable supplies and equipment are being used can help an athletic trainer justify financial resource deployment. For example, treatment records are an excellent source of information about how often and on whom therapeutic modalities are being used. Many computer software packages can help develop statistical reports.

Purchasing Supplies, Equipment, and Services

After the sports medicine budget has been approved, the process of budget implementation can begin. **Purchasing** is the process that athletic trainers use to implement the budget plan. Methods of purchasing supplies, equipment, and services are critical to the cost-effective operation of the sports medicine program. Creative purchasing strategies can reduce expenditures for sports medicine supplies by up to 40% (Ray 1991).

Basic Steps in the Purchasing Process

Athletic trainers should be familiar with the basic components of the purchasing process. These include, but may not be limited to, a request for a quotation, the negotiation process, a requisition order, a purchase order, receiving the purchase, confirmation of appropriate functioning order, and accounts payable. Each is a critical element in organizing a well-supplied sports medicine program. Today it is common to complete the entire bidding and purchasing process through an online procedure.

PEARLS OF MANAGEMENT

Athletic trainers implement the budget when they purchase equipment, supplies, and services for the sports medicine program. Although bidding is usually the most cost-effective purchasing method for consumable supplies, other purchasing options can be more effective for capital equipment and services.

Basic Steps in the Purchasing Process

1. Request for a quotation
2. Negotiation process
3. Requisition order
4. Purchase order
5. Receiving the purchase
6. Confirmation of appropriate functioning order
7. Accounts payable

Request for Quotation

The first step in the purchasing process is to send a request for quotation to a variety of vendors. A **request for quotation (RFQ)** is a document that accompanies a bid sheet and provides instructions for vendors to bid on the supplies, equipment, and services needed by a sports medicine program (see figure 5.4). The use of RFQs is known as **bidding**, and it is the most effective way to reduce costs for expendable sports medicine supplies (see figure 5.5). Certain questions should be considered before distributing supply bid sheets to vendors:

- *Will brand names be specified or are generic products acceptable?* Products for which a brand name is required should have a "no substitute" notation clearly marked on the bid sheet.

- *How many and which vendors will be invited to bid?* The suggested minimum is three. Vendors who have a reputation for excellent service should be considered over those who do not.

- *Will the institution or the vendor be responsible for paying shipping costs?* Most suppliers of consumable products are willing to pay shipping if it's specified on the bid.

- *What types of products will be purchased via bidding?* Consumable supplies and some types of durable equipment are good candidates for bidding. Most services should be bid only with great caution because the quality of service may be reflected in lower prices.

- *When should RFQs be sent to vendors?* This depends on the institution's purchasing process. If athletic trainers are required to purchase supplies through a central purchasing department, a minimum of three months from RFQ to delivery should be allowed.

Negotiations

Negotiations (the process of bargaining) are an important part of the purchasing process because their effective use can help safeguard the interests of a sports medicine program. Athletic trainers should negotiate in the following three categories of purchases.

1. *Capital equipment.* This is the expensive, durable equipment that often makes up the bulk of the rehabilitation and therapeutic modality inventory for a sports medicine program. Purchases are infrequent and costly.

2. *Medium-priced annual rebuys.* These are usually purchases of services that require annual renegotiation. Examples include salaries, physician consulting fees, ambulance services, and athletic medical insurance.

3. *Lower-cost consumable supplies.* These items constitute the bulk of the sports medicine supply budget. Although some supplies will have to be reordered throughout the year, careful planning will allow the athletic trainer to place only one major supply order for the entire year. This method will strengthen the athletic trainer's negotiating position because of the discounts normally associated with quantity purchasing.

Although negotiation on the price of a supply, a piece of equipment, or a service is common, athletic trainers should also consider other areas in which they can realize cost savings through negotiation. The athletic trainer should also negotiate the way in which the goods will be supplied, their quality, shipping costs, and support after the purchase.

- *Price.* Price is the most obvious point for negotiation in purchasing sports medicine goods and services. The use of the RFQ is the first step in price negotiation for consumable supplies, but it isn't the only option. Vendors are often willing to negotiate price reductions after submitting the RFQ. However, if athletic trainers use excessive price negotiation after vendors have returned the RFQ, a poor working relationship and higher prices in subsequent years are likely to result. Athletic trainers have an ethical responsibility to avoid the practice of playing one vendor against another to achieve the lowest possible price. Most vendors understand that they will be most competitive if they keep their prices low. In addition, they understand that athletic trainers will use bidding to try to keep their costs as low as possible. Playing one vendor against another after the bids have been

GRANT PUBLIC SCHOOLS

Department of Sports Medicine

Request for Quotation
(This is not an order)

Submit bid to: Stan Curtis, Head Athletic Trainer
                  Grant Public Schools
                  Municipal Stadium
                  Grant, CA 98201

If additional information is required, contact Stan Curtis at 415-555-7708.

Date Mailed: April 11, 2018   Closing Date: May 2, 2018

Goods must be able to be delivered before: August 1, 2018   Billing not before: July 1, 2018

To receive consideration, one copy of the Request for Quotation, with your bid properly filled in, must be signed and returned by the specified closing date.

All prices and conditions, including freight charges, must be shown. Additions or conditions not shown on this bid will not be allowed.

Contracts or purchase orders resulting from this quotation may not be assigned without the consent of the head athletic trainer at Grant Public Schools.

The seller agrees to protect the purchaser from all damages arising from alleged infringements of patents.

Unless otherwise specified, the right is reserved to accept or reject all or any part of your proposal.

Delivered FOB to specific address in Grant, California 98201. Seller assumes all freight and delivery expenses.

If given an order for item(s) specified on the attached Grant Public Schools Sports Medicine Bid Request, bidder agrees to furnish the items at the price(s) specified and under the conditions indicated.

Bidder to Complete

Bidder's name and address: Prices will be good for _____ days.

_____   Delivery will be made _____ days after receipt of order.

_____

_____   Signed by: _____

Telephone number: Printed name: _____

1-800-_____ and/or   Title: _____ Date: _____

Area code (___) _____

Figure 5.4   Sample request for quotation form to accompany bid sheet.

GRANT PUBLIC SCHOOLS SPORTS MEDICINE BID REQUEST

Please complete and return within three weeks of receipt to Stan Curtis, Head Athletic Trainer, Grant Public Schools, Grant, CA 98201.

Phone 415-555-7708 or fax 415-555-7922

All bid prices should include the following factors:

  Cost of shipping to Grant, CA

  Billing no sooner than 7/1/18

*If listing a substitute item, please specify brand name, packaging quantities, and product codes. If no brand is specified in the item column, please specify the brand you are bidding in the substitute column.

Item	Item no.	*Substitute	Quantity	Bid price/unit	Total
1.5-inch J & J coach tape (32 rolls/case) (no substitute)	26-2514	No Substitute	110 cases		
3-inch elastic tape (16 rolls/case) (Elastikon or substitute)	23-6485		10 cases		
2-inch elastic tape (24 rolls/case) (Conform or substitute)	89-8787		10 cases		
3-inch underwrap (48 rolls/case)	21-2336		5 cases		
6-inch elastic wraps with Velcro closure (irregular if available)	66-89907		20 dozen		
3-inch elastic wraps with Velcro closure (irregular if available)	66-89006		4 dozen		
1/8-inch adhesive felt (6" × 36")	34-3689		20 pieces		
1/8-inch adhesive foam (5" × 72")	43-3320		10 pieces		

Figure 5.5 Sample bid sheet to accompany request for quotation.

Types of Services Commonly Purchased by Athletic Trainers

- Team physician
- Consulting physician
- Ambulance
- Liability and malpractice insurance
- Athletic accident insurance
- Drug screening
- Laboratory and radiology
- Equipment service contracts
- Nutritional consultation
- Counseling
- Radiology
- Pharmacology
- Durable medical equipment

returned is frowned upon and is sure to damage relationships with vendors. Price negotiation is usually the most effective when one is purchasing services, for which bidding is less common.

- *Supply.* Among the most common points for negotiation between athletic trainers and vendors are delivery and payment schedules for purchased goods. Because many educational institutions have fiscal years that begin on July 1, common practice is for athletic trainers to order supplies for the next school year in May, take possession in June, and defer billing until after July 1. This allows athletic trainers time to restock and prepare for their fall seasons during one fiscal year and pay for the supplies during the subsequent year. Negotiation over delivery and billing is even more important for sports medicine clinics, where fluctuations of cash flow have a greater effect. For larger purchases, some vendors will allow the payments to be over three fiscal years, which can simply be over 14 months for the vendor if the AT makes payments in June, July, and then the following July.

- *Quality*. Athletic trainers typically negotiate for the quality of the goods they purchase by specifying brand names or generics on the bid sheet. A point of negotiation particularly applicable to large capital improvement items is the warranty. Although an **implied warranty**, the unstated understanding that the vendor will "make good" if the product is faulty, should accompany every product, the athletic trainer is free to negotiate an **express warranty** that affirms the performance characteristics of the product. See figure 5.6 for an example of an express warranty.

- *Shipping*. The two primary points for negotiation of shipping purchased goods are payment of shipping costs and the freight-on-board (FOB) point.

Negotiable Points in Sports Medicine Purchasing

The following elements of a purchase can be negotiated:

- Price
- Supply
- Quality
- Shipping
- Technical support

The wise athletic trainer will include a statement in the RFQ stipulating that the vendor will assume all costs associated with shipping and handling the product. This common practice clarifies the cost of supplies for athletic trainers by allowing vendors to factor the costs of shipping into their bids. The **FOB point** specifies the place at which title for the sports medicine supplies will pass from the vendor to the purchaser. Generally, athletic trainers should specify their institutions or clinics as the FOB point to provide greater protection against loss or damage during shipping.

- *Support*. Negotiation for technical support is especially important for high-tech capital improvement items. Computers and isokinetic testing and rehabilitation devices are two examples of the type of equipment for which athletic trainers might require technical support. The cost of this support is often negotiable and will become an important factor in the overall cost during the life of the equipment.

Requisition

The next step in the purchasing process is completing and submitting a **requisition** for needed supplies, equipment, or services. This step can be formal or informal depending on the authority level of the athletic trainer in the overall institutional bureaucracy. The requisition is simply a written request to the institution's or department's purchasing approver to expend institutional funds for needed resources (see figure 5.7).

Period	What we will replace at no cost to you:
One year from the date of the original purchase	Any part of the ultrasound unit that fails because of a defect in materials or workmanship. During this one-year period we will also provide, free of charge, necessary labor to replace or repair the defective component.
Five years from the date of the original purchase	Any part of the generator or crystal that fails because of a defect in materials or workmanship. During this five-year period we will also provide, free of charge, necessary labor to replace or repair the defective component.
Seven years from the date of the original purchase	Any part of the plastic housing that fails because of a defect in materials or workmanship. During this seven-year period we will also provide, free of charge, necessary labor to replace or repair the defective component.

What this warranty does not cover:

- Improper installation
- Failure of the product if it is abused, misused, or used for a purpose other than that for which it was intended
- Damage to the unit caused by flood, fire, or natural disasters
- Damage to circuit breakers or electrical systems
- Incidental damage caused by failure of this unit
- Routine maintenance or calibration

Figure 5.6 Example of an express warranty for an ultrasound unit.

Grant Public Schools — Purchase requisition

Suggested vendor				Previous supplier? Yes ☐ No ☐	Date	
Ship to:			Attn:		Date needed	
Quantity	Description				Unit	Total
Requested by:	Requested for:			Acct. no.	Approved by:	
For purchasing department use only						
Date ordered	P.O. No.	Ordered from:			Ship via:	

Figure 5.7 Sample purchase requisition form.

Purchase Order

Once an athletic trainer has approved requisitions in hand, purchase orders can be produced and sent to vendors. A **purchase order** is a document that formalizes the terms of the purchase and transmits the intentions of the buyer to purchase goods or services from the vendor (see figure 5.8). It is the actual order for the items you are purchasing. The purchase order should be completed and transmitted only after the RFQs have been received from the vendors. An important decision is whether to award purchase orders to vendors based on the low bid for the entire supply order or to make the award based on the low bid for each item. Athletic trainers will save the most money if they make the award based on each item. This method, however, has drawbacks. Most vendors have a minimum-order policy. A vendor awarded a purchase order for $4.95 out of a possible $10,000 RFQ will be unlikely to negotiate favorable terms in the future. One possible solution is to award purchase orders only for amounts over a certain critical level, usually around $500. This procedure breaks the total supply order into packages that will save the athletic trainer money and ensure a reasonable profit margin for the most competitive vendors.

Receiving

Receiving is the process of accepting delivery of goods purchased from vendors. When goods are received, they should immediately be checked to make sure that the packing slip matches the contents of the shipping container and to determine whether all the goods specified in the purchase order have been received. All goods should be inspected for damage. If damage is discovered, it should be reported to the vendor immediately. Most vendors have a policy of replacing damaged goods only if reported within a given period. It is a good idea to save the packing slips when an item is received to serve as institutional records in case proof of receipt is ever requested.

Vendor's copy

Grant Public Schools

Purchase order no.

To:

This number must appear on all invoices

↓ Ship to Grant Public Schools, Grant, CA

☐ Memorial Stadium, 225 Stadium Dr.

☐ Central Administration, 321 Pine St.

☐ Physical Plant, 5436 Elm Ave.

Bill to: Grant Public Schools
           Grant, CA 98201

Account number:	Order date:	Ship via:		
Quantity	Description		Unit price	Amount
Please send duplicate invoices.	Approved by:			

Figure 5.8   Sample purchase order form.

Accounts Payable

Payment for sports medicine supplies and equipment is usually due within a specified time period after the receipt of the goods or the invoice, whichever occurs last. Athletic trainers who work in educational, professional, or industrial settings should submit invoices to their respective business offices as soon as they receive them to take advantage of early-payment discounts offered by most vendors. Those athletic trainers who work in independent sports medicine clinics should evaluate the terms of the early-payment discount. If the finance charge is lower than the current cost of money, stretching the payments as far as possible into the payment term would make sense. For example, assume that you are in charge of an independent sports medicine clinic that needs to borrow money from a bank to cover supply purchases during certain times of the year when cash flow is predictably slow. If a particular vendor charged 0.5% per month (6% annual percentage rate) on the unpaid balance of your account and the bank was charging you an annual rate of 8%, you could pay off your account with the vendor over the maximum time allowed and spend the 2% you will save on another program need.

Alternative Purchasing Strategies

Besides the traditional method of bidding for sports medicine supply purchases and paying for them with institutional funds, athletic trainers should consider three other potential sources of cost savings: pooled buying consortia, alumni and booster organizations, and external funding organizations and programs.

Pooled Buying Consortia

A **pooled buying consortium** can be an effective method for purchasing certain types of sports medicine supplies. Schools that are members of an athletic conference or contracted through the same hospital or clinic should consider pooling their adhesive tape orders, for example, to receive a quantity discount. This method can be effective for many types of supplies, including bandages, ice bags, paper cups, elastic wraps, and crutches. Coaches and athletic directors have used pooled buying consortia for many years to purchase balls and other athletic equipment for less than it would cost to purchase such supplies individually. This method can provide cost savings when administered at the districtwide administrative level. One disadvantage of this method is that the athletic trainers employed at different schools must agree on the supplies being purchased.

Alumni and Booster Organizations

Alumni and booster organizations can be helpful in offsetting the costs of large capital expenses that would usually lie outside the normal budget of the sports medicine program. Treatment and rehabilitation devices are expensive items that booster clubs are often willing to buy for the sports medicine program. Athletic trainers, however, must work in conjunction with the institutional development officer when making such requests of booster clubs. Many institutions have policies designed to ensure that all philanthropy passes through the development office to maximize the ability of the institution to obtain such gifts. In some cases, programs can establish naming rights to facilities in an effort to raise funds for a sports medicine program. For example, universities might have procedures in place whereby a donor can contribute money in a restricted manner toward an athletic training program and in return, the program will name its educational classroom or athletic training clinic after the donor.

External Funding Organizations and Programs

Many organizations and agencies provide money to help offset the costs of research and education for a variety of needs related to sports medicine. Grants from organizations generally pay for expenses associated with specific projects and are not intended to fund the routine expenses associated with operating a sports medicine program. For example, a college with an accredited athletic training education program that wants to begin a lecture series might consider applying to a funding agency to help offset the cost of the series for a specific period. An athletic trainer who needs a particular piece of equipment to conduct a research project might also consider applying for a grant. External funding often supports the purchase of automated external defibrillators or initiation of drug and alcohol education programs.

Athletic trainers seeking a grant from a funding agency must prepare a comprehensive grant application according to the exact specifications

External Funding Sources

Contact the following sources for information on external funding:

- National Athletic Trainers' Association Research and Education Foundation
- American College of Sports Medicine
- Gatorade Sports Science Institute
- National Institutes of Health
- National Science Foundation
- National Operating Committee on Standards for Athletic Equipment

The Foundation Center is an outstanding source of information for people who want to apply for financial support from one of the thousands of public or private funding sources. See its website for complete online information about how to get started, how to develop a proposal, where to apply, and other important information on grant proposal development.

Reasons Grant Proposals Fail

Writing a grant proposal can be a tedious and lengthy process, with no guarantee of acceptance. Grant proposals do not receive funding for many reasons. The granting agency will probably reject a late or incomplete application. Similarly, if the proposal does not meet the granting agency's specifications or is poorly written, it will likely be rejected. Even well-written proposals that are submitted on time may be denied if the granting agency doesn't believe the project will advance the field. If the budget is unrealistic or the proposed methods are inappropriate, the granting agency is unlikely to fund the request. Additionally, the grant application may fail if the project is a low priority for the granting agency. Finally, in challenging economic times, competition from investigators seeking external funding is likely to increase.

outlined in the application instructions. Most grant programs are competitive, and only the most worthy projects receive funding. An athletic trainer should select a funding agency whose goals are consistent with the project for which she is seeking support. Some organizations and agencies support funding programs that are national in scope. Many states, cities, and local school districts also have either public or private foundations that support worthy projects. Most universities staff an office dedicated to helping their employees identify potential sources of external funding for specific projects.

Capital Equipment —Buy or Lease?

Once a decision has been made to acquire an expensive piece of equipment, the athletic trainer and the organization's business manager must decide whether to purchase the equipment or lease it. Many expensive rehabilitation devices and other therapeutic modalities can be leased rather than purchased. Each method presents advantages and disadvantages. The primary advantage of purchasing over leasing is cost, especially if the equipment is being purchased outright as opposed to being financed. The other advantage of purchasing is that the sports medicine program owns the equipment. Ownership can become a disadvantage, however, if the equipment relies on technology that becomes obsolete before the equipment is fully depreciated. Because of the speed at which technology advances, athletic trainers should carefully assess the advantages and disadvantages of buying and leasing. One of the advantages of leasing is that an institution can use its capital in other ways because it has not devoted large amounts to equipment purchases.

Relative Merits of Leasing

Advantages
- Possible tax advantages
- Decreased risk of obsolescence
- Lower initial costs
- Possible repair service

Disadvantages
- Higher overall costs
- No ownership
- Higher effective interest rate than traditional financing

In addition, some tax advantages may be available to sports medicine clinics when they lease their equipment rather than purchase it.

Purchasing Services

Purchasing services is different in several ways from purchasing supplies or equipment. The first, and most obvious, difference is that the quality of a service can be more difficult to assess than the quality of a product. It is important to monitor all service-related contracts for quality assurance (Kujawa and Short 2005). Athletic trainers should keep meticulous records of the services performed and repairs or upgrades made. This should include the dates and the names of the technicians who performed the work.

For example, assume that a large university sports medicine program contracts with a local radiology clinic for all its X-ray, MRI, CT, and nuclear medicine needs. The athletic trainers at the university will probably find it more difficult to determine the quality of these diagnostic services than they would, for example, the quality of the athletic tape they buy. This circumstance arises, in part, because they have to rely on the professional judgment of another person in the case of the radiology services. They don't have the expertise to make an informed judgment on the quality of every aspect of the service. The problem can become more acute if only one radiology service is available in the community. The athletic trainers cannot compare the service they receive from one radiology practice with what another might be able to offer. Athletic tape, on the other hand, is easier to evaluate. Many brands and styles are available from many vendors. A straightforward exercise can determine which brand is best for the money.

Nevertheless, athletic trainers can employ several methods to take some of the uncertainty out of purchasing services:

- *Try to get the service free of charge.* Most team physicians volunteer their time. Many ambulance companies are willing to park at the site of an athletic contest free of charge. Some service providers are willing to donate their time in exchange for an advertisement in the game program.

- *If you can't get the service free of charge, try to employ cost sharing whenever possible.* For example, your team physician might not be willing to see injured athletes in his office for free, but he might be willing to accept only what the athlete's insurance will pay.

- *When more than one provider is available for a particular service, be sure to evaluate in advance what each is willing to provide and at what price.* For example, if two ambulance services operate in your community, speak with both to find out how much they charge for event standby and transport. Find out which hospitals they are willing to transport patients to. Ask them about their mean response time. Will they participate in your emergency plan drills? How often do they anticipate having to leave the game if another emergency occurs in the same city?

- *Investigate the service provider's reputation with other athletic trainers.* If you are searching for an orthopedic surgeon to serve your athletes, ask other athletic trainers whom they use and why. Discussions with other athletic trainers can also help you attain equitable services.

- *Develop a contract or memorandum of understanding that specifies your expectations of the service provider.* This document can help improve communication between the sports medicine program and the service provider and prevent problems in the future. The contract should specify a period, usually no more than two years, for which the contract will be in effect. It may also include termination clauses and renewal options.

- *Develop a database for each service provider.* How many injured or ill athletes did your team physician see last year? How long do your athletes have to wait before the orthopedic consultant sees them? What is the rate of false-positive drug screens reported by the laboratory you employ? Only by answering those kinds of questions and comparing the answers with the cost of retaining the services will you be able to judge the value of this aspect of your program.

- *Involve other departments.* It is possible that other departments at your institution or organization may be using the services of the same vendor as the sports medicine department. Communication between departments can bring about greater awareness and possibly contribute to collaborative service benefits.

- *Perform annual reviews.* To ensure ongoing satisfaction with services, it is a good idea to perform annual reviews of service agreements. Any concerns should be addressed formally.

Inventory Management

Inventory management is the practice of overseeing and controlling the ordering, storage, and use of a program's products. Key considerations for accurate inventory management include, but are not limited to, the following:

- Acquiring an adequate supply and variety of inventory to meet production and sales needs
- Providing safety stocks to meet unexpected demand or delays in inventory replenishment
- Investing in inventory wisely so that excessive capital is not tied up, excessive space is not required, and unnecessary borrowing and interest expense are not required
- Maintaining accurate and up-to-date records to help identify and prevent shortages and to serve as a database for decisions

PEARLS OF MANAGEMENT

Athletic trainers have a financial responsibility to maintain control over the inventory of sports medicine equipment and supplies. They can usually accomplish this by inventorying regularly, centralizing storage of supplies, automating the inventory process, restricting access to storage areas, and implementing reminder systems.

Inventory management, one of the most important aspects of increased efficiency in a sports medicine program, is equally important for large and small operations. Large operations, such as professional athletic teams and universities with National Collegiate Athletic Association Division I football programs, make significant investments in sports medicine supplies, and they should manage them wisely and prudently. Larger programs are more likely to operate multiple facilities, making the control and distribution of sports medicine supplies more difficult and requiring more attention to inventory techniques.

Inventory control is important for small programs as well, because errors in inventory and supply management result in more financial hardship for programs with smaller budgets. Another problem athletic trainers in smaller programs face is that coaches, athletic administrators, and physical education teachers often have access to the athletic training room and the sports medicine supplies in it; this can lead to unnecessary use and poor inventory control.

Stiefel (2002) describes an inspection and prevention maintenance program (IPM) consisting of five key elements:

1. Maintain an up-to-date list of all equipment owned or leased.
2. Inspect only those items that actually require periodic inspection.
3. Inspect all equipment before its first use, and record identifying information, purchase order number, cost, warranty information, physical inspection, electrical inspection, and applicable performance tests.
4. Establish an inspection schedule for each piece of equipment based on its failure rate.
5. Keep track of completed inspections.

The following suggestions should help athletic trainers improve their ability to track the location and rate of use of their supplies.

- *Inventory regularly.* Compile a complete inventory of expendable supplies at least once a month. Institutions that operate multiple athletic training rooms should inventory the stock in each facility every week. Compile the inventory reports for these satellites in the primary athletic training room and use them to develop the monthly inventory report.

- *Centralize storage.* Wherever possible, centralize the storage of sports medicine supplies to make them easier to manage. If you need to stockpile supplies in several locations, send the smallest amount that will suffice for a reasonable period, preferably one week. This system requires athletic trainers to be attentive to inventory levels and helps prevent sudden or unexpected shortages.

- *Automate the inventory process.* Develop and implement a continuous monitoring system that allows for a quick check of inventory levels at any time. One effective method uses a computerized inventory record based on standard spreadsheet software. When removing supplies from the central storage site, the athletic trainer fills out a small form indicating the date, type, and amount of supply being taken and the amount remaining after the withdrawal (see figure 5.9). At the end of each day, a student or administrative assistant enters the information on the forms into the computer record. This system allows the athletic trainer to track the status of the inventory daily.

- *Restrict access.* Unauthorized access to the athletic training room and the supply room where sports medicine supplies are kept is the primary cause of inventory control breakdown. Institutions should develop policies and procedures that specify who has access to the sports medicine facility and under what circumstances. As few people as possible should have keys to the facility; access should be limited to those who are responsible for and have a legitimate need to use it. Policies should clearly state the responsibilities of anyone issued keys to the facility. Having locked supply cabinets and closets within the athletic training clinic can also help reduce inventory control issues.

- *Keep a reminder system.* Each type of supply should be marked with a sign that reads "Reorder when X amount remains." to remind athletic trainers

SPORTS MEDICINE SUPPLY CHECKOUT FORM

Date _____

Supply type _____

Quantity _____

Supply destination _____

Amount remaining in storage _____

Person taking the supplies _____

Person recording the withdrawal into the computer _____

Figure 5.9 Sample inventory control form.

to reorder supplies when they reach a critically low level.

Summary

Budgeting is a process designed to coordinate resources and expenditures and also serves as a tool for estimating receipts and disbursements. Several formal types of budgeting exist: zero-based, fixed, variable, lump-sum, line-item, and performance budgeting. Each of these methods can help athletic trainers plan the financial activity of their programs.

Performing a needs assessment assists with setting budgetary priorities and the allocation of resources. Purchasing supplies, equipment, and services can be a regular task for athletic training managers. Purchasing involves bidding, requisitions, and other legal steps that are required to appropriately obtain goods and services. Once items are purchased, an accurate inventory should be maintained that reflects an adequate supply of items to meet an organization's needs. Proper maintenance of inventory and service agreements requires accurate and up-to-date records.

Learning Aids

Case Study 1

Tamika had just arrived at Los Ranchos College after being appointed the school's first certified athletic trainer. It was mid-June, and Tamika knew she had quite a bit to do to get ready for the arrival of the fall-sports athletes in August. She decided to start by approaching the athletic director.

"Coach," Tamika began, "I need to order the sports medicine supplies as soon as possible if we expect to be ready to go in August. I need to know a few things. First, how much money do I have to work with? Second, are there specific purchasing procedures I need to follow? I'd like to get busy with this today if I could."

The athletic director informed Tamika that she didn't have a specific budget for sports medicine supplies. In the past, sports medicine supplies were paid for out of the general athletics budget, which he controlled. "You just put your list together, and I'll take a look at it," he told her. "Oh, I almost forgot," the athletic director continued, "I wanted to make sure we at least had the tape here in time, so I went ahead and ordered it. It should be delivered sometime in July."

Although Tamika was uncomfortable about not having a specific budget, she knew she wouldn't be able to change everything right away. She spent the rest of the day compiling an inventory of the supplies on hand. That evening she put together a list of the supplies she thought she would need to get through the first year, along with an estimate of each item's cost.

When she presented it to the athletic director the next day, he told her she would need to cut the proposal by 25%. "I think this list is fairly modest," Tamika said. "I'm not sure I can cut that much out of it." After further discussion, the athletic director told Tamika that the cost of the tape, when added to the total cost of her supply list, was just more than he could afford. When Tamika asked how much he had paid for the tape, she was astonished to find out that it was 100% higher than the price she paid at the school where she used to work. "Where did you order the tape from?" asked Tamika. The athletic director replied, "We get all our supplies from Acme Sporting Goods downtown. We always have. Anything you need, just call them and they'll take good care of you. The owner is a big supporter of the college." Tamika suddenly realized that she had her work cut out for her!

Questions for Analysis

1. What budgeting system does the Los Ranchos College sports medicine program use? Is it optimal for the conditions? What system would you implement? Why?

2. Why was Tamika so distressed when she found out how the tape had been purchased? What is the likely effect of this purchasing system on Tamika's program? How should she alter the purchasing system?

3. If Tamika changes from direct purchasing at Acme Sporting Goods to a system of competitive bidding, what would be the likely result?

4. What can Tamika do to lower her costs for sports medicine supplies while maintaining the supportive relationship the college enjoys with the owner of Acme Sporting Goods?

5. If you were in Tamika's position, would you have taken the same approach to purchasing supplies? If not, what would you have done differently? Why?

Case Study 2

Diversified Physical Therapy Services (DPTS) is a large rehabilitation services corporation that operates a string of clinics in a 10-county area in eastern Iowa. Besides operating the clinics, DPTS supplies rehabilitation professionals to 12 hospitals. DPTS recently acquired contracts at 15 high schools to supply sports medicine services. The contracts provide an athletic trainer for each school for 1,000 hours per year. As an additional service, DPTS purchases all sports medicine supplies for the schools up to a maximum of $2,500 per school.

At a recent meeting of the DPTS partners, one of the owners expressed concern over the plan to provide the schools with sports medicine supplies. Although he liked the idea in general, he was concerned about waste and cost effectiveness. He also pointed out to the other partners that if each school used less than the $2,500 allotment, the company would come out ahead.

The DPTS partners decided to create a central storage site for all 15 high schools. The athletic trainers would be allowed to take what they needed for a two-week period. When they exhausted those supplies, they would have to come to the central storage site, housed in a clinic in the geographic center of the schools' service area, and check out enough for another two weeks. The business manager in the clinic where the supplies were stored would be responsible for auditing supply requisitions to ensure that each school remained below the $2,500 limit.

Questions for Analysis

1. What are the strengths of the central supply plan adopted by DPTS? What are the weaknesses?

2. What are alternatives to the central supply plan? Would they be superior? If so, why?

3. What are the strengths and weaknesses of the plan to provide up to $2,500 in supplies to each school? Is this a service that most schools would want? Why or why not?

Key Concepts and Review

Understand the different kinds of budgeting processes and apply them to an athletic training setting.

A budget is a plan for the coordination of resources and expenditures. It helps ensure that needed services are delivered effectively and on time and that financial resources are expended in accordance with the institutional mission. The six most common types of budgeting systems are zero based, fixed, variable, lump sum, line item, and performance. An organization can use each in either a spending-ceiling (or incremental) or a spending-reduction model. Careful consideration of which funds will support the various activities of the sports medicine program enhances budget development. Budgeting for the first year of the sports medicine program is the most difficult because of a lack of previous spending patterns. Budgeting for capital improvements is more difficult than for consumable supplies because of the expense involved. Budget evaluation is an important but often neglected activity that will help athletic trainers make informed decisions on how to expend program resources.

Coordinate the purchasing of athletic training equipment, supplies, and services to maximize the use of program funds.

Purchasing is the process of budget implementation. The seven most common steps in the purchase of sports medicine supplies include request for quotation, negotiation, requisition, purchase order, receiving, confirmation of appropriate functioning order, and accounts payable. Athletic trainers should attempt to negotiate with vendors over price, supply, quality, shipping, and technical support. Alternatives to purchasing by bidding include pooled buying consortia and the use of alumni and booster organizations. Athletic trainers should consider the relative merits of leasing over buying when shopping for expensive capital equipment.

Manage the athletic training program's inventory of equipment and supplies.

Inventory management is an important aspect of administration for athletic trainers. Mistakes in inventory management can have drastic consequences for both large and small programs. Athletic trainers should always be aware of the status of their supply inventory so that they can deliver sports medicine services in a timely manner.

Facility Design and Planning

Objectives

After reading this chapter, you should be able to do the following:

- Understand and defend the importance of the design phase in planning and constructing new sports medicine facilities.

- Understand the facility design and construction process in sports medicine settings.

- Understand the common design elements of a woll-planned sports medicine facility.

- Describe the sports medicine facility in terms of its specialized-function areas.

- Discuss principles associated with marketing a sports medicine facility and practice.

As athletic trainers become more involved in administrative leadership roles and experience increasing potential for remuneration for services, the development of sports medicine programs may involve the planning of a facility. Planning a sports medicine facility is not a task for an inexperienced athletic trainer. A variety of elements must be considered during the earliest planning stages (Knowles 1997). The opportunity to be involved in the planning, design, and construction of a sports medicine facility usually comes only once during the career of most athletic trainers, who typically have little or no experience in facility planning. Most buildings are designed and constructed to provide service for decades; decisions made during the planning, design, and construction phase of the sports medicine facility are, for all practical purposes, permanent. Hence, it is understandable but unfortunate when expensive and uncorrectable mistakes occur. This chapter will help athletic trainers understand the basic processes of planning, designing, and constructing a sports medicine center. Keep in mind that while there may be differences in planning when considering a facility that is in a university or high school setting versus a private free-standing facility, many of the concepts are in fact similar and equally important to address.

Conceptual Development

The most important phase in constructing a new sports medicine center is developing an appropriate concept for its design. Whether the facility is intended to serve a school or a professional or private sports medicine clinic, the conceptual development process is essentially the same despite the important differences in layout and funding strategy between these facilities.

At least two arguments support paying careful attention to the conceptual development of the design of the sports medicine center. First, this is the only stage of the project that involves review by the people who will actually use the facility. After the project has begun, many reviews will occur, but primarily construction professionals and municipal employees such as plumbing and electrical inspectors will carry them out. The athletic trainer has input during the design phase of a facility construction project. The construction of a new building is a political act that involves making choices about how to use limited resources. The time for athletic trainers to exercise their influence is during the design phase.

The second argument for paying attention to design development relates to permanency and cost. Buildings are intended to last a long time. Once the foundation is poured and bricks and mortar are in place, changes based on new thinking about the way the sports medicine facility should be designed become expensive to implement. Although the owners of private sports medicine clinics can always sell the building if they become dissatisfied with its design, school and university officials generally do not have this option because most campus-based sports medicine centers are part of large, multipurpose buildings.

KEY POINT

The design process is a critical time for athletic trainers to influence the final form of the sports medicine facility. Elements of the process include needs assessment, institutional approval, selecting a construction process, selecting an architect, developing schematics, securing funding, bidding construction, bid analysis, and beginning and monitoring construction.

Design Process

Most athletic trainers will never be involved in selecting an architect. As mentioned before, however, many will be responsible at some point in their career for input into the design of new sports medicine centers. Understanding the processes normally used by institutions during the design and construction phases of a new building can help athletic trainers avoid making mistakes. Although the steps described in the following paragraphs are not the only way to design, plan, and construct a new facility, they represent the most common elements of the construction process.

Planning Committee

The **planning committee** is a group of individuals appointed to work with the architect to develop the design of a new building. Members of the planning committee should have a vested interest in the usage of the facility. The most appropriate person to act as chair of the planning committee is the person who leads the department or discipline most responsible for use of the new facility. This person may or may not be an athletic trainer. Hence, athletic trainers must effectively communicate their needs so that the overall design will incorporate them.

PEARLS OF MANAGEMENT

Most athletic trainers do not have the opportunity to design an athletic training facility. If the opportunity exists, be sure to consult with others who have done so and learn from them what they thought they did well and what they would do differently.

Step 1: Conduct a Needs Assessment

The first step in designing a new sports medicine facility is a comprehensive assessment of future program needs. The process of needs assessment might seem tedious, but without it, a competent job of planning for future space needs cannot be accomplished. The needs assessment is usually conducted at the departmental or program level and

Phases of Design and Construction of a Sports Medicine Center

1. Conduct a needs assessment.
2. Seek approval for the project.
3. Select a construction process model.
4. Select an architect.
5. Develop schematics.
6. Secure the required funding.
7. Bid the construction.
8. Analyze bids and take action.
9. Begin construction.
10. Monitor construction.

Sports Medicine Facility Needs Assessment

Question	Where to look for answers
What is the current clinic caseload? How is it likely to change?	Annual reports, interviews with staff and administrators
Is the current facility adequate? Why or why not?	Building codes, national design standards, literature review, peer consultation
Is the current facility suitable for implementing the strategic plan?	Program and institutional facility strategic plans
Which program problems are related to facilities?	Critical incident reports, interviews with staff, accreditation reports
Can the facility benefit from additional use by other tenants or providers?	Class space, community education programs

involves asking and answering a series of questions. If the administrator of a sports medicine program has been doing a good job of programmatic self-study, the needs assessment will be much easier to complete

Step 2: Seek Approval for the Project

After the needs assessment has been completed, assuming it justifies the need for a new sports medicine facility, the people with financial control of the institution must be convinced that the project is necessary. This step is important whether the sports medicine program is in a school, professional, or private clinic setting. Every organization has a person or a group of people who must ultimately decide whether to spend the vast sums required for new construction. An athletic trainer must be willing to document the need for such facilities in detail. Even after presenting documentation, however, the athletic trainer should not be disappointed if it takes months, or more realistically, years, for a project to gain approval.

Step 3: Select a Construction Process Model

Construction of new facilities usually occurs in one of three ways. **Lump-sum bidding**, the most traditional method, is often used for governmental units like public schools and colleges. In lump-sum bidding, the architect submits schematic drawings to several general contractors. The contractors study the plans and quote a cost based on the instructions provided by the architect. Because some contractors might intentionally underbid a project to secure a contract, it is wise to screen the contractors in advance and send bids only to those with proven

records. The importance of this step can't be over-emphasized. The temptation to accept the lowest bid without regard for the reputation of the contractor is powerful. The differences in the bids can amount to many thousands of dollars. You might eventually have to spend this money, however, if the workmanship is shoddy or if the contractor has cut corners. A prudent approach is to visit at least one building that each of the contractors has constructed to determine the quality of the work. Be sure to spend some time alone with the owners so that you will feel free to ask questions about the experiences they had with the contractor. Although negative responses to some of the following questions would not necessarily reflect on the contractor's skill, it would be wise to find out whether

- the contractor worked well with the architect,
- the project was completed on time,
- the project stayed within the budget,
- all the building systems functioned properly when the project was finished,
- the construction was of high quality,
- the contractor was willing to require subcontractors to correct mistakes,
- the owners would make changes to the building if given the chance, and
- the owners would hire this contractor again.

Another construction model that may be used is **construction management**. The construction-management approach uses the general contractor as part of the design team; that is, the contractor is on board from the beginning of the project, rather than coming in near the end of the design phase.

Advantages and Disadvantages of Lump-Sum Bidding

Advantages

- Results in the lowest possible price.
- Ensures fairness.
- Complies with state and federal statutes.

Disadvantages

- Contractors might underbid.
- Owner has less control.
- Contractor might cut corners.

The construction manager can then advise on building materials, schedules, cost analysis, and necessary subcontractors. A drawback to using the construction-management approach is the manager's fee, which can approach 5% of the total project cost (Snider 1982).

The third construction process method is **design–build**. This system uses only one firm to both design and build a sports medicine center. As with the other construction models, there are advantages and disadvantages to the design–build concept. The obvious advantage is that the owners communicate with just one firm. They can take any problems that arise to a single source for redress, allowing for more rapid and potentially cost-saving approaches to solving problems that arise during the construction phase of the project. The streamlined approach used in design–build is also its weakness. This method involves fewer checks and balances among the various firms normally involved in a construction project. The integrity of the entire project rests on

Advantages and Disadvantages of Construction Management

Advantages

- Construction manager is part of the design team.
- More advice on materials, costs, and schedules is available.

Disadvantages

- Construction manager charges a fee.
- No direct control over subcontractors exists.

Advantages and Disadvantages of Design–Build

Advantages

- Easier communication
- Ability to fast-track problems

Disadvantages

- Fewer checks and balances
- Greatest potential for major problems

the ability of one firm—specifically on the ability of a few people in one firm. This is a good reason to screen design–build proposals even more carefully than a more traditional construction process model.

Step 4: Select an Architect

The owner of a clinic or the chief executive officer of an institution retains an architect to create building designs. The architect should be available to provide advice and guidance from the beginning of a project until the keys to the new facility are handed over to the users. Although the selection of an architect is listed as the fourth step in this text, it frequently comes earlier in the process. In fact, an architect can help with many of the previous steps.

Several methods can be used for selecting an architect (American Institute of Architects n.d.). The first and easiest way is to contract with a firm recommended by friends or colleagues. For obvious reasons, this might not serve a sports medicine program well. A better method is to develop a list of architectural firms with a variety of attributes—big and small, local and distant, and so on. Interview each firm to determine whether it would be suitable for and interested in taking on the project. A site visit to at least one project each firm has completed is recommended. A third method for selecting an architect is to commission a design competition. This method is typically used only on very large projects because it is costly in terms of money and time.

Whichever method is used, a good match between the client and the architect is essential for a successful outcome. Architects for sports medicine facilities should be selected based on their openness to suggestions and their previous experience in designing similar facilities. *Athletic Business* magazine showcases architects that have experience in designing athletic facilities. Many of these architects have designed sports medicine facilities as a part of these larger projects.

Three Methods for Selecting an Architect

- Ask friends and colleagues.
- Screen several architectural firms.
- Commission a design competition.

For more information on how to find an architect, contact the American Institute of Architects.

Step 5: Develop Schematics

The architect will develop **schematic drawings** that reflect the relationships among the principal functions of the sports medicine center.

Determining Space Needs Secor (1984) created a formula that athletic trainers can use to plan space requirements based on the number of athletes and other physically active patients they expect to serve during peak caseloads:

(Number of patients at peak / 20 per table per day) × 100 square feet = Total square footage

Even though this formula is more than 30 years old, it still provides a good starting point for determining space needs, and athletic trainers charged with the design of a new sports medicine center must take into account that varied functions will take place in the sports medicine center and that each of those functions will have different space requirements. It is always best to consult with peers who have been through the experience of designing a facility, and learning from them what they felt worked well and what they might do differently.

Many factors influence the overall space requirements of a modern sports medicine center:

- Type of setting (secondary school, hospital, college)
- Age of patients (youth, geriatric)
- Total number clients using the facility
- Types of services provided

One important thing to keep in mind is planning for future growth and trends. Anticipated growth of a program, for example, that may add sports teams in the future, is a necessity. Otherwise, you will outgrow the size and needs of a facility too soon. It is also important to consider as best one can where trends are headed. Will hydrotherapy be a necessity for everyone? Will manual treatment space or functional rehabilitation space be important to plan for? Although difficult to predict at times, inquiring with others in the profession may be critical in planning for future needs of a facility.

In summary, the following factors influence the space requirements of a sports medicine facility:

- Number of clients to be served
- Type of clients to be served
- Type of services to be offered
- Amount and kinds of equipment needed
- Number and qualifications of staff
- Projected growth of the program
- Specialty rooms (e.g., physician examination, private, wet, storage)

Traffic Patterns When working with the architect to develop the schematic drawings, the athletic trainer should determine anticipated **traffic patterns** based on the relationships between the subfunctions of the sports medicine center. This step in the design phase is crucial. Attractive, functional sports medicine facilities are characterized by smooth traffic flow through all parts of the facility. If the design does not anticipate the traffic patterns that develop once the facility is built, the result is likely to be a sports medicine center that seems noisy, congested, crowded, or all three.

Step 6: Secure the Required Funding

All construction projects require a source of funding. Many funding options are available for sports medicine center construction depending on the type of institution. Private sports medicine clinics generally have fewer options than do public-sector institutions like high schools, colleges, and universities. Even professional athletic teams have greater flexibility in financing sports medicine facilities than private clinics do, because many of the stadiums that house them are constructed at least in part with public tax dollars. The owners of most private sports medicine clinics will have to secure loans from a bank for new construction.

Athletic trainers who approach a financial institution for a loan should remember that banks are more likely to make loans for the construction of multipurpose buildings. For example, the athletic trainer who wishes to build a sports medicine clinic as part of a larger medical arts building will probably have a better chance of securing a loan than will the person who wants to build a health club that offers sports medicine services. The medical arts building can serve many purposes, whereas the health club would probably require extensive remodeling before resale should the bank need to foreclose. In general, bankers perceive medical practitioners as good risks.

At least two things are usually required of an athletic trainer who applies for a **commercial loan** from a bank for new construction of a private sports medicine facility: an assignment of life insurance (this protects the bank against loss in the event the athletic trainer dies before paying off the debt) and a **business plan**. The business plan is essential because it contains information that the bank will need to project whether or not the clinic is likely to succeed. A business plan for a sports medicine clinic would include the following items:

- A statement of the activities that the clinic will engage in
- A **market analysis** detailing the clinic's competitive advantages, analysis of the competition, pricing structure, and marketing plan
- The credentials of the principal owners and operators of the clinic
- Historical and projected financial statements of both cash flow and income
- A breakdown of costs associated with the project based on the schematics developed by the architect
- The amount of personal equity being committed by the athletic trainer
- The amount of the loan being requested

KEY POINT

Many online resources are available to help you develop an effective business plan.

Sports medicine facilities in the public sector, including private educational institutions that receive state and federal assistance, can be funded in at least three ways other than by a commercial loan. One of the most common fund-raising methods is the **capital campaign**. A capital campaign is a major institutional response to several needs that the institution intends to remedy over three to five years. People at the very top of the institutional hierarchy usually authorize and direct capital campaigns. The goal of a capital campaign is to secure pledges of financial support from a broad institutional constituency including alumni, faculty and staff, foundations, affiliated institutions such as churches, and friends. Funds for a new sports medicine center will usually be a small fraction of the overall goal for a capital campaign. Nevertheless, an athletic trainer might be heavily involved in helping secure pledges under the direction and supervision of the institutional development officer.

Another way in which public-sector institutions and some hospitals secure funding for the construction of sports medicine facilities is through the sale of **tax-exempt bonds**. The sale of such bonds is usually authorized either by public vote (as in the case of public school construction) or by a bonding authority established by the states. Bonds are usually sold in one of two ways: publicly, usually to friends of the institution, or privately to a bank or other financial institution as part of its investment portfolio. A common practice is for similar institutions to pool their projects and sell bonds together under one issue. This practice is useful because it lowers the overhead costs associated with conducting a bond issue.

The third common method that institutions use to finance new sports medicine facilities is to borrow internally from their **endowments**. An institution's endowment is the sum of its assets in cash and investments. Institutions usually hesitate to borrow from endowments because the interest earned from an endowment can account for a significant percentage of the annual operating budget. If the endowment is large, however, and the sports medicine building project is relatively modest in relation to it, this is probably the easiest method of financing such a project.

Step 7: Bid the Construction

If an athletic trainer is using the lump-sum bidding model, this is the time to bid the construction. Before the actual bids are sent to the contractors who will compete for the job, the architect will develop the **construction documents** (American Institute of Architects n.d.). The construction documents are

Methods for Funding Public-Sector Sports Medicine Facilities

- Capital campaigns
- Bond sales
- Borrowing from endowment
- Commercial loans

highly detailed technical drawings that the contractors will need to determine a realistic estimate of construction costs. The construction documents are the drawings that the contractor will use to guide construction of the new sports medicine center.

The architect will then prepare and send a packet of **bidding documents** to acceptable contractors. The bidding documents include an invitation to bid, the bid form, and special instructions from the architect. The bidders must submit their bids within a specified time, and all bids are opened at the same time. Normally, administrators hire the contractor who submits the lowest bid. In many states, law requires public institutions to allow all qualified contractors to bid for new construction projects. In addition, a certain percentage of the construction budget might have to be reserved for contractors of historically underrepresented minority groups.

Step 8: Analyze Bids and Take Action

After the sealed bids have been opened, the planning team must carefully analyze each one. First, the athletic trainer–architect team must make sure that the information on the returned bids is consistent with the project described in the bidding documents. If a contractor changes any item of the project, producing a lower bid, and the change goes unnoticed, legal problems could result. Another reason to screen the bids carefully is to ensure that the costs quoted by the various contractors are somewhat consistent. If one contractor's quotation is significantly lower than all the others, the athletic trainer and architect should ask for an explanation. Obviously, the quality of the finished facility will suffer if the contractor cuts corners to secure the contract.

If the returned bids exceed the available funding, five possible courses of action can be pursued:

1. Negotiate a more cost-affordable price with those who supplied bids.
2. Delay the project until additional funds can be raised.
3. Modify the original plan to one that more closely fits the budget of the proposed bids.
4. Request a rebidding process and explain to the contractors that all bids are too high.
5. Cancel the proposed project.

Step 9: Begin Construction

This step is self-explanatory. After the contractor's bid has been accepted, the architect works with the athletic trainer's (or the institution's) attorney to draw up the construction contract. The architect will have access to several standardized contract forms for this purpose.

Step 10: Monitor Construction

Several people play important monitoring roles during construction. The first is the **general contractor**, who is responsible for coordinating the work of the various **subcontractors** and for ensuring the quality of their workmanship. The architect represents the athletic trainer or the institution and ensures that construction is proceeding according to the standards developed by the architect. If the workmanship does not comply with the standards enumerated in the contract and construction documents, the architect has the authority to reject the work (American Institute of Architects n.d.).

The athletic trainer and the planning committee have important roles to play during the construction phase. They should be present on the job site as often as possible to make sure that the design features agreed on are being implemented. The frequent presence of the athletic trainer at the construction site can ensure that the contractor and subcontractors are implementing the details as planned. The athletic trainer should know the sports medicine facility better than anyone else.

PEARLS OF MANAGEMENT

Log on to the Board of Certification website to launch a web-based facilities principles assessment.

If the athletic trainer suspects that the contractor or subcontractor is not properly implementing the architect's design, she should quickly inquire into the situation. The athletic trainer must address all concerns to the architect, not to the contractor or subcontractors. As the agent of the athletic trainer or the institution, the architect will investigate and mediate a solution to the problem. However, in some cases, the athletic trainer may need to communicate her concerns through an administrator at the institution, rather than directly to the architect.

Elements of Sports Medicine Facility Design

Athletic training facilities should meet the standards of any modern health care facility (Accreditation Association for Ambulatory Health Care n.d.). An athletic trainer must consider numerous elements when working with an architect to design a new sports medicine facility: size, location, ergonomics, electrical systems, plumbing systems, ventilation systems, lighting, flooring, line of sight, specialized-function areas, and accessibility (see figure 6.1). The section on developing schematics discussed size and space estimates. This section addresses the other eight design elements.

Location

A sports medicine center that is intended to serve the general population should be located near other health care providers. Patients will appreciate, for example, not having to travel far for X-ray or laboratory services. Proximity to referring physicians is another practical feature. The ideal location for a private sports medicine clinic is in a medical office building that houses other health services: physicians, laboratory, and X ray.

Having athletic facilities nearby is useful for observing a rehabilitating patient's functional capacity in running or other sport skills. If the clinic sees many student-athletes, a location close to the school makes travel convenient for students.

As mentioned earlier, school-based sports medicine centers for student-athletes are usually housed in large multipurpose athletic, physical education, or recreation buildings. The placement of the sports medicine center within the facility is an important decision. Facilities should be close to locker rooms, and if at all possible playing venues. Although some suggest that each locker room have direct access to the sports medicine center, problems of security and privacy may intervene. Athletes and other physically active patients should not have to cross through another activity area to reach the sports medicine

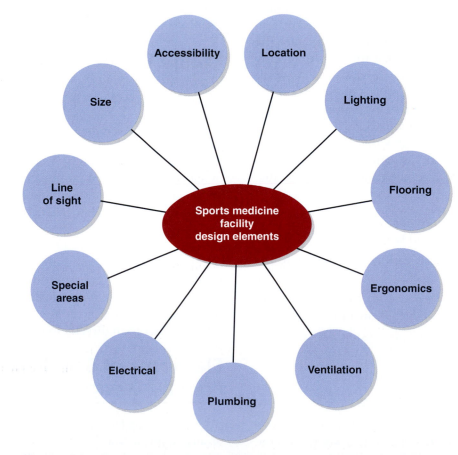

Figure 6.1 Elements in the design of sports medicine facilities.

center, although this may not always be possible if multiple teams use the same athletic training clinic. Efficiency and function are important when considering the ideal location.

Another consideration is access to the sports medicine center from the outside. An injured athlete should not have to walk or be carried through multiple doors—ideally, a door should lead directly from the outside playing fields into the sports medicine center. Wherever the center is located, it should have extra-wide doors that will accommodate two people assisting a nonambulatory athlete. (Wide doors will also be able to accommodate a stretcher, spine board, and gurney.) Some facilities also have doors wide enough to allow a small cart to be driven directly into the room.

In a multistory building, a ground-floor location is most accessible to clients who ambulate with difficulty. If the sports medicine center cannot be located on the ground floor, it should be close to an elevator.

Locating an institution's facilities for health services and sports medicine services adjacent to each other provides several advantages. First, cooperation can be enhanced if athletic trainers and other health professionals work together daily. Second, placing these two facilities next to each other means that they can share certain operations, often resulting in savings of time or money. For example, if health services and sports medicine services are adjacent, medical records can be stored in a single location (the health services file room). Assuming that procedures protecting student confidentiality are upheld (see chapter 7), medical records are thus more conveniently available and more complete.

Proximity among facilities also enhances the referral process. A student-athlete who reports to the athletic trainer with an illness can be referred immediately to health services (increasing the likelihood of compliance). Likewise, if a student who is not an athlete comes to health services with an orthopedic injury, the athletic training staff is readily available for consultation. Perhaps the ultimate argument for this arrangement, however, is financial—costs may decrease because facilities, supplies, and services need not be duplicated. If health services contains private examination rooms, they don't have to be included in the sports medicine center. Health services and the sports medicine center can share clerical support and insurance billing staff, as well as certain types of equipment and supplies, such as cast saws and suture kits. Locating health services adjacent to the sports medicine center also

eliminates the need for athletic trainers to store or dispense medications; health service personnel can more properly handle that function.

Although this concept generally functions well on small campuses, larger schools might find it difficult to implement because athletic facilities are typically located on the periphery of the campus, whereas student health services are more centrally located. However, a combined facility should be considered whenever possible in light of the many advantages.

Ergonomics

The International Ergonomics Association (IEA) defines **ergonomics** as the "scientific discipline concerned with the understanding of interactions among humans and other elements of a system, and the profession that applies theory, principles, data and methods to design in order to optimize human well-being and overall system performance." Ergonomists contribute to the design and evaluation of tasks, jobs, products, environments, and systems in order to make them compatible with the needs, abilities, and limitations of people (International Ergonomics Association n.d.).

The purpose of considering ergonomics in the design of a sports medicine center is to enable athletic trainers to work more productively, safely, and comfortably. Athletic trainers do not perform all their work in the sports medicine facility, of course. They perform a variety of tasks requiring a sound ergonomic basis on the field, in the gym, and in the office. Athletic trainers employed in industrial settings are frequently called on to suggest workstation design changes based on ergonomic problems. The discussion here is especially important for industrial settings. Many ergonomic considerations are beyond the scope of this text.

One of the prime tenets of ergonomic design is to consider the fact that each sports medicine facility is vastly different, and therefore the design of each should include spaces, furniture, and fixtures that are as adaptable as possible. Although other sections of this chapter cover some ergonomic considerations in the design of a sports medicine facility (see the sections on lighting and ventilation, for example), a few ergonomic design issues do not fit neatly into other sections and so are included here.

- *Tables.* Treatment and taping tables typically come in one height, even though the size of the athletic trainers using the tables varies greatly. Consider installing taping tables of different heights. If a taping counter is planned, consider three sections ranging in height from 32 to 40 inches (81-102 cm). The ideal treatment table, from an ergonomic standpoint, would be adjustable so that the user could raise or lower it depending on the task to be accomplished (just as a dentist's chair can be raised or lowered depending on the height of the patient and the procedure to be performed).

- *Shelves and cupboards.* Equipment should be stored on shelves or in cupboards that are easy to reach. It should not be stored on the floor where the athletic trainer will have to stoop to lift it. Some equipment can be hung on pegs fixed to the wall. Step stools should be available near the equipment storage area so that shorter athletic trainers can access the equipment without having to reach too far overhead. Heavier supplies should be stored on lower shelves with lighter items such as prewrap stored in higher shelves.

- *Stools.* Adjustable-height stools should be available at every treatment station so that athletic trainers can administer treatments from a sitting position if necessary. Adjustable-height stools are especially important when treatment tables are not adjustable, as most are not, and the athletic trainer is tall.

- *Carts and dollies.* Rolling carts, dollies, and laundry bins should be available so that athletic trainers can move equipment and supplies from one place to another with minimum effort.

Flooring

The kind of flooring installed in the athletic training facility has consequences for both the patients and the staff. The harder the surface, the more difficult it will be for staff to stand for long periods. Floors that have an excessively high or low coefficient of friction will present slipping or tripping hazards. Flooring can be expensive and should be carefully planned for in the budget. Similarly, the shelf life of flooring should not be overestimated: these facilities typically experience high volumes of traffic at all times of the year. And they may be host to mud, dirt, and other common elements of the outdoors brought in on athletes' or physically active patients' shoes.

In the athletic trainer's office, carpet is usually the most appropriate floor covering. Likewise, the best type of floor covering in the rehabilitation center is also carpeting. The largest part of the rehabilitation area might consist of nothing but carpeted floor to allow for a variety of functional and closed kinetic chain rehabilitation activities. When patients use dumbbells or other free weights, a carpeted floor absorbs the shock and noise more effectively when equipment is dropped. Specially designed rubber mats can also be used in areas that experience a lot of wear and tear caused by activities such as lifting free weights or jumping. Many sports medicine facilities incorporate a functional field or artificial turf area so that athletes can perform weight-bearing activities on a return-to-play surface. If the rehabilitation room is located anywhere other than the ground floor, the architect might need to specify a reinforced floor to support heavy equipment.

Line of Sight

Line of sight refers to the athletic trainer's ability to safely see patients at all times. Special consideration and attention should be paid to wet rooms and areas that house the ground tubs and pools. Glass windows should be installed in the walls to help keep patients in sight at all times when using such equipment. Mirrors on the walls of L-shaped facilities help with the line of sight around corners.

Electrical Systems

The electrical system is one of the few elements that, if improperly installed, could cause injury or death. Three-pronged hospital-grade plugs and electrical outlets (characterized by a green dot), along with circuit breakers, are useful in preventing damage to electrical equipment. Because electrical shock can cause severe burns or cardiac arrest, all electrical outlets in a sports medicine center should also be equipped with a **ground fault interrupter (GFI)**, designed to interrupt the flow of electricity if a surge of 5 milliamps or more is detected. Ground fault interrupters can act in as little as 0.025 seconds as a circuit breaker, limiting the total amount of energy flow through a body to a safe level (Knight and Draper 2012). Ground fault interrupters can be installed either as part of the electrical outlet or as part of the circuit breaker, and they are required in rooms in public and private buildings where water is present. Some medical and therapeutic durable equipment, such as isokinetic machines, may require a different voltage output (220 volts) rather than the typical 110 volts.

Another issue in electrical design is the location of electrical outlets. Given how much electrical technology is used today, a practical recommendation is to build in as many electrical outlets as possible in an effort to accommodate future needs. It is always easier and less expensive to build them in at the beginning than to find out later that more outlets are needed. This also gives the athletic trainer the flexibility to move equipment as the program changes. To reduce the probability of overload, a single circuit should service a limited number of modality outlets. The quantity will depend on the type and number of appliances that will be used simultaneously. Outlets can be placed within a support beam or on the floor if the open area is too large to permit use of wall-based outlets for equipment that is best located in the center of the open space.

Many sports medicine centers, especially those located in hospitals, have designed treatment stations with pull cords that patients can use to shut off electrical power. This feature is especially useful when patients' electrical stimulation treatments become painful. Rather than wait for the athletic trainer to cross the room to adjust the dosage, the patient can simply pull the cord and stop the flow of electricity to the modality. Athletic trainers can also choose to place remote power switches for hydrotherapy units in their offices to prevent accidental shock. An extension of this concept would be to have a master switch in the athletic trainer's office for every outlet to which a therapeutic modality is connected for rapid shutoff in case of emergency.

Keep in mind that some equipment problems are caused by operator error. All electrical equipment should be carefully checked during setup, and the operator's manual should be reviewed before service calls are initiated. However, equipment should be immediately removed from patient use in the case of electrical shock, a burning odor, or smoke coming from a device.

Plumbing Systems

Placement of water outlets and drains is an important consideration in the design of a sports medicine center. A mistake in the design of the plumbing system, which is usually installed inside walls and under floors, is expensive to correct.

Like the electrical system, plumbing systems should be designed to be easily expandable. As a sports medicine program grows and changes, the need for water or drainage in different parts of the facility might change as well. Outlets for both hot and cold water should be provided in every section of the sports medicine facility. Some of these outlets should drain into sinks, and others should be free standing to fill hydrotherapy tubs. Floor drains should be placed at several strategic points in the facility. The percentage of floor sloping should be evaluated by professionals in coordination with the athletic training staff who can convey the usage and likely displacement of water during the busiest times.

If the facility is to contain an ice machine, a separate cold-water line and floor drain should be provided for it. Whenever possible, the built-in drain of each hydrotherapy tank should connect directly to a dedicated floor drain. The drain faucet of tanks that use a pump drain should be connected to a **standpipe drain** by a hose or similar device to prevent splashing. In every case, a hydrotherapy tank should have an overflow prevention drain.

A plumbing contractor will be able to offer a variety of fixtures. **Plumbing fixtures** used in a sports medicine center can be relatively simple and inexpensive, but athletic trainers might find three exceptions desirable. The first is a **mixing valve**, which allows precise water temperature by combining hot and cold water and eliminates the need for separate controls. Mixing valves often have built-in thermometers and are especially useful for filling hydrotherapy tubs. Another plumbing enhancement athletic trainers might choose is a foot-pedal activator or touchless, automatic faucets for hand-washing stations. These devices are especially useful for athletic trainers who use massage and perform other activities in which their hands are covered with lotions, ointments, or similar products. Finally, the athletic trainer might choose to connect hydrotherapy tanks directly to the water source. The advantage of having a dedicated source of water for hydrotherapy is that accidental spills are much easier to prevent. On the other hand, using hoses to fill hydrotherapy tanks provides greater flexibility for each water outlet.

A common mistake is to pay a great deal of attention to designing the plumbing systems and then overlook associated accessories. For instance, built-in liquid soap dispensers and air hand drying stations next to hand-washing stations are extremely useful. Paper cup dispensers are desirable. The planning team could choose paper towel dispensers and wastepaper containers that are recessed into the wall—they're usually more expensive, but they save space and are more attractive. Finally, a drinking fountain will require a dedicated water line and drain and an electrical outlet so that the water can be chilled.

Planning for installation of plumbing systems should include consideration of areas such as bathrooms, physician examination room, changing and locker rooms, and possible drug-testing rooms or facilities. Each of these types of rooms would require a sink or shower area. Even minor renovations of health care spaces can result in substantial upgrades of mechanical, electrical, and plumbing systems (Kesler and Fagan 2005).

Ventilation Systems

Little has been written about the ventilation of sports medicine facilities. However, if a sports medicine center is improperly ventilated, working conditions can become extremely uncomfortable. The two most important ventilation concerns are temperature and humidity control. Because most athletic trainers do not possess sufficient knowledge of these controls, they should communicate early with administrators during the planning and budget phases and with the contractors during installation to ensure adequate temperature and humidity control within the environment.

A sports medicine center should have its own temperature control system in place. A common mistake in designing ventilation systems is to use a common temperature control for the sports medicine center and adjacent areas, such as locker rooms and shower areas. The result is that the sports medicine center is usually too warm to work comfortably in. If the sports medicine center has several rooms, it is optimal to have separate thermostats that can be operated with the most contemporary form of technology.

The other major ventilation concern is humidity. Excessive humidity not only diminishes comfort, but it also creates hygiene issues. Viruses, fungi, and bacteria survive more easily on moist surfaces than they do on dry ones. Areas where water is used extensively, such as the hydrotherapy section, should be equipped with exhaust fans that are strong enough to keep humidity to reasonable levels. This is especially important if glass walls separate the hydrotherapy section from the rest of the facility because high humidity levels in the hydrotherapy room may fog the glass.

Whether or not to provide air-conditioning is an important decision because it is expensive to install and use. In many areas of the United States, however, the temperature and humidity are so extreme at the times that the sports medicine center is used most heavily that air-conditioning is essential. Because air-conditioning cools the air by removing moisture, it is an important feature for both comfort and hygiene. Air-conditioning becomes even more

important as fall preseason practices start earlier in the year and many teams hold formal conditioning and youth sports camps during the summer.

Lighting

Adequate lighting is another critical element that requires proper planning in a sports medicine center design. How bright should the sports medicine center be? Common sense dictates that different sections of the sports medicine center have different illumination requirements. Areas devoted to taping, bandaging, and wound care require more lighting than storage or hydrotherapy areas do. The areas designated for physician examination and treatment of injured athletes and other patients probably require the most intense illumination. Floor lamps can supplement lighting in these areas to provide extra illumination for procedures such as wound debridement and suturing. It is also important to consider the overall location of the facility. Some locations are well suited to an athletic training facility with numerous windows that can provide natural lighting during the day, while other locations make windows inappropriate, thereby limiting their use. When planning to use windows for natural lighting, it is important to consider privacy issues that may be affected by who is able to view inside the athletic training facility.

In addition to artificial lighting, **natural lighting** from either skylights or windows, and light colors on reflective surfaces such as ceilings, walls, and floors, can significantly brighten a sports medicine center. The design of school sports medicine centers has traditionally lacked windows because of concerns about student-athletes' privacy. The sports medicine center, however, is not a locker room. All patients should be dressed properly when entering the facility, and they should be draped appropriately when receiving treatment. With natural lighting supplied by windows, appropriate drapery or blinds must still be considered for the purposes of patient confidentiality of care. In particular, when care is provided during evening hours when lights are on inside the facility, outsiders can see into rooms with ease. Even though patients are wearing proper dress, privacy of medical care must be considered. Windows that open can also provide additional ventilation and airflow when needed.

Specialized-Function Areas

Eight specialized-function areas are common to most sports medicine facilities: office, taping and bandaging, hydrotherapy, general treatment, rehabilitation, storage, lavatory and changing area, and private examination (see figure 6.2). Many factors determine how much space to devote to each of these functions, including the types and numbers of sports to be served, the number of athletes and other physically active patients to be served, the qualifications and expertise of the sports medicine staff, the operational budget, and the type of client to be served. See figures 6.3 through 6.6 for examples of how to arrange special-function areas for different types and sizes of programs.

Office

In most situations, the athletic trainer's office is located within the sports medicine facility. The athletic trainer's office should serve several purposes. First, it should serve as the central repository for all program records, including patients' medical files (unless they are kept in an adjacent health service records room or in an electronic database), budget information, correspondence, insurance information, product information, and educational materials for students and patients. The athletic trainer's office can also be used for private examinations (although this presents several problems; a separate private examination area is ideal) and counseling if space is limited or unavailable. Finally, the office serves as an administrative work area for the athletic trainer. Adequate office space should be available to accommodate all staff athletic trainers. A common

conference area within the office is a useful place for meetings or for students to do their work.

Several design features are important for the athletic trainer's office. First, the athletic trainer should have a clear view of the entire sports medicine facility from the office; windows should allow supervision of activities at all times. If the office must also serve as a private examination and consultation room, it must be equipped with an exam table and blinds for the windows. The office should contain a desk, filing cabinets, bookshelves, and a telephone. **Data ports** or secure Wi-Fi with adequate bandwidth (or both) should be included as well. The office should also have enough comfortable seating to accommodate several people at one time for those occasions when the athletic trainer must consult with patients, parents, coaches, physicians, and others in groups.

Taping and Bandaging

In school-based sports medicine centers, the taping and bandaging section is often one of the busiest, especially just before practices and games. For this reason, athletic trainers designing school sports medicine centers should carefully consider the location and space devoted to this function. Private and hospital-based sports medicine clinics generally perform much less taping and bandaging, so the area they devote to these needs is usually minimal.

Several design elements are important for a functional taping and bandaging area. First, it must

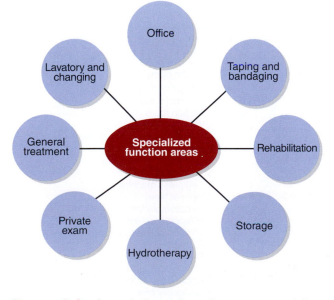

Figure 6.2 Specialized-function areas of the sports medicine center.

Figure 6.3 Floor plan for a small college sports medicine facility.

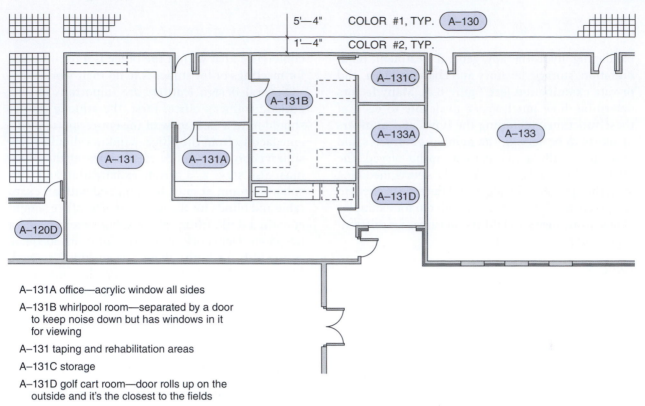

A–131A office—acrylic window all sides

A–131B whirlpool room—separated by a door to keep noise down but has windows in it for viewing

A–131 taping and rehabilitation areas

A–131C storage

A–131D golf cart room—door rolls up on the outside and it's the closest to the fields

A–133A not part of the athletic training room

Figure 6.4 Floor plan for a high school sports medicine facility.

Courtesy of Ann Arbor Pioneer High School, Lorin Cartwright.

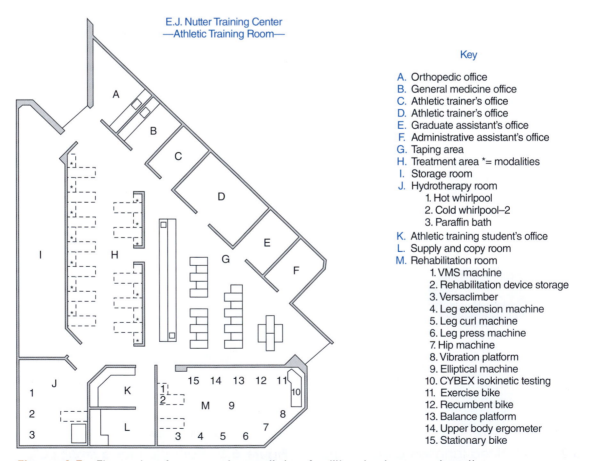

Figure 6.5 Floor plan for a sports medicine facility at a large university.

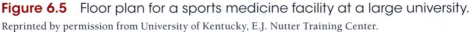

Reprinted by permission from University of Kentucky, E.J. Nutter Training Center.

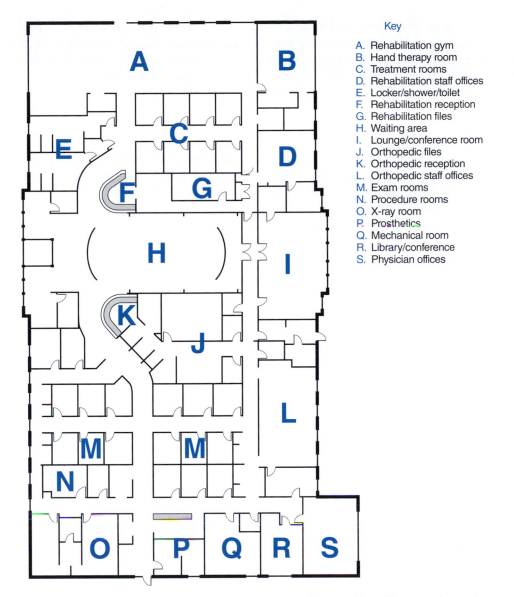

Key

A. Rehabilitation gym
B. Hand therapy room
C. Treatment rooms
D. Rehabilitation staff offices
E. Locker/shower/toilet
F. Rehabilitation reception
G. Rehabilitation files
H. Waiting area
I. Lounge/conference room
J. Orthopedic files
K. Orthopedic reception
L. Orthopedic staff offices
M. Exam rooms
N. Procedure rooms
O. X-ray room
P. Prosthetics
Q. Mechanical room
R. Library/conference
S. Physician offices

Figure 6.6 Floor plan for a combination orthopedic office and sports physical therapy clinic.

Reprinted with permission from Horizon View Development, L.L.C. Designed by Eckert/Wordell Architects, Kalamazoo, MI.

include an adequate number of taping stations. Taping stations can be individual tables or large platforms that accommodate several people at one time, and nowadays they can be custom designed to one's preference. Whichever arrangement is chosen, the taping table should be a minimum of 36 inches (91 cm) high, although some athletic trainers will be better served by taping tables that are shorter or taller. Athletic trainers should inquire about specific taping tables and stations early in the process to better plan for spacing needs.

Another important design element of the taping and bandaging area is adequate counter space. The counter should have an easily cleaned surface like Formica, should be large enough to allow easy access for all athletic trainers working in the area, and should have electrical outlets every 4 feet (1.2 m). Although the traditional placement of the counter is along a wall, an attractive alternative is an island counter in the middle of the taping and bandaging area—the island provides taping stations on both sides, allowing easy access for twice as many athletic trainers. The taping and bandaging area should include cupboards and drawers with locks for secure short-term storage of supplies needed routinely.

Finally, choosing the type of floor covering to use in the taping and bandaging area can be difficult. Both adhesive sprays and petroleum-based ointments can permanently stain carpeting and vinyl tile. For that reason, it might be wise to contract with a company that provides carpet runners for doorways and entrances. When the runners become soiled, the company will replace them with clean ones.

Hydrotherapy

The hydrotherapy section of the sports medicine center is the one specialized-function area that should be physically separated because of water spills and the noisy turbines used to power whirlpool baths. The ideal design would include a glass enclosure around the area, which will contain noise, heat, humidity, and accidental spilling or flooding while allowing the athletic trainer to monitor the activities from another section of the facility.

In addition to the sloped floor and expandable plumbing mentioned earlier, athletic trainers should consider other important features when planning the hydrotherapy area. Adequate space should be available for all equipment that uses water, including hydrotherapy tanks, steam pack units, ice machines, freezers, and paraffin baths. In school sports medicine centers, water coolers and portable ice chests are usually stored here as well. Although expensive to construct, operate, and maintain, multistation submersed whirlpools and two-lane training pools can be included in hydrotherapy areas. If so, plans must also include filtration units and water heaters. Ceramic tile similar to what is found in a shower room or toilet area should cover the floor of the hydrotherapy area. The walls can be constructed from cinder block if they are painted with a high-gloss epoxy paint that can be easily cleaned. Some athletic training clinics have purchased hot tubs made for personal home use because they can be maintained with chlorine and do not require frequent filling and draining like a typical therapeutic whirlpool. Some newer models also allow for cold or hot water immersion. From the outset, budgeting for hydrotherapy areas should take into consideration the cost of ongoing daily and long-term maintenance of the equipment being planned. In the absence of adequate budgeting for required maintenance, athletic trainers will need to modify their annual sports medicine program budgets to offset the costs incurred by the hydrotherapy equipment (Stiefel 2002).

General Treatment

The general treatment area usually contains treatment tables and electrotherapeutic equipment and is therefore one of the largest spaces in the facility. You can estimate the square footage, or area, needed for this space by determining the peak caseload at the busiest time of the day and estimating the number of treatment tables necessary to accommodate these patients simultaneously.

Allow approximately 30 inches (76 cm) between tables for placing three-shelved carts holding therapeutic modalities. Place an electrical outlet next to each treatment table. Provide a light immediately above each table, each with its own light switch. Make sure that at least some of the treatment tables have sliding drapes for privacy during treatment. Some treatment tables should be adjustable so that swollen extremities can be elevated. Treatment tables can double as storage cabinets if you fit them with cupboards, drawers, or shelves.

Materials for walls and floor coverings for this area should be light colored and easy to clean. Vinyl tile works well for this purpose, but it is slippery when wet. Carpet is difficult to clean, but provides a warmer, quieter atmosphere (see previous discussion of flooring ergonomics).

Rehabilitation

In most athletic training settings, the rehabilitation area is another section that requires a great deal of space; it might take up most of the space in private and hospital sports medicine clinics. A few commonly used pieces of equipment to rehabilitate injured physically active patients—isokinetic equipment, treatment and exercise tables, treadmills, upper and lower extremity ergometers, stair climbers, and isotonic weight machines—can easily fill a large area. In addition to the space for the equipment, adequate space must exist between exercise stations for safety purposes. Some athletic training clinics are intentionally positioned adjacent to the weight room so that the larger equipment can be housed in the weight room, saving space in the athletic training clinic.

The location of the rehabilitation area can be problematic. Most athletic trainers agree that it should not occupy the same space as the treatment or taping functions. Many athletic trainers have moved the rehabilitation function to a general-purpose weight training facility. Although this offers some advantages, exposing unsupervised patients to expensive and potentially harmful devices is not recommended. The best arrangement gives the rehabilitation area its own room within the confines of the sports medicine center, especially if the institution's weight training facility is nearby in the same building. This scheme allows for careful, supervised rehabilitation of injured physically active patients while maintaining a quiet atmosphere in the general treatment area. When these patients are ready to advance to heavier weights and general-purpose strengthening devices, they can go to the weight room.

Walls should be constructed of a material that allows insertion of hooks and screws so that rehabilitation tools can be stored by hanging them on the wall. A full-length mirror gives patients visual feedback when they perform rehabilitation exercises. The facility's ceiling height should always be considered in the early phases of planning based on the intended use of space. If the area will also encompass functional rehabilitation and sport-specific types of activities, a higher ceiling should be considered.

Storage

The storage area of the sports medicine center is commonly overlooked; administrators may believe that building a large, empty space is a waste of money. But this space for storing everyday items is important and should be included in the plans. Given the cost, several important considerations apply to storage rooms. The storage room should be located within the sports medicine center itself if possible. In addition, the closer the storage room is to the taping and bandaging section, the more convenient it will be for the athletic trainer to restock depleted expendable supplies. The storage room must remain cool and dry at all times. Many expendable supplies commonly used in sports medicine, especially adhesive tape, deteriorate in warm, humid environments. The storage room should have plenty of shelves and cupboards. To maximize storage space, shelving should be placed as high as possible; a ladder will enable access to lesser-used items. Access to the storage room should be strictly controlled to prevent unauthorized removal of supplies. Additionally, it is important to consider the pharmaceutical requirements that the storage room must meet. Storage rooms need to provide a secure environment for both prescription and nonprescription medications that are housed for athletes and patients. Prescription medications must be stored in compliance with state laws as described in chapter 14.

Lavatory and Changing Area

Although many older athletic training facilities lack a lavatory and changing area, this highly desirable feature is commonly included in newer facilities. This area can be designed to serve both the athletic training staff and the patients who use the sports medicine facility. It should include an accessible toilet and sink, along with a shower and lockers. The area should have a shelf for storing towels and a bin for disposal of soiled laundry. In some programs, this area may also be used during drug-testing procedures.

Private Examination

Many situations in sports medicine call for private examination of an injured client to preserve modesty or provide a calm environment. Although the private examination area of the sports medicine center does not need to be large, it should provide a comfortable environment for the client and the athletic trainer or physician. Private examination rooms should include an examination table, a mobile lamp, a sink for washing hands, and a counter and cupboards to hold commonly needed supplies. Any supplies or equipment that the team physician frequently uses should be readily available in the private examination room, as should gowns and drapes for clients. As already mentioned, the private examination room can be combined with the office if necessary.

Accessibility

Title III of the Americans with Disabilities Act of 1990 (ADA) "prohibits discrimination on the basis of disability by public accommodations and requires places of public accommodation and commercial facilities to be designed, constructed, and altered in compliance with the accessibility standards." The law applies to virtually every kind of facility, including public and private educational institutions, health care facilities, and other places of business. The ADA applies to all buildings, requiring access to people with disabilities except where such alterations would be structurally impractical. Common design elements that help ensure accessibility include ramps, special parking spaces, railings, modified door handles and automatic opening devices, elevators, lowered drinking fountains, and toilet stalls wide enough to accommodate a wheelchair. Architects, construction managers, facility designers, and building code officials all have training in the elements of ADA compliance. Working with a well-qualified architect who is sensitive to the needs of people with disabilities is the best way to ensure that the sports medicine facility will be able to serve a broad range of patients.

Traffic Patterns

Important to all of the areas previously discussed in the planning of a new facility is the overall traffic pattern. This refers to the number of people who will use the facility and, more specifically, the areas of the facility that will be used the most. Having a general knowledge and ability to predict traffic patterns will allow you to predict the rate of wear and tear in certain areas and structures. For example, knowing that the taping station will see high volumes of people daily lets you predict that the flooring in that area will wear down quickly and thus need to be replaced more frequently than flooring in other areas. Using additional runner-type industrial carpets would lengthen the life of the carpet in that area. The types of sports served and the gender of the athletes can also determine which services are more likely to be provided frequently and which pieces of equipment will undergo heavier use. It is also prudent to store the coolers and water bottles near the door so that water is not dripped across the room when they are taken in and out of the clinic.

KEY POINT

The Board of Certification (BOC) has developed a guiding document for athletic training facilities in an effort to standardize and promote appropriate compliance and regulation. The document can be accessed on the BOC website.

Marketing a Sports Medicine Facility and Practice

As a provider of health care services, the sports medicine program and its facility should strive to be recognized as an operation of high quality, appearance, and reputation. In a not-for-profit environment, such as most secondary schools, colleges, universities, and professional team settings, obtaining such status is often achieved simply through the quality of care and interpersonal skills. This is because the practitioners already have a customer base that intends to use their service, which is mostly free (excluding auxiliary consultations and services), is easily accessible, and is offered for the sole purpose of providing care for the athletes. The circumstances are entirely different in a for-profit program, such as a private practice sports medicine center. When your fiscal survival relies on a business model for

remuneration for services, you must successfully recruit a clientele base and provide a level of care and services that has all of the hallmarks of a thriving operation. One of the main tasks in operating a successful for-profit sports medicine program is planning and implementing a marketing strategy. Clover (1997) has outlined the following 11 critical elements that encompass a marketing strategy, and even though this list was developed more than 20 years ago, the principles still apply:

1. *Name.* The name of a business is important. Some names will be easier than others to market. For example, naming a facility using the owner's last name, such as Clover's Sports Medicine Center may make it easy to remember. However, if the owner's last name is difficult to pronounce or remember, it may not be as easy to market. Catchy logos, slogans, and colors are all part of the naming process that should be considered from a marketing perspective. Names should always be protected through copyright and trademark procedures. The following is a list of examples that an AT named Janet could consider for naming a sports medicine facility in Tampa, Florida:

   Owner's name: Janet's Sports Medicine Center

   Location: Tampa Sports Medicine Center

   Specialty identification: Sports Injuries Specialists

   Acronyms: Tampa Injury Specialists, TIS

   Naming a business is always a risky proposition and should be carefully thought out before planning formal operations. The name that is eventually chosen will be branded in such a way that every association with the business will link back to the name. Each of the options just listed for naming a business has strengths and weaknesses. Using a person's name may mean that developing a known identify around town will take time. However, if the person already has a reputation for expertise in sports medicine, a business title inclusive of the person's name will be beneficial. Use of a subspecialty term in the title to describe the type of expert services provided may draw the attention of clients with those injuries. However, it may give potential clients with other types of injuries the impression that the practice does not have expertise in other areas.

2. *The strategic planning team.* It is always helpful to gather the assistance of stakeholders who can offer objective viewpoints. Those developing

a marketing plan should consider including individuals who are viewed as stakeholders in various levels of the organization, although not all of them need to be employed by the business. Aside from clinicians employed by the business, area athletic directors, referring physicians, and others who are familiar with either the community or health care in general can offer significant support to your effort to achieve success.

3. *The decision-making team.* This team comprises a few key people who have the ability to extrapolate all of the input of a marketing plan and turn it into a long-term vision that can be implemented in a practical and cost-effective manner. If a decision-making team is too large, members may find it difficult to agree on a final plan.

4. *Environmental assessment.* An environmental assessment looks at both internal and external factors related to the marketing plan. Internal environmental factors include the organization's strengths and weaknesses, the types of services provided, staff skill sets, the geographical location of the business, financial status, and staff morale. External environmental factors are those controlled by people and forces outside of an organization. These may include, but are not limited to, consumer needs, competitors' strengths and weaknesses, third-party payer influences, referral patterns, and population and commercial business growth within the surrounding community.

5. *Market segmentation.* The total number of people in a surrounding area is not a good overall indicator of potential business. Instead, a marketing plan should be able to identify various segments of the population that need services and match the services offered to those in need. Specializing in youth sport injuries in a predominantly retirement-based community may not bode well for a business. Market segmentation is essentially about supply and demand.

6. *Objectives, strategies, and goals.* Establishing goals and objectives enables formulation of a process for the organization or business to follow in an effort to measure success. For a sports medicine marketing program, objectives that can be measured in terms of a time line, as well as quantitative and qualitative perspectives, are best suited to decision making.

7. *The marketing mix.* The marketing mix is the fun part of the plan. However, if it is not taken seriously and carefully thought out, it can turn into an overhead expense with no return on investment.

Marketing mix involves using products or gadgets to promote your sports medicine practice. There is much more to it than placing a logo on a T-shirt to promote a business. Price assessment, product durability and usage, locations, and forms of promotional advertising are all included in the marketing mix. Promotional ideas along with their strengths and weaknesses are listed in the following sidebars.

8. *Positioning.* Positioning is a simple yet daunting process to create a certain type of image or reputation. Positioning includes all thoughts at all times for the purpose of defining an end product that will be implemented within the overall marketing plan.

9. *Patient relations.* Patient relations is an ongoing process that involves more than good interpersonal exchanges with patients. Additional actions that have an effect on positive patient relations include timely responses to physician inquiries, a flexible schedule for patients, objective responses to complaints or concerns, and maintenance of short waiting room times.

10. *Finalization of plan and review.* Prior to the implementation of a marketing plan, the entire plan and its objectives should be reviewed with all stakeholders. This is important for ensuring that everyone involved has a clear understanding of the investment and expected return.

11. *Evaluation.* Periodic evaluation of the marketing plan should be performed and tracked to determine how all parts of the plan are working. Changes can be made if necessary based on findings from the evaluation that would have an effect on the plan as a whole.

Private Practice

Entrepreneurial athletic trainers who own their own business face additional considerations when planning a facility.

- *Business structure.* Health care providers understand that providing their services forms a business operation, and therefore, their business must operate under the legal structure typically defined by individual states. **Legal structure** is a process that regulates the business operations; identifies who the business owner is; and ensures a method for tax collection, employee wages and protection, and fair practice acts. Although individuals may own their own business as a self-proprietor, many register their business as a corporate entity. As a self-proprietor, one assumes all risk and liability associated with the business, and personal assets can be used against any debt or claim against the individual and the business. With corporate status, an individual becomes a corporate officer, and any claim against the business does not affect her personal assets. Different types of corporations involve various leadership and ownership structures.

- *Taxes and licenses.* All businesses must register with their state for a business license. In some locations, city or county business licenses (or both) are also required. Part of business license registration is a description of the types of services one provides. Health care-related services often fall under "professional regulation." Both state and federal registration of a business are required for the purpose of collecting governmental tax revenue. Various forms of taxes may need to be paid based on the type of tax structure, the number of employees one has hired, and the amount of claimed revenue versus expenses of the business operation. Incentives often

Ideas and Techniques to Promote and Advertise the Clinic

- Social media (e.g., Facebook, Twitter, Instagram)
- Digital marketing and targeting through search engines, eblasts, and so on
- Brochures
- Newsletters
- Educational pamphlets (e.g., what to do for a sprained ankle, how to access your medical group given the type of insurance you have)
- Direct mail (e.g., special educational programs coming up)
- Media exposure (e.g., well-written news releases about what the clinic is doing)
- Presentations to clients (e.g., physicians, coaches)
- Exhibits (e.g., at health fairs, road races)
- Special service events (e.g., chamber of commerce, Junior League)
- Speaker's bureau (e.g., being available to speak on sports medicine–related topics)
- Public education forums (e.g., bringing in athletic trainers from the area to go over face mask removal using the Trainer's Angel, doing a series on injury prevention for different sports, presenting a taping clinic)
- Phone book (advertisement should stand out on a crowded page and be found in all related parts of the phone book)
- Advertising in a program, magazine, or newspapers (e.g., information, reply mechanism)
- Cable television ad
- Radio (e.g., spot advertisement: "Snow report brought to you by . . .")
- Signs (e.g., at ball parks)
- Education (e.g., high school, adult learning, college, first aid training)
- Sponsorship of teams, individuals, athletic events
- Participation in athletic events (e.g., corporate challenge, road races)
- Establishing a tradition (e.g., all-star football game, scholarship)
- Vehicle advertising (e.g., signs on a company van)
- Receptions for physicians
- Barbecues for coaches
- Equipment demonstrations (e.g., types of knee braces, types of shoulder pads)
- Membership in athletic organizations (e.g., sports medicine consultant)
- Membership in local athletic groups (e.g., Chamber of Commerce, athletic council)

Reprinted from J. Konin, "Possible ideas and techniques to promote and advertise the clinic," in *Clinical athletic training* (Thorofare, NJ: Slack Inc., 1997), 116. By permission of J. Konin.

Strengths and Weaknesses of Advertisement and Promotional Approaches

Television (public or cable)

Strengths

- High impact
- Audience selectivity
- Schedule when needed
- Fast awareness
- Sponsorship available
- Merchandising possible
- Must be local

Weaknesses

- High production cost
- Uneven delivery by market
- Up-front commitment required
- If not a local station, may have no impact on area

Radio

Strength

- Low cost per contact
- Audience selectivity
- Schedule when needed
- Length can vary
- Personalities available

Weaknesses

- Nonintrusive medium
- Audience per spot small
- No visual impact
- High total cost for good reach

Social Media

Strengths

- Cost efficient
- Potentially large audience
- Very broad audience
- Popular mode of communication
- No waste
- Customer interaction

Weaknesses

- Restricted audiences
- Less formal
- Bad public relations spreads fast

Magazines

Strengths

- Audience selectivity
- Editorial association
- Long life
- Large audience per insert
- Excellent color
- Minimal waste
- Merchandising possible

Weaknesses

- Long lead time needed
- Readership accumulates slowly
- Uneven delivery by market
- Cost premiums for regional or demographic editions

Newspaper

Strengths

- Large audience
- Immediate reach
- Short lead time
- Market flexibility
- Good upscale coverage
- Information advertising

Weaknesses

- Difficult to target
- High waste
- High cost for national use
- Minimal positioning
- Clutter

Posters, Billboards

Strengths

- High reach
- High frequency of exposure
- Minimal waste
- Can localize
- Flexible scheduling

Weaknesses

- No depth of message
- High cost for national use
- Best positions already taken
- No audience selectivity
- Minimum one-month purchase

Reprinted from J. Konin, "Strengths and weaknesses of advertisement and promotional approaches," in *Clinical athletic training* (Thorofare, NJ: Slack Inc., 1997), 117. By permission of J. Konin.

are provided to small-business owners and minority business owners to encourage business growth and operations.

- *Business development team.* No athletic trainer should assume that he knows everything there is to know about starting a private sports medicine practice. Despite the fact that athletic trainers possess creative skills and a strong work ethic, some areas of business development require consultation with experts to ensure a better chance of success. Legal advice on real estate guidelines, business registrations, and contractual document preparation can be beneficial to the planning of a new facility. Accountants can be of assistance in determining what type of tax structure a business should operate under. The process of identifying a good location for building a facility can benefit from the expertise of a real estate agent.

- *Insurance.* Athletic trainers are familiar with liability insurance as health care providers. Operating a facility also entails risk; thus, risk management plans should include insurance coverage for the facility. This would include protection against adverse conditions related to the property or equipment and even financial loss that could ultimately lead to business failure. If the business will employ staff, health insurance offerings will become an expense that must be planned for. Additionally, if third-party reimbursement will be sought for services, contractual relationships will need to be formed with insurance companies.

Summary

Athletic trainers work in a variety of settings that often are already in place when they begin employment. However, it is not uncommon for an athletic trainer to be involved in the planning of a new facility or the renovation of an existing sports medicine center or space. The most effective sports medicine facility is one that has undergone comprehensive planning before building and development. The process of planning includes, but is not limited to, design elements such as spacing, lighting, and accessibility. It is important to consider optimal function in terms of the traffic that will characterize the facility and the use of equipment. Planning, designing, and constructing a sports medicine center will involve the collaboration of internal and external stakeholders and contractors, as well as financial planning. Once a sports medicine center is built and ready for use, key factors in promoting and marketing the facility will be considered.

Learning Aids

Case Study 1

Deanna is the athletic trainer for a large high school in Wisconsin that offers 20 sports for 750 student-athletes. The voters of the school district recently approved a bond issue to build a new $60 million high school. The planning committee asked Deanna to meet with the architect to discuss her ideas for the new athletic training room. Before the meeting, Deanna carefully considered the features she wanted to see incorporated into the new facility. She drew a sketch of the layout she desired and made a list of all the design features she wanted, including

- total size of 2,500 square feet (232 sq m);
- separate but connected rooms for taping, treatment, rehabilitation, office, storage, and private examination;
- a hanging ceiling with acoustical tiles to reduce noise;
- one treatment and taping table for every 10 athletes she would have to service during peak service hours;
- floor coverings of vinyl tile (for the taping, treatment, and storage areas), ceramic tile (for the hydrotherapy area), and carpeting (for the office and private examination room); and
- air-conditioning, with separate thermostats for each of the six rooms.

After considering Deanna's suggestions and attempting to incorporate them into the overall design of the athletic and physical education portion of the building, the architect informed her that the new sports medicine center was too expensive as proposed and that they would have to reduce its cost by one-third.

Questions for Analysis

1. Did Deanna employ the proper planning process when developing her ideas for the new athletic training room? What should she have done differently? How could she build a stronger case for her ideas?
2. What additional features should Deanna include in her list? How can she justify these features?
3. Which features should Deanna modify or eliminate to meet the architect's requirement?
4. Place yourself in Deanna's position and produce your own schematic drawing of the athletic training room you would propose for the new high school. Justify each of the features that you would include.

Case Study 2

Russ operates a successful seven-year-old physical therapy and sports medicine practice. His caseload nearly doubled when three new orthopedic surgeons moved into town a couple of years ago. When the local high school proposed a contractual relationship in which Russ would provide athletic training services for a fee plus referrals, he decided the time had come to expand out of his rented, cramped facility into his own building. Russ consulted a friend who had recently built an auto parts store for advice about hiring an architect. "I know just the architect you want," his friend told him. "He did a great job for me, and I'm sure you'll like him." Russ decided to take his friend's advice, and he made an appointment to see the architect. When they met a couple of weeks later, Russ was pleased with his friend's advice. The architect listened carefully to Russ' ideas and offered many helpful suggestions that Russ had not considered. Toward the end of the meeting Russ asked the architect how he should go about locating a contractor to build the new clinic. "You wouldn't necessarily have to find anyone," the architect replied. "My firm could coordinate the construction internally. You'd only have to deal with one person, and we could probably speed the whole construction process up quite a bit." Russ decided he liked the idea, and several weeks later, after reviewing the project with his attorney and a loan officer from the bank, he signed a design–build contract with the architect's firm.

Questions for Analysis

1. What advantages will Russ have in owning his building? What disadvantages?
2. Did Russ make mistakes in hiring an architect? What could he have done to avoid those mistakes?
3. Russ chose to use the design–build model for developing his new building. Was this a wise decision? What kinds of problems is he likely to encounter? What advantages will he realize?
4. What factors should Russ consider in the location of his new practice?

Case Study 3

Following the first month at your new job at Ramo Sports Medicine Clinic, the owner, Mr. Ramo, has asked you to lead a team of employees to develop a new and innovative comprehensive marketing plan. The major goal is to take advantage of the skills and expertise of the staff clinicians and increase the number of clients who would seek Ramo Sports Medicine Clinic for rehabilitation. All of the clinicians have an interest in manual therapy skills and injury prevention methods.

Mr. Ramo has annually attempted to reignite his staff's enthusiasm toward marketing efforts. However, he believes that the majority of them have a greater interest in simply treating patients, and that they feel the business side of marketing the clinic is not their responsibility. Knowing this, your task is to propose a plan that is inclusive of the staff yet isn't entirely reliant on their efforts.

While Mr. Ramo is not paying you additional money for your role of coordinating the marketing plan, he has agreed to release you from 5 hours per week of treating patients. He has not informed you of any budget limitations; all he said was that he wanted you to keep the overhead costs within reason and create a financial plan that would demonstrate how your return on investment will cover all of the marketing costs.

Questions for Analysis

1. What challenges will you have marketing the name of the clinic? With respect to positioning, what type of information would you need to gather before making suggestions regarding how the clinic should be portrayed by the community?

2. How would you plan to incorporate the ideas and input of the current staff?

3. Which key stakeholders within the community should you consider using in an advising capacity?

4. If Mr. Ramo informs you during your planning process that he has decided to allot you a total of $10,000 for marketing expenses, which can be spent over the course of six months, in what ways do you think it would be best to promote the clinic?

5. Based on your choices for promoting the clinic, what methods would you put into place to measure the success or failure of the marketing efforts?

Key Concepts and Review

Understand and defend the importance of the design phase in planning and constructing new sports medicine facilities.

The design and construction of new sports medicine facilities is a task that athletic trainers carry out infrequently but is expensive and important. It is at the design stage of such projects that athletic trainers can exert the greatest influence over the final product. Mistakes during the design phase will increase the facility's cost or decrease its function.

Understand the facility design and construction process in sports medicine settings.

Most athletic trainers will work with planning committees consisting of program specialists and high-level administrators to design a sports medicine center. The design process involves 10 steps: assessing needs, approving the project, selecting a construction model, selecting an architect, developing schematic drawings, securing funding, bidding the construction, analyzing bids and reacting to them, commencing construction, and monitoring construction.

Understand the common design elements of a well-planned sports medicine facility.

Eleven factors must be considered in the design of a sports medicine center: size, location, ergonomics, electrical systems, plumbing systems, ventilation systems, lighting, flooring, line of sight, specialized-function areas, and accessibility.

Describe the sports medicine facility in terms of its specialized-function areas.

The specialized-function areas of most sports medicine facilities include an office; areas for taping and bandaging, rehabilitation, general treatment, hydrotherapy, storage, and lavatory and changing; and a room for private examination of patients.

Discuss principles associated with marketing a sports medicine facility and practice.

Principles associated with marketing a sports medicine facility and practice include the following: establishing a name; forming a strategic planning team; forming a decision-making team; performing an environmental assessment; assessing market segmentation; developing objectives, strategies and goals; identifying the marketing mix; determining positioning; establishing patient relations; finalizing a plan and reviewing it; and performing periodic evaluations.

Information Management

Objectives

After reading this chapter, you should be able to do the following:

- Understand the importance of documentation as part of a complete information management system in sports medicine.

- Understand and describe the different methods of athletic injury and treatment documentation.

- Understand and describe the different types of information to be managed in a typical sports medicine program.

Most athletic trainers perceive their primary mission as providing high-quality health care to injured student-athletes and physically active clients. This chapter provides athletic trainers with the basics on information management in the athletic health care setting. We are working in an information society in which athletic trainers will increasingly be expected to be effective managers of information. The rapid pace at which technology changes and the nature of a litigious society require athletic trainers to be meticulous consumers of information related to their professional responsibilities.

As health care professionals, we do not have the luxury of deciding whether or not we will manage information. The question is not "Will I choose to manage information and communicate effectively?" but rather "What skills and tools do I need to manage information and communicate effectively?" For many reasons, athletic trainers are expected to document every patient care activity and the response to it. Athletic trainers must gather and disseminate the information necessary to accomplish a variety of goals, including improvement of patient care, professional development, and improvement in education and counseling. Finally, athletic trainers are increasingly expected to be competent leaders of the sports medicine programs in their institutions. Athletic trainers who lack the information management skills necessary to assume these leadership positions will quickly become frustrated. Their jobs are likely to be characterized more by problems than by creative solutions.

Why Document?

Although documentation is only one of the information management tasks that athletic trainers must accomplish, it is common to all employment settings. Why is this skill so important? Why should busy athletic trainers concern themselves as much as they do with this task? There are many reasons.

1. *Legal protection.* Medical documentation helps protect the legal rights of the physically active patient, the athletic trainer, and the employer by providing a written record of the care that the athletic trainer provided. Medical records are often the only defense that athletic trainers have when aggrieved patients take legal action. The adage "If it isn't written down, it didn't happen" is an increasingly appropriate guiding principle for all athletic trainers (Panettieri 2000).

2. *Memory aid.* Medical documentation acts as a memory aid for athletic trainers and other professionals involved in the care of injured athletes and other physically active patients. Human memory is a poor substitute for accurate recording of medical facts, especially because a patient's medical record might not need to be referred to for months or even years.

3. *Legal requirements.* In many cases, the law requires medical documentation. For example, athletic trainers in professional sports are required to document player injuries for the Occupational Safety and Health Administration (OSHA). Athletic trainers in various practice settings might be required to provide medical documentation for legally mandated workers' compensation insurance. Most state practice acts also require athletic trainers to maintain appropriate documentation.

4. *Professional standards.* Medical documentation is required to meet professional **standards of practice**. The Board of Certification (BOC) Standards of Professional Practice requires documentation of physician referral, initial evaluation and assessment, treatments, and dates of follow-up care for all athletes cared for in a service program typical of most educational settings. The requirements for athletic trainers working in direct service programs, typically in sports medicine clinics, are more rigorous. Besides meeting the service program standards, an athletic trainer in this setting must provide a program plan with estimated length, methods, results, revisions, and a discontinuation or discharge assessment and summary. Other professional organizations follow different documentation standards. For example, the Joint Commission publishes minimum standards for health care documentation that apply to athletic trainers who work in hospitals and similar health care institutions (Joint Commission 2010). Furthermore, professional associations like the National Athletic Trainers' Association (NATA) publish many consensus and position statements that identify professional standards of care for given circumstances (e.g., emergency action planning, lightning safety) that require specific components of documentation.

5. *Improved communication.* Medical documentation improves the quality of communication among the various professionals involved with the patient's case (Kettenbach 2003; Konin and Frederick 2018). Often, the only communication an athletic trainer has with the team or family physician is in writing. If the quality of the documentation is poor, either in content or in writing style, misunderstandings can result between athletic trainer and physician. Additionally, **standing orders** should be established between the directing physician and the athletic trainer for interventions necessary in the absence of the physician being on-site or in direct communication with the athletic trainer. By definition, a standing order is when a physician provides operational directions in writing for an athletic trainer to adhere to (Konin and Neal 2017).

6. *Insurance requirements.* Reimbursement decisions by third-party payers, such as insurance companies and health maintenance organizations, are based on medical documentation. This rationale is especially relevant for private or hospital-based sports medicine clinics, but it can also be important in professional, high school, and college sports medicine programs.

7. *Discharge decisions.* Medical documentation should be part of the basis for deciding when to discharge a patient from an athletic trainer's care (Kettenbach 2003; Konin and Frederick 2018). The medical record should act as a map to guide a reader unfamiliar with the case through the entire injury, treatment, and rehabilitation process. The reader, whether a physician, athletic trainer, or physical therapist, should be able to determine by reading the record whether the patient is ready to be discharged.

8. *Improved care.* When properly organized, medical documentation helps direct the athletic trainer to deliver better care. Well-written and well-organized medical documentation should serve as a tool for problem solving in difficult cases (Makoul, Curry, and Tang 2001).

9. *Injury surveillance.* Thorough documentation allows an athletic trainer to review medical records and tally findings as they relate to the types of injuries reported, sports associated with more injuries, body parts injured most, and many other indicators of trends in injury incidence and intervention.

10. *Outcomes assessment.* As discussed in chapter 3, the formal assessment of outcomes plays a critical role in determining one's effectiveness. Effective documentation can be designed to serve as a vehicle for assessing the interventions by athletic trainers, including the effectiveness of sports safety equipment (Hrysomallis and Morrison 1997).

PEARLS OF MANAGEMENT

Athletic trainers should refer to the most current best practices for documentation established by NATA. For the complete text of the BOC *Standards of Professional Practice,* visit its website. For the Joint Commission standards related to documentation, visit its website.

Medical documentation forms the raw material for program quality assessment. An athletic trainer should set both short- and long-term goals for the care of every injured patient. If the medical record shows care inconsistent with these goals, athletic trainers should be concerned that injured athletes and other physically active patients are being discharged without receiving all the care they need to function competitively.

Two Kinds of Information

Athletic trainers must differentiate between medical records and program administration records. The two types of records are separate entities and, with a few exceptions, little overlap should occur between them.

KEY POINT

Athletic trainers must manage two kinds of information: medical records and program administration records. Each is produced, maintained, and disseminated in different ways.

Medical Records

A patient's medical record is a written outline of her health history during the time she was under an athletic trainer's care. Medical records are patient specific, and only data that relate directly to the patient's health should be included. Information not related to health, such as news clippings or academic information, has no place in the medical record and should be stored elsewhere. Regardless of whether medical records are stored in written or electronic format, everyone should follow certain guidelines to minimize risk and maximize documentation effectiveness. The following are guidelines for written medical records (Konin and Frederick 2018):

- Write legibly or print neatly. The record must be readable.
- Use permanent ink (appropriate ink color depends on hospital policy).
- Black ink is preferred for clarity when copying.
- For every entry, identify the time and date, sign it, and provide your title.
- Describe the care provided and the patient's response.

- Describe findings objectively (that is, in terms of behaviors).
- Write entries in consecutive and chronological order with no skipped lines or gaps.
- Write entries as soon as possible after care is provided.
- Be factual and specific.
- Use patient (or family or caregiver) quotes.
- Document patient complaints or needs and their resolution.
- Use only standard and accepted abbreviations.
- Chart only the care that you provided.
- Promptly document a change in the patient's condition and the actions taken based on that change.
- Write the patient's, family's, or caregiver's response to teaching.
- If you make an error, cross out, initial, and date.
- With electronic records, only view those you have the appropriate rights to view.
- Do not give out your password or leave a medical record open when not attending.
- Be sure to log out of all electronic medical records (EMR) as soon as you are finished with a patient's record.
- Errors can be corrected in electronic medical records because they are time stamped.

When documenting for medical records purposes, athletic trainers should work closely with their administration and legal advisors to determine the extent to which patient encounters should be documented. By definition, a **patient encounter** is any interaction that an athletic trainer has with a patient that is related to that patient's medical history. This could include an actual assessment, treatment intervention, or consultative advice. It is expected that athletic trainers will document formal injury assessments and daily rehabilitation sessions. Many athletic trainers, however, do not document every ankle that is taped before a team practice, every gauze pad that is given out for a small cut, a warning of side effects while preparing to deliver an ultrasound treatment, or even a conversation that may occur in the hallway regarding how one should elevate a recently swollen knee. However, each of these situations, and many others, would by definition constitute a patient encounter, and could potentially result in an adverse outcome. An adverse outcome absent appropriate documentation places the athletic trainer at higher risk of malpractice. Identifying what is reasonable and expected to be documented should be established and placed in writing as part of a policy and procedure for every athletic training setting.

Where and how should medical records be stored? The answer, of course, depends on the environment in which the sports medicine program operates. It also depends on whether we are referring to paper or electronic medical records. Two principles are fundamental:

1. The athletic trainer must be able to access medical records easily at the time they are most needed—when the injured athlete or physically active patient is present in the sports medicine facility.

2. Medical record storage should be centralized to the greatest extent possible so that all those with a need to access the records are able to do so.

These two principles can be difficult to reconcile in certain environments. For example, a university sports medicine program might operate several facilities on a campus covering a large geographic area. Similarly, a hospital-owned satellite sports medicine clinic might be part of a larger rehabilitation services department but be physically located many miles from the hospital. How can a university athletic trainer working in an arena have immediate access to a basketball player's medical record when the files are maintained in the central athletic training room in the stadium? How can an athletic trainer in a sports medicine clinic access his patient's records when they are maintained in the central records depository of the hospital 5 miles (8 km) across town? Regardless of how these challenges are overcome, privacy of information should always be considered and medical records should be stored securely, which includes locking file cabinets and using secure passwords for electronic records. These remain important considerations for programs using written medical records in part or full.

A more common approach to medical records is electronic record keeping. Various formats exist that must be compliant with the Health Insurance Portability and Accountability Act of 1996 (HIPAA) and be secure with proper encryption. Files are maintained in a computer database that anyone with authorization can access from computers linked to the central computer network. Entries into the record are made in one of three ways:

1. Dictated directly into the system through telephone links or by voice recognition software from one of the computers linked to the records network.
2. Entered into existing electronic forms built into the computer database.
3. Scanned into the medical record. (This is most applicable to records that do not lend themselves to either of the previous methods, such as communications from physicians.)

The advantage of electronic medical records is that authorized users can easily access records from a variety of locations. More and more software programs are being developed to meet the specific needs of the athletic trainer. These systems also have disadvantages. They can be expensive to operate and maintain through regular system upgrades. Despite the fact that the electronic medical record is becoming more of the accepted norm, computer technology is evolving at such a rapid pace that systems quickly become obsolete. Another concern is that computerized medical records require scrupulous attention to security measures. The confidentiality of this information is only as safe as the systems designed to prevent unauthorized access. Finally, computerized record keeping has the potential to decrease the quality of athletic trainer–patient interaction. The athletic trainer with a file folder in his hands can easily review a patient's history while asking questions regarding the patient's current complaint. This discussion is more difficult when the medical information is stored on a computer in another part of the room or in the athletic trainer's office.

Regardless of the type of medical records used, the information they should contain is the same. Examples of the types of information contained in the medical record follow.

Physical Examination Forms

The physical examination results (see chapter 13 for more comprehensive detail) should come first in the medical record. The physical exam normally occurs first chronologically, and the results can be a quick reference for athletic trainers or physicians. Some states mandate the use of specific physical examination forms for high school student-athletes. In other states and settings, athletic trainers can choose from a wide variety of forms. The form chosen should call for the following information:

- Personal data (e.g., name, address, date of birth, e-mail, cell phone)
- Health history (past and current, family)
- Vital signs
- Physician's review of systems
- Medications
- Special procedures (e.g., blood and urine analyses, X rays, echocardiograms)
- Functional and special tests (e.g., joint strength, aerobic capacity, neurocognitive tests)
- Statement of clearance signed and dated

Injury Evaluation and Treatment Forms

Injury evaluation and treatment records should provide a concise account of the athlete's or physically active patient's progress from the time of injury until the time of discharge. These forms often constitute the bulk of the medical record. Although many athletic trainers maintain separate records of injury evaluations and treatments, each treatment should be easily linked to a documented injury. Athletic trainers can choose from five methods for documenting injury evaluation and treatment data. Keep in mind that historically, many athletic trainers have only followed the SOAP note format (described later), despite the multiple options for documenting. Additionally, electronic documentation prompts data input according to the software's fields and screens, not necessarily according to a specific documentation style. Athletic trainers should become familiar with a variety of styles of writing because software programs they learned as a student or in a job may be specific to that setting (Konin and Frederick 2018).

Problem-Oriented Medical Record (POMR)
The **problem-oriented medical record (POMR)** is a system of medical record keeping that organizes information around the physically active patient's specific complaints and has been shown to increase the quality of note documentation (Mehta et al. 2016). A cover sheet in the POMR summarizes the patient's past medical, social, and family history, as well as personal habits that might affect the patient's health. A list of the patient's problems, along with a brief description of the plans implemented to ameliorate those problems, is also on the POMR cover sheet (see figure 7.1).

PROBLEM-ORIENTED MEDICAL RECORD COVER SHEET

Database

Past Medical Hx.	Family Hx.
Social Hx.	Habits Tobacco: Alcohol: Drugs: Seat belts: Exercise: Nutrition:

Problems	Dates											
1												
2												
3												
4												

Plans	Dates											
1												
2												
3												
4												

Follow-up: See SOAP notes in record.

Figure 7.1 Cover page for problem-oriented medical record.

Another important component of the POMR is the **SOAP note** (see figure 7.2). The POMR cover sheet should reference each SOAP note. *SOAP* is an acronym for the following documentation parameters:

S: *Subjective evaluation of the patient's problem.* The subjective portion relates to how the patient conveys symptoms. It would include recording the patient's statement "My right knee popped and gave out." The subjective portion may also reflect statements of others who may have seen an injury occur.

O: *Objective evaluation of the patient's problem.* The objective portion of the evaluation includes physical data observed and measured by the athletic trainer during evaluation. It would relate information such as the presence of intra-articular effusion, 2+ Lachmann sign, and AROM –15 degrees in extension.

A: *Assessment of the patient's problem.* Assessment is the athletic trainer's judgment and professional opinion of the nature of the problem (i.e., their diagnosis) based on the subjective and objective evidence. Using the same knee injury case, a reasonable assessment of the problem would be internal derangement of the right knee with probable anterior cruciate ligament disruption. Statements of both short- and long-term goals for the athlete or physically active patient should be included for quality assurance.

P: *Plan of action that the athletic trainer will implement to resolve the problem.* This section should emphasize specific treatment interventions to be performed, as well as identify precautions or contraindications for future clinicians to adhere to. The plan may also include statements regarding interval progressions.

Focus Charting Focus charting is a less cumbersome alternative to the POMR medical record-keeping method and was first described and used in the nursing profession (Lampe 1997, Wolters Kluwer Health 2008). Typical focus-charting forms

INDIVIDUAL INJURY EVALUATION AND TREATMENT RECORD

Name: Jones, Mike   **Sport:** Basketball   **Body part:** R-ankle

Date injury occurred: 2/5/18   **Date injury reported:** 2/6/18

Primary complaint: R-ankle pain   **Secondary complaint:** None

Subjective data: Pt. inverted R-ankle while playing basketball. Reports "a loud snap." No previous hx. of ankle injury. Otherwise normal medical hx. Pain w/ walking is 5/10. Pain at rest is 3/10. Pain to palpation over the ant. talofibular ligament. No other bony or soft tissue tenderness noted.

Objective data: Moderate swelling over lateral malleolus. No discoloration or deformity. Ankle is warm to touch. Lacks 5 deg dorsiflexion and 10 deg plantar flexion in both AROM and PROM compared to L-ankle. Strength is 4+/5 for DF, PF, Inv. & Ev. compared to 5/5 for L-ankle. Anterior drawer test is remarkably positive w/ mushy end point. Talar tilt test equivocal due to swelling. Neg. Kleiger's test. Pt. walks w/ a noticeable limp and cannot bear wt. on the R-foot w/out assistance. Applied an ice wrap for 20 minutes. Issued compression sleeve and ankle brace. Fitted crutches and provided instruction in crutch walking. Educated pt. on RICE techniques for home program. Provided pt. w/ ankle home care brochure. Pt. indicated he understood instructions.

Assessment: Probable 3° ATF sprain

Goals: Decrease pain, decrease swelling, protect from weight bearing

Plan: Will refer to Dr. Smith. Appt. arranged for 3:00 p.m. today. Continue to use ice bag and ace wrap for 20 minutes every 2-3 hours, a compression sleeve, and ankle brace. Continue to keep elevated when possible, wear compression sleeve and ankle brace except when icing, and remain non-weight bearing for home program.

Evaluator's signature: David Black

Date	Treatment and progress
2/6/18	Ice bag with ace wrap × 20 min. Instructions for home care program. Crutches w/ instructions. Compression sleeve and ankle brace. Pt. tolerated tx. well. Pain at rest 2/10. Swelling reduced. DB

Figure 7.2 Sample evaluation and treatment form using SOAP note format.

list pertinent data about the injury in the first column, describe the action the athletic trainer will take in response in the second column, and present the response to the athletic trainer's action plan in the third column (see figure 7.3). As in all other forms of medical charting, each entry should be signed and dated, and time notations should be entered if appropriate.

Charting by Exception   Charting by exception, as its name implies, is a method in which only patient responses that vary from predefined norms

SPORTS MEDICINE FOCUS CHART

Name: Jones, Mike		Sport: Basketball	
Date	Data	Action	Response
2/6/18	Probable 3° R. ATF sprain	RICE × 20 min. Compression sleeve, ankle brace, crutches issued.	Pain decreased to 2/10. Patient understood home care instructions.
2/7/18	3° R. ATF sprain	Cold whirlpool with AROM × 20 min. Form walking × 10 min. JOBST compression pump × 30 min.	Decreased limp with walking. Increased DF ROM to 5°.
2/8/18	3° R. ATF sprain	Cold whirlpool with AROM × 20 min. BAPS in PE in seated position. JOBST compression pump × 30 min.	Discarded crutches. Swelling reduced to minimal level. PF/DF ROM equal to L. ankle.

Figure 7.3 Sample focus chart for use in recording injuries (data), treatments (action), and progress (response).

are noted on the record (Murphy and Burke 1990, Kerr 2013). This method was also first described in the nursing profession, used by surgical nurses in an effort to make record keeping more efficient and less time-consuming. Although charting by exception is inappropriate for recording an initial injury evaluation, it has many potential uses for recording treatments and rehabilitation. This method, however, requires maintaining tightly controlled and frequently monitored treatment protocols. Another concern with using this type of documentation is that it lacks the level of detail that is often needed for liability purposes.

Computerized Documentation The use of computers for keeping sports medicine records in athletic training settings was described as early as 1982 (Abdenour 1982), and the products available to athletic trainers have been increasing in number and utility ever since. As the power and capacity of computers have increased and their price has decreased, athletic trainers have gradually shifted from using large, centralized mainframe computers toward using stand-alone and networked personal computers. Most recently, iPads, tablets, smartphones, and other devices have been used to assist with documentation. While these devices make electronic documentation of medical record information more practical, arrangements for proper storage, transmission, and legal privacy protection must be in place before implementing their use in any circumstance.

Athletic trainers see computerized record keeping as a way to decrease time spent documenting athletic injuries and treatments, thereby increasing time available for hands-on care of injured patients. The switch to a computerized system of medical record keeping will probably result in an initial increase in time spent on record keeping. Athletic trainers will need time to learn to use the computer software. In addition, record keeping and procedural changes will probably have to occur to adapt to the new technology, not to mention upgrades, potential transitions from one software program to another, and integration of external documents (Allan and Englebright 2000).

Another potential problem of computerized records is maintaining confidentiality. Safeguarding digitally stored data is more difficult than safeguarding data on paper in locked file cabinets. The use of passwords can sometimes slow unauthorized retrieval of medical records, but thwarting a motivated computer hacker is extremely difficult. Finally, depending on the limitations of the computer software, computerized record keeping can limit the athletic trainer's ability to describe the case as fully as might be desirable. An industry standard is to keep files under two locks, such as a password-protected laptop in a locked office. This becomes more challenging with portable and handheld devices, so there should be one password or fingerprint to open the device and a second password to enter the software. Passwords protecting electronic medical records should be strong (including numbers and symbols), changed regularly, and not used for other accounts such as personal e-mail accounts.

Nevertheless, athletic trainers should welcome the computer as a tool for effective and efficient medical record keeping in sports medicine. Computers allow athletic trainers to retrieve only those parts of the medical record desired for a specific purpose—we no longer need to search physically through a 100-page medical record for a single entry. Nonprofessional clerical staff can perform some of the data entry, freeing the athletic trainer to spend more time with injured athletes and other physically active patients. This is important because all patient-related interactions should be documented to include all preventive and therapeutic taping procedures (Lam et al. 2016). Athletic trainers can pull information from many individual medical records for writing reports. By using this feature, they can quickly prepare year-end injury and treatment summaries that used to take weeks to complete.

When planning to incorporate an electronic documentation system for medical records, additional considerations should be taken into account. First, what is the life expectancy of the software program? Will it require upgrades anytime soon? How frequent are the upgrades, and will they be provided at no cost or will they carry additional fees? Some software programs can be purchased at a lower cost for smaller facilities that have a limited number of users and needs, while other packages can save larger institutions money by allowing for an unlimited number of users and all functions for a single package price. Second, institutional policies or procedures may exist regarding the addition of software to a network or computer. The athletic trainer should always consult with the information technology department to seek its expertise in purchasing and installing a new software program and to be sure the software meets security guidelines.

Although a few institutions may use their own custom-designed electronic medical records for computerized documentation, the majority of athletic training settings purchase a commercially established program. In doing so, individuals may become comfortable with a single program or system and benefit from the features of that program while also being limited to what that particular program offers. Therefore, in addition to becoming familiar with a computer-based program in your employment setting, it is imperative to understand all aspects of documentation in order to gain comprehensive skills and practice optimal risk management.

Narrative Charting **Narrative charting** involves a more lengthy prose entry into the medical record. This is the most traditional method of medical record keeping. Athletic trainers make entries in paragraph form preceded by the date and time of the entry, relying little on abbreviations or medical shorthand (see figure 7.4). **Dictation** is useful in narrative record keeping. Although clerical transcription can be expensive, dictation can significantly reduce the amount of time required to document injuries, treatments, and progress notes. Voice recognition software is now available that allows health care professionals to dictate directly to an electronic file in their computer through a microphone, thus avoiding the expense of using a transcriptionist.

Dictation, like writing, is a skill that takes practice to perfect. The following suggestions will help improve the effectiveness of dictation:

- Organize the data to be dictated by taking notes in medical shorthand while interviewing the patient. Use these notes to dictate a more comprehensive entry into the medical record.
- Speak clearly and slowly into the dictation machine. If possible, avoid dictating in a noisy room.
- Spell all proper names and medical terms that are used infrequently. This practice is especially important if the transcriber is inexperienced in medical transcription. Consider providing a medical dictionary to the transcriber.
- Review and initial all dictated narrations before filing them in the medical record.
- If you are planning to use voice recognition software, be sure to buy a package designed for medical environments. Allow plenty of time (up to several hours) for the software to imprint your voice patterns and thereby reduce the number of errors.

Reports of Special Procedures

Reports of all special procedures should be included in the medical record. Although special-procedure reports should be entered into the medical record chronologically, each should be annotated to refer the reader back to an initial injury or illness assessment report. Special procedures include, but are not limited to, the following:

- Isokinetic strength tests
- Blood tests

- Urinalysis
- X rays or other imaging procedures
- Surgical reports
- Cardiac assessments (echocardiogram, graded exercise tests, thallium uptake scans, and so forth)
- Neurocognitive testing

Communication From Other Professionals

An athletic trainer commonly receives written documentation of a patient's medical status from physicians, physical therapists, and other health care professionals involved with the case. One type of documentation is the referral form sent with an injured athlete when she goes to the physician's office or the emergency room (see figure 7.5). The injured athlete referral form provides legally defensible proof that the athletic trainer consulted with a physician as required by the BOC *Standards of Professional Practice* and, in many states, by law. In addition, it improves communication between the athletic trainer and the physician by taking the burden of relaying information off the injured athlete.

The referral form should include the athlete's name, sport, injury date, and appointment date and time. It should allow space for the athletic trainer to document the initial evaluation findings. The form should provide space for the physician to write a diagnosis and orders for treatment or rehabilitation. The athletic trainer and physician should date and sign their notes. Finally, the form should include a section that complies with the Health Insurance Portability and Accountability Act (HIPAA) (see the later section, Release of Medical Information). The athlete signs the form, authorizing the physician to share the athlete's medical information with the athletic trainer or other members of the sports medicine team. Athletic trainers have three means of ensuring that referral forms are returned:

1. The most direct is to ask the injured athlete to bring the form to the next appointment.

2. Athletic trainers can ask the physician to mail the form back, but this method delays direct feedback from the physician.

Sugimoto, Haruto

April 7, 2018

Haruto is a sprinter on the school's track team. He came in today to be evaluated for pain that he has been experiencing in his anterior shins for the past three weeks. He has been icing his shins prior to and after every track practice in order to relieve the pain, but the problem has progressed to the point where it is very uncomfortable to run. He also experiences some pain when he walks. He has some pain while lying in bed at night. The pain is a dull ache unless the anterior shin is touched, when it becomes a sharp pain.

Visual examination is unspectacular. No swelling, discoloration, or deformity is noted. Palpation reveals point-specific tenderness over the anterior surface of the distal one-third of both tibias. A mild elevation in local temperature is palpable. No crepitus is noted. The gastroc and soleus are both tight bilaterally, allowing only 6° of passive dorsiflexion.

It is my impression that Haruto may be suffering from bilateral tibial stress fractures. Haruto is a member of an HMO and his physician while he is in college is Dr. Van Notten. I called Dr. Van Notten this morning to discuss Haruto's case and was instructed to obtain a bone scan of Haruto's tibias bilaterally. Haruto is scheduled for the bone scan at Holland Community Hospital tomorrow morning at 9:30. He will be kept out of practice until Dr. Van Notten reviews the bone scan. He was placed on crutches and instructed to apply ice to his shins for 20 minutes every 2 hours while awake. He was told to return to the athletic training room tomorrow after his bone scan.

Signed: _____

Figure 7.4 Example of the narrative charting method of injury documentation.

3. The athletic trainer could ask the physician to fax a response, which provides the information quickly and gets around the possibility of the athlete's losing or forgetting the form.

Electronic medical records may also be used to transmit referrals and acknowledge informed consent by the patient.

A second method for communicating with other health care professionals is through the common professional courtesy of sending letters or copies of office notes to referring health care colleagues. Athletic trainers should enter these notes, often a useful source of information and documentation of the injured athlete's status, into the medical record. Athletic trainers should request a letter from all physicians and other health care professionals to whom they frequently refer injured athletes. Systems that connect an interprofessional health care team with all forms of documentation can be beneficial, but often they are difficult to establish because of the complexities of each system using different employers and organizations for care.

Emergency Information

Athletic trainers in high schools and colleges must frequently contact an injured student-athlete's parents or guardians, which is an urgent responsibility if the athlete has had a serious accident or illness. To do so, the athletic trainer usually uses the emergency information form in the medical record (see figure 7.6). This form should include athlete information, such as name, address, phone number or numbers, date of birth, and Social Security or student identification numbers. The form should also include

---

NUJAX HIGH SCHOOL STUDENT-ATHLETE REFERRAL

Name: _____ Sport: _____

Date: _____ Contact e-mail: _____ Contact cell: _____

Parent/guardian name: _____ Relationship: _____

Parent/guardian cell: _____ Physician: _____

Athletic training assessment: _____

_____

_____

Athletic training recommendation: _____

_____

_____

Physician order: _____

_____

_____

_____

Next visit: _____

Physician signature: _____ Date: _____

Figure 7.5 Sample medical referral form.

Developed by Jeff G. Konin.

parents' or guardians' names, addresses, and telephone numbers (home, cell, and business). This form should be readily accessible in the medical record, perhaps affixed to the inside cover of the athlete's folder; this information will also be stored electronically for those programs using electronic medical records. Emergency information forms could also be organized according to sport and placed in three-ring binders that teams take with them wherever they go. Some athletic injury and treatment database programs have the capability to store this information on a laptop or handheld device as well.

Permission for Medical Treatment Forms

A widely recognized legal principle is that people (or their parents or guardians in the case of minors) must consent to medical treatment. Consent forms should be maintained in the medical record (see figure 7.7). Although the use of such forms has been standard operating procedure in most hospital sports medicine programs, their use in other settings has been limited. Consent forms are especially important in the high school setting because most of these injured student-athletes are still minors.

Athletic trainers should also remember that some college athletes are also still minors.

Along with permission forms, signed releases from patients or their parents or guardians that waive all future legal claims against the athletic trainer or the employing institution are commonly used. However, these **exculpatory clauses** may or may not be legally upheld (*Atkins v. Swimwest Family Fitness Center* 2005; *Powell v. American Health Fitness Center* 1998; Stolle and Slain 1997). The primary legal argument against them is that such clauses are contrary to public policy and are therefore legally invalid. Because the public has a stake in quality health care, the courts have been hesitant to allow negligent practitioners to hide behind prospective waivers. In addition, in many states, parents cannot sign away the rights of their children. Any athletic trainer planning to use a prospective waiver with exculpatory language should first have an attorney and liability insurance carrier thoroughly evaluate it.

Release of Medical Information

Another commonly understood legal principle is that health care providers may not release a person's medical records without consent. This principle has been written into the federal legal code in the form

EMERGENCY INFORMATION

Name: _____ Sport: _____

Gender: _____ DOB: _____

Mailing address: _____ Cell phone: _____

Parents or guardian: _____

Relationship to student: _____

Mailing address: _____

Cell phone: _____

Best person to contact in case of an emergency: _____

Relationship to student-athlete: _____ Cell phone: _____

Name of primary insurance company: _____

Name of insured person: _____

Policy/group numbers: _____

Figure 7.6 Sample emergency information form.

PERMISSION TO PROVIDE MEDICAL TREATMENT AGREEMENT

I HEREBY give my permission for my son/daughter, _____, to undergo medical treatment for any injury or illness he/she may sustain or acquire while engaged in interscholastic athletics at Eagletown High School. I understand that the medical personnel of Eagletown High School, including athletic trainers, nurses, and team physicians, will perform only those procedures that are within their training, credentialing, and scope of professional practice to prevent, care for, and rehabilitate athletic injuries. In the event that more serious medical procedures are required, such as surgery or other invasive procedures, I understand that attempts will be made to contact me for my consent. I understand that if my child suffers a potentially life-threatening injury or illness, and in the event I am unable to be contacted within a reasonable period of time, that I authorize any duly licensed medical practitioner to perform such procedures as may be medically necessary to alleviate the problem.

I have had the opportunity to ask questions regarding this release, and all of my questions have been answered to my satisfaction. Having understood the above agreement, I freely sign this Permission to Provide Medical Treatment Agreement.

_____   _____

Date   Signature of Parent or Legal Guardian

Figure 7.7 Sample agreement form for the parents or guardians of minors to grant permission to provide medical treatment.

of two laws: the Family Educational Rights and Privacy Act of 1974 (FERPA or sometimes referred to as the *Buckley Amendment*) and the Health Insurance Portability and Accountability Act of 1996 (HIPAA).

Family Educational Rights and Privacy Act

The **Family Educational Rights and Privacy Act (FERPA)** requires educational institutions to receive formal written consent from students (or, in the case of minors, their parents or guardians) before they can disclose educational records to a third party. The law also requires educational institutions to make available to students all records relating to their enrollment unless they specifically waive the right on a case-by-case basis. Several exceptions to the rule exist. For example, employees of educational institutions may legally disclose information regarding students, without their consent, to safeguard their health in an emergency. Health records created or maintained by a physician, psychiatrist, psychologist, or other recognized professionals or paraprofessionals are not considered educational records under FERPA and are therefore not covered by the law. Student-athletes do not have a legal right under FERPA to access the content of their health records. Nonetheless, good practice in health care includes receiving informed consent from patients before sharing information regarding their health with a third party.

Health Insurance Portability and Accountability Act

The **Health Insurance Portability and Accountability Act (HIPAA)** was enacted to help employees transfer their health insurance when they switched employers, to ensure that their health information would remain private, and to give people more access to their own health care information. The privacy portion of the law was, in part, a reaction to the fact that much health care information is now transmitted electronically and is therefore more vulnerable to unauthorized release. HIPAA applies only to "covered entities." The law may cover athletic trainers in some settings but not those in other settings. However, even if the athletic trainer is working in a setting that is not a covered entity, it would be wise to follow the general principles of HIPAA to protect the privacy of the patients and athletes he or she treats. In general, athletic trainers work in environments subject to HIPAA rules when each of the following three conditions applies:

1. The person, business, or agency furnishes, bills, or receives payment for health care in the normal course of business.
2. The person, business, or agency conducts covered transactions. Covered transactions are those activities normally associated with billing.

3. The covered transactions are transmitted in electronic form.

Athletic trainers working in covered entities should be most attentive to seven areas with regard to HIPAA rules:

1. *Obtain consent for treatment.* Athletic trainers must provide patients with a written Notice of Privacy Practices that delineates the manner in which the health care agency intends to use and disclose a patient's health information. Patients must acknowledge in writing that they received this information, except in emergencies that render the patient unable to provide written acknowledgment.

2. *Obtain authorization to release health information.* Athletic trainers working in covered entities must receive written authorization to share a patient's health information with people who are not part of the chain of health care providers, including coaches, athletic administrators, scouts, and the media. The athletic trainer must obtain authorizations for each instance of information release; a blanket release signed at the beginning of the year or even at the initiation of the treatment will not suffice (for athletic trainers not covered by the law, a blanket authorization is permissible). A valid authorization must include

- a description of the information to be disclosed,
- the persons authorized to disclose information,
- the persons to whom the information may be disclosed,
- the purpose of the disclosure,
- the expiration date of the authorization,
- the patient signature and date, and
- if signed by a representative, a description of his or her authority to act for the patient.

Furthermore, authorizations are not valid under the HIPAA rules unless they include each of the following:

- A statement that the individual may revoke the authorization in writing, instructions on how to revoke the authorization, and a reference to the Notice of Privacy Practices mentioned earlier
- A statement that treatment, payment, enrollment, or eligibility for benefits may not be conditioned on obtaining the authorization, or, if such services are conditioned on the authorization, a statement that details the consequences of refusing to sign the authorization
- A statement that informs patients that the persons to whom the information is being provided could disclose their health information

3. *Release only the minimum necessary information.* HIPAA requires that athletic trainers and other covered entities limit the amount and frequency of information released to the minimum required to accomplish the purposes for which the information is being released. Although this part of the rule does not apply to health care providers involved in the chain of an individual's care, it definitely applies to nonmedical entities such as coaches, administrators, and insurance companies.

4. *Safeguard patient information.* Although HIPAA allows for certain incidental disclosures of patient information (for example, someone in the clinic overhearing a conversation between two athletic trainers regarding a patient case), the rules require that reasonable efforts be made to safeguard such information. Good practices require maintaining charts and other patient documents in a secure manner.

5. *Observe state laws governing the treatment of a minor's health information.* Because HIPAA defers authority for access to the health records of minors to the individual states, athletic trainers must be familiar with their state's laws governing minors and their health records.

6. *Do not combine authorizations except for research purposes.* The HIPAA rules generally require that the patient sign a separate authorization for each purpose for which patient information will be used or released. This rule does not apply when the information will be used for research purposes.

7. *Business associates must safeguard patient information.* Athletic trainers who refer patients to other entities must ensure that the entity to whom the referral is being made has policies in place to safeguard the patient's health information. The athletic trainer must have contracts with these entities that specify the nature of the safeguards. For example, if an athletic trainer refers patients to a private practice dietitian, the AT must have a contract with the nutritionist specifying that the dietician may not release the athlete's health information without written authorization from the athlete.

Many parties will want access to the athlete's medical records, including parents, coaches, the press, insurance companies, and professional sports organizations. Before providing information, the athletic trainer should make certain that the athlete has formally agreed to the release by signing a properly formatted authorization. If the athlete is a minor, a parent or legal guardian must also sign the waiver. The athletic trainer must be certain to release only the information authorized by the athlete. Prior to releasing information to parents or guardians of minors, athletic trainers should also verify that the individual is the custodial parent or guardian. Each time an athlete's medical information is released, the medical release form should show the content, purpose, and receiver of the information (see figure 7.8).

Insurance Information

Financial documents such as patient invoices and insurance claim forms are not medical records. They have different purposes and uses, and the laws governing confidentiality protect them in different ways. Correspondence with insurance companies and other third-party payers should be maintained separately from the medical record. Letters and copies of insurance forms often contain information directly related to the description of the injury circumstances. Copies of medical records used to document claims should not be maintained in the insurance folder; to protect confidentiality, a note referring to the supporting portion of the medical record should be used. This method protects the confidentiality of the medical record by ensuring that unauthorized individuals do not gain access through the insurance claims process. Electronic medical records should ensure similar protection, with password-protected information made available only to those who would need to access specific records.

Program Administration Records

Much of the information that athletic trainers must manage is administrative. Whereas medical records are specific to only one athlete or physically active patient, **program administration records** are more general and are usually organized around subfunctions of the sports medicine program. The absolute standards for confidentiality that apply to medical records are usually, but not always, significantly relaxed for many types of program administration records. Whenever program administration records deal with specific individuals, however, confidentiality should be maintained. Examples of various types of program administration records follow.

Reports to Coaches

A common practice of most athletic trainers who work in professional, high school, and college settings is to provide coaches with daily written reports of the health status of their athletes (see figure 7.9). Daily reports can help improve communication between the athletic trainer and the coach. Coaches appreciate timely information about the health status of their athletes because they can then plan more effectively. Another important benefit of the daily report to coaches is that athletic trainers can easily document recommendations for participation status. For example, assume that the athletic trainer recommends in the daily report that an athlete be limited to noncontact football drills because of a resolving neck injury. If the coach allows the athlete to participate in a full-contact scrimmage and the athlete is reinjured, the athletic trainer can at least document that she recommended a reduced activity level for the injured athlete.

Should athletic trainers be concerned about violating their legal and ethical duty to hold athlete's medical information and health status in confidence—even from their coaches? This is a thorny issue for a variety of reasons. First, as mentioned in the section on HIPAA, the legal responsibilities associated with confidentiality of a patient's record will vary depending on whether the athletic trainer is a covered entity under HIPAA. Second, although athletic trainers have an ethical responsibility to obtain authorization from the athlete before disclosing information to a coach, common practice in school, collegiate, and professional sports for many years has been for athletic trainers to report on the health status of athletes to their coaches (for all the reasons enumerated in the previous paragraph) even in the absence of explicit authorization. Many injury situations occur in such a way that the coach is a witness to the injury or is the agent of referral to the athletic trainer. In situations like these, the coach is already an informed party. Even when the coach doesn't know about an injury, most athletes

---

RELEASE OF MEDICAL INFORMATION AUTHORIZATION

I, _____, DO/DO NOT give consent for the team physician, athletic trainer, or other medical personnel employed by _____ College to release such information regarding my medical history, record of injury or surgery, record of serious illness, and rehabilitation results as may be requested by either the representatives of any professional or amateur athletic organization seeking such information.

I understand that the representatives of a professional or amateur athletic organization have made representations to the team physician, athletic trainer, or other medical personnel employed by _____
College that the purpose of this request for my medical information is to assist the organization being represented in making a determination as to offering me employment.
I understand that a record will be kept of all individuals requesting information and the date of the request. This information is normally confidential and except as provided in this Release will not be otherwise released by the custodian of the information. This Release remains valid until revoked by me in writing.
I have had an opportunity to ask questions regarding this Release and the process by which my medical information may be released. All of my questions have been answered to my satisfaction. Having read and understood the above, I freely sign this Release of Medical Information Authorization.

_____   _____
Date   Signature of Student-Athlete

_____   _____
Date   Signature of Parent or Legal Guardian (for minors)

_____   _____
Date   Signature of Parent or Witness

— —

Date of release	Released to	Form of release	Content of release	Released by
1.				
2.				
3.				
4.				

Figure 7.8 Sample authorization form and log for release of medical information.

just assume that the athletic trainer will speak to the coach about the situation. Conversely, most athletic trainers have had cases in which athletes have specifically requested that the athletic trainer not inform their coaches about an injury or illness—for a variety of reasons. The question is complicated even further when athletic trainers, as agents of management of professional athletic organizations, are required by the terms of their contracts to disclose the health status of all athletes to a coach or general manager.

All athletic trainers establish a policy that clearly outlines and informs all parties how protected health information will be shared within and among the organizational stakeholders. In the absence of these written agreements, the athletic trainer should hold all information in confidence. In addition, the following guidelines are recommended for dealing with this issue:

• Inform all athletes in writing that you will share with the coach health information that

DAILY COACH'S REPORT

Sport: Football

Date: October 14, 2018

Name	Injury	Date injured	Date reported	Comments
Smith, Tim	L-wrist/old fx. pain	10-12-18	10-12-18	Seen by Dr. West
Funk, Roger	L-shldr. sublx.	10-12-18	10-12-18	See by Dr. West, rest
DeHaan, Dirk	R-AC contusion	10-12-18	10-13-18	Treatment, seen by Dr. West
Russell, Bob	R-ankle sprain	10-12-18	10-13-18	Treatment, rest
Fernandez, Scott	Neck strain	10-12-18	10-13-18	Seen by Dr. West, treatment, play as able
Jones, Rick	L-arm contusion	10-10-18	10-11-18	Seen by Dr. West, rest

No participation	Play as able	Remove from list
Funk, Roger DeHaan, Dirk Russell, Bob Jones, Rick	Smith, Tim Fernandez, Scott	Nick, Art Rio, Manny

Figure 7.9 Example of a computer-generated daily coach's report.

affects athletes' ability to participate fully in team activities or when their safety might be at risk, except when an athlete makes a specific request to withhold the information. Obtain athletes' written consent for this at the beginning of each season (see figure 7.10). Remind athletes during their initial assessment that as part of their treatment plan you will discuss their status with their coaches. If HIPAA classifies you as a covered entity, obtain written authorization for this.

- Counsel athletes who are reluctant to allow you to discuss their case with a coach about the advantages and disadvantages of withholding the information.
- If athletes request that you hold information in confidence before you have had an opportunity to evaluate the information ("I want to tell you something, but you have to promise me you won't tell the coach"), inform them that you can't make that promise and that you'll have to hear what they tell you first. If they won't tell you without your assurance, offer to refer them to another health care provider not associated with the team or institution.

- Disclose to coaches only the information they need either to plan team activities or to structure a safe participation environment for the athletes in question. Suppose, for example, that an athlete has a sexually transmitted disease and must see the physician at 4:30, thus having to miss practice. We recommend that you tell the coach only that the athlete is ill and will miss one day of practice.
- Document in the medical record the extent of disclosure made to a coach. In cases in which the athlete will not authorize disclosure, document this as well.

Budget Information

Athletic trainers with financial authority must maintain accurate records of all financial transactions. In school, college, and professional settings, financial reports usually include monthly budget statements (produced in-house or sent from the institutional business office), purchase orders, and invoices. Documents that support budgetary decisions and **requests for proposals (RFPs)** should also be maintained in the program administration record system.

SOUTHWEST UNIVERSITY HIPAA PRIVACY AUTHORIZATION FORM

1. Authorization

I _____ authorize the athletic trainers and team physicians at Southwest University to use and disclose my protected health information to the coaching staff of my team.

2. Effective period

This authorization for release of information covers the period of athletic participation and health care at Southwest University from:

a. ❏ _____ to _____

OR

b. ❏ All past, present, and future periods

3. Extent of authorization

a. ❏ I authorize the release of my complete health record including any health conditions that may affect my participation in my sport at Southwest University (including records relating the mental health care, communicable diseases, HIV or AIDS, and treatment of alcohol or drug abuse).

OR

b. ❏ I authorize the release of my complete health record with the EXCEPTION of the following information:

   ❏ Mental health records

   ❏ Communicable diseases (including HIV and AIDS)

   ❏ Alcohol or drug abuse treatment

Other (please specify): _____

4. This authorization shall be in force and effect until _____ (date or event), at which time this authorization expires.

5. I understand that I have the right to revoke this authorization, in writing, at any time. I understand that a revocation is not effective to the extent that any person or entity has already acted in reliance on my authorization.

_____	_____
Name of Athlete	Sport(s) at Southwest University
_____	_____
Signature of Athlete	Date
_____	_____
Name of Witness	Title of Witness
_____	_____
Signature of Witness	Date

Figure 7.10 HIPAA Privacy Authorization Form

Nonmedical Correspondence

Nonmedical correspondence comprises letters and memoranda not associated with a specific patient's health status. Unlike medical correspondence, which must be meticulously recorded and preserved, much of the routine nonmedical correspondence can be discarded after action is taken. Nonmedical correspondence that must be retained should be filed according to subject matter instead of putting all letters together in a file labeled Correspondence.

Equipment and Supply Information

Equipment and supply inventories and catalogs from medical supply vendors form another kind of program administration record. Institutions often require administrative units to keep an inventory of nonexpendable capital equipment on file. This inventory usually includes the type of equipment, the amount or number of units, and the serial numbers. Some institutions assign their own identification numbers for nonexpendable equipment, which should also be included as part of this record. Athletic trainers in all settings are frequently called on to purchase or recommend the purchase of sports medicine products. A well-organized file of appropriate catalogs can be useful. Warranties and equipment maintenance records should also be filed in the program administration records.

Personnel Information

Information on sports medicine staff members' employment constitutes an important part of the program administration record-keeping system. Like an individual's medical record, the personnel record is confidential, and only those with a documented need for the information should be able to access it. Personnel information should be kept in a secure place, preferably a locked filing cabinet. Records on athletic training students' performance should be treated similarly. Examples of the kinds of records normally associated with the personnel function include

- performance evaluation records;
- salary and promotion records;
- employment application information, including application forms, resumes, and letters of recommendation; and
- employment contracts.

Reporting Information

Athletic trainers are often responsible for documenting the activities of a sports medicine program either for institutional or for outside accreditation purposes. The information required to compile such reports constitutes another aspect of the program administration record-keeping system. Documentation of patient caseloads and summaries of special program accomplishments are often compiled in an annual report. Accreditation agencies require access to different kinds of information, depending on their purpose. Hospital accreditation agencies generally request summary statistics on patient outcomes and evidence of compliance with professional standards of practice. Agencies that accredit educational programs require data related to student outcomes such as graduation, certification, and employment rates.

Reporting is required by law to show compliance with **OSHA's Bloodborne Pathogen standard**. Part 1910 of Title 29 of the Code of Federal Regulations requires that employers develop programs that protect employees, including athletic trainers, from occupational exposure to bloodborne pathogens (Occupational Safety and Health Administration 2016). These rules require significant record keeping. Records kept to comply with the OSHA rules must be retained for three years. Documents that must be entered into the employee's medical record, however, must be maintained for the duration of the employee's employment *plus* 30 years.

KEY POINT

Training materials and forms related to compliance with OSHA's Bloodborne Pathogens standard are available online.

Patient and Student Education Information

All athletic trainers should maintain an up-to-date database of article reprints, handouts, and other educational materials that they can provide to both patients and student athletic trainers. The maintenance of this database, which serves as another type of program administration information, is important because the body of knowledge in athletic training and sports medicine changes rapidly.

Evaluating Electronic Medical Records

As technology continues to advance, it is likely that more and more athletic training settings will implement some form of electronic medical records. Electronic medical records are critical to the documentation and record-keeping process of any athletic trainer. The following list is an example of things to consider when evaluating electronic medical records to purchase and implement in one's setting.

- *Security and compliance (HIPAA).* No electronic medical record software or system should be used unless it meets all HIPAA requirements and security acceptance within one's organization.

- *Ease of application.* Documentation in general can be a time-consuming task. For the clinical athletic trainer, it is essential that the chosen system exemplify an ease of application that supports efficient time management.

- *Web based.* When choosing a system, consider where and how the data will be stored. Programs that are Web based support backup systems and greater storage capacity.

- *User fees and associated costs.* Consider start-up, annual, and training costs, especially if your program has a large staff, because fees are typically user based.

- *Upgrade potential and associated costs.* Software programs are upgraded frequently. It is important to inquire how often upgrades are planned and if there will be any associated costs.

- *Customization potential.* Standardized software programs offer many advantages, yet most organizations like to customize the program to their specific needs. If this is your preference, find out how easily the program can be customized and what the associated costs would be if applicable.

- *Reputation of vendor (reviews, ratings, and experiences of current and past users).* You have many options to consider when choosing documentation software. When determining which program to purchase, ask for references and for a list of others who use a certain program to help you review a vendor's reputation in the athletic training profession and documentation software industry.

- *Service and accessibility of salesperson.* Part of a vendor's reputation is based on its accessibility and responsiveness when you have troubleshooting concerns.

- *Database and outcomes potential.* Documentation software that has the capability to query data in an effort to help the athletic trainer assess outcomes, injury patterns, and other pertinent data is beneficial.

- *Functional and necessary features.* Some documentation software programs were first developed for other health care industry professionals, and are thorough relative to one's respective discipline. Be sure that what you are purchasing is not only thorough for athletic training practice but also functional in terms of your specific needs.

Summary

Athletic trainers now practice in a society overwhelmed with information. The need to document in a timely and accurate manner is essential for all athletic trainers regardless of the setting they practice in. Documentation of information typically falls under one of two categories: medical records and program administration records. Reasons for the importance of documentation include legal protection and requirements, professional standards, communication, insurance company requirements, outcomes measurement, and overall potential for improved delivery of care. The Family Educational Rights and Privacy Act of 1974 (FERPA) and the Health Insurance Portability and Accountability Act of 1996 (HIPAA) are examples of legislation that specifies certain privacy standards related to documentation of information. Various methods can be used to document, including problem-oriented medical records (POMR), SOAP notes (subjective, objective, assessment, plan), and narrative formats, to name a few.

Learning Aids

Case Study 1

When Carlos, the athletic trainer at Eagletown High School, met with his student staff at the beginning of each school year, he always covered documentation procedures for injuries and treatments. He required all students to use the following procedures:

- Injury evaluation forms are to be completed only by the head athletic trainer. Students are expected to file the forms in individual medical files every Monday, Wednesday, and Friday.

- All treatments are to be recorded by students on the daily treatment log as soon as the treatment is administered. On Monday, Wednesday, and Friday afternoons, the students are to copy all treatments from the daily treatment log onto the bottom half of the injury evaluation report. After a page of the log has been transferred, it is thrown away.

One day Carlos was surprised to find a subpoena in his mail for all medical records related to a former student-athlete who had graduated five years earlier. At first, Carlos could not find the student's file. Finally, after several hours of digging through boxes in a storage closet in the gymnasium, he found the file. When he looked up the injury evaluation form for the case in question, he was shocked to see that the treatment records were sloppy, often not dated, and usually illegible because they had been written with a fountain pen that had left blotches of smeared ink on the page. Although Carlos complied with the subpoena and submitted all the requested records, he had an uneasy feeling about the quality of those records.

Questions for Analysis

1. What are the advantages of the injury and treatment recording system used at Eagletown High School? What are the disadvantages?

2. What kinds of problems is the Eagletown High School system likely to foster? How could those problems be overcome? What kinds of resources would be required to implement these solutions? How much would it cost?

3. What are the legal implications for this record-keeping system? Which legal issues should Carlos address when considering changes in the system?

Case Study 2

Andrea is an athletic trainer for an AA minor league professional baseball team. Besides her duties as athletic trainer, Andrea is also equipment manager and traveling administrative assistant for the team. Because of her many duties, Andrea doesn't have a lot of time for record keeping. She usually discusses the health of individual players with the team's manager over coffee and rolls each morning. Andrea informs the manager of new injuries, and the manager can ask questions.

One day in August, as the playoffs were rapidly approaching, Andrea was unable to have coffee with the manager and the other coaches because she had to make arrangements for an upcoming trip. During the game that night, the star pitcher's knee suddenly buckled after a pitch, and he fell to the ground. He had to leave the game, and the team physician evaluated him in the locker room. After the game, the physician told the manager that the knee would be fine in a couple of days but that in the future, the manager should rest players for a day or two following an accident like the one the pitcher had suffered. "What accident?" asked the manager with a puzzled look. The physician related that during his exam the player told him he had twisted his knee in the parking lot the previous evening. He had gone to the athletic trainer and gotten some ice for it, and in the morning the knee felt better. The manager immediately went to Andrea and demanded to know why he hadn't been informed.

Questions for Analysis

1. Why is the manager so upset with Andrea? Is his anger justified?

2. What steps could Andrea have taken to prevent this situation? How should Andrea modify her information management system to avoid problems like this in the future?

3. What legal risks does Andrea's system pose, both for the club and for herself?

4. If Andrea decides to use a computer to help her with her information management needs, what kinds of hardware and software might serve her best?

Key Concepts and Review

Understand the importance of documentation as part of a complete information management system in sports medicine.

To succeed as professionals in an information society, athletic trainers must manage and communicate information effectively. Documentation is a central task in the athletic trainer's information management role. Medical documentation helps ensure legal rights, acts as a memory aid, satisfies laws and professional standards, and provides data with which to make informed decisions.

Understand and describe the different methods of athletic injury and treatment documentation.

The five methods for documenting injury evaluation and treatment data are problem-oriented medical records, focus charting, charting by exception, computerized documentation, and narrative charting.

Understand and describe the different types of information to be managed in a typical sports medicine program.

Information in sports medicine is usually made up of medical records and program administration records. Medical records are confidential and should contain injury and treatment reports, physical examination data, reports of special procedures, communications from other health care professionals, emergency information, permission to treat and medical waiver forms, release of medical information forms, and certain kinds of insurance records. Program administration records include reports to coaches, budget information, nonmedical correspondence, equipment and supply information, personnel information, patient and student education information, and information required for writing self-studies and other kinds of evaluative reports.

Revenue for Health Care Services

Athletic administrators have long felt a moral responsibility to prevent the cost associated with athletic injury from barring access to school sports programs. However, minimizing the cost of health care associated with playing sports results in passing these costs to the schools and organizations sponsoring the activity. The costs of prevention and care at any level continue to rise, placing burdens on families and administrators to pay the medical bills. Possessing a strong knowledge of the entire process associated with the administrative costs and revenue generation related to athletic health care has become an essential role for every athletic trainer (Garner 2016).

The cost of health care became an important political issue during the early and mid-1990s. In 1997, the federal government passed the Balanced Budget Act, which launched the system that we know today as *managed care*. Managed care was a major transition for both health care providers and patients. In an effort to control costs and better manage a single person's overall health care, a "gatekeeper" approach was established whereby a primary care physician served as an entry point for a patient regardless of the type of condition, signs, or symptoms that he or she possessed. It became the responsibility of the primary care physician to serve as the initial consult for a patient interaction and to determine what, if any, further specialty care consultation or ancillary work (laboratory, imaging) would be necessary. The goal of this reform was to enable a single provider to make the best judgment and coordinate a patient's care, thereby avoiding multiple practitioners providing a person with unco-ordinated services. This approach had the potential to prevent patients from seeking their provider of choice if they were required to use only providers who were contracted to a specific insurance pro-vider. This also placed an increased burden on the primary care physician.

KEY POINT

A summary of health insurance terms can be found on the Bureau of Labor Statistics website.

More recently, in 2010, the Patient Protection and Affordable Care Act (PPACA), commonly referred to as the Affordable Care Act (ACA) was enacted. This act was designed to reform the health insurance industry and the American health care system as a whole. The law includes provisions that increase the rights and protections of the insured and expands access to affordable quality health care to those who are uninsured. The law required all American citizens to possess health insurance by 2014 (U.S. Department of Health and Human Services 2015). While short-term feedback has revealed both advan-tages and disadvantages of this reform, it is too early to assess the long-term impact on overall health care services and reimbursement.

Today, schools and colleges face greater financial risks from medical costs than at any time in the past. In addition, many athletic trainers find themselves employed in clinical out-patient and orthopedic phy-sician settings. Although little research is available regarding the use of athletic trainers in the latter type of setting, Nicolello reported that the clinical efficiency in terms of relative value units (RVUs) improved with the addition of an athletic trainer by 4.3 per day and 3.8 patients (21%) per 6.5-hour day (Nicolello et al. 2017). This chapter therefore provides athletic trainers with the information they need to manage insurance systems and more effectively safeguard the resources of the institu-tions they represent while living up to the moral responsibility to remove financial barriers from the nation's playing fields. In addition, the chapter examines the third-party reimbursement process to help athletic trainers working in hospitals and clinics understand how they receive payment for what they do, and it looks at the emerging trend of cash for service.

Insurance Systems

Medical insurance is a type of insurance that a patient purchases in the form of a policy from a health insurance company for the purpose of covering medically related expenses (illnesses and injuries). Health insurance, on the other hand, is generally more comprehensive, because it often includes provisions for maintaining good health rather than simply paying for illnesses and injuries.

Both of these insurance classifications should be distinguished from the type of policy most edu-cational institutions buy for their student-athletes: athletic accident insurance, which is primarily intended to supplement a student's family insurance plan and reimburses the cost of athletic accidents only (Dixon 2015). The insurance industry defines accident differently from the concept of injury as understood by most athletic trainers, coaches, par-ents, athletes, and other physically active patients. To an insurance company, accidents usually include acute, traumatic injuries, independent of any other cause or preexisting condition, that occur during practices and games. Specific exclusions in most accident insurance plans include injuries caused by overuse (tendinitis, bursitis, stress fractures, and so on), illnesses, and degenerative conditions. Some athletic accident insurance companies offer riders to cover the costs of chronic conditions, but riders generally increase the premium significantly. A pre-mium is a baseline periodic payment one submits to an insurance company in return for coverage.

KEY POINT

Among the many kinds of insurance are medical, health, athletic accident, cata-strophic, and disability. Athletic accident insurance comes in one of three forms: pri-mary coverage, secondary coverage, and self-insurance.

A fourth type of coverage is catastrophic insur-ance, which usually takes effect after the first $75,000 (in some cases $90,000) in medical bills has been reached and provides lifetime medical, reha-bilitation, and disability coverage for athletes who have suffered long-term or permanent disabilities as a result of athletic injuries (National Collegiate Athletic Association n.d.). Member institutions of the National Collegiate Athletic Association (NCAA) have received catastrophic insurance at no cost since 1991. Catastrophic insurance is also available to non-NCAA institutions and high schools through their national governing organizations.

KEY POINT

For a complete description of NCAA-sponsored insurance programs, visit the Resources section of the NCAA website.

Disability insurance is also available through many companies. This type of insurance is designed to protect athletes against future loss of earnings because of a disabling injury or sickness that occurred while they were engaged in sport activities. The definition of a disability differs depending on the amount of time that has elapsed following the injury. To be eligible, an individual must have suffered irrevocable loss of speech, hearing in both ears, sight in both eyes, use of both arms, use of both legs, or use of one arm and one leg, or have severely diminished mental capacity caused by a brain stem or other neurological injury such that a person is unable to perform normal daily functions. Additional criteria that one must meet can be reviewed on the NCAA website. For example, one must be an active member of a qualifying intercollegiate sport, or QIS (varsity status, administered by participating NCAA Institution, and student-athlete eligibility). Additionally, student coaches, student managers, and athletic training students are covered under the QIS definition. These policies also set a maximum level of payment provided: Some are capped by the participating sport (men's and women's basketball, football, baseball, men's ice hockey) and others are determined on a case-by-case basis. Insurance underwriters offer what is referred to as a loss of value insurance policy to further protect athletes who are likely to have promising professional careers and lose potential long-term earnings as the result of a disability. The NCAA also sponsors a special assistance fund program that may be used to pay for some medical and dental expenses for Division I student-athletes. Finally, some insurance companies provide coverage for specific kinds of health-related problems. Dental insurance and vision insurance are two examples. These policies can be bought separately or added to broader health care plans as riders.

Experimental Therapy

Despite the type of insurance coverage an athlete possesses, policies today do not include terms that will cover **experimental treatments** and procedures. A variety of medical and surgical techniques now common in sports medicine began as experimental therapies. Physicians, athletic trainers, and other health care professionals frequently experiment with new methods to help patients return to physical activity earlier and more safely. Unfortunately, the insurance industry often determines that a therapeutic method has made the transition from experimental to conventional several years after the medical profession has. Insurance companies define *experimental* in different ways, the best way being simply to list in the policy what they consider experimental procedures. Another method that companies sometimes employ is to list the criteria by which they will determine whether a procedure is experimental. This method is less exact and more difficult to defend in the courts. The final, and most common, method that insurance companies use is to decide on a case-by-case basis which methods are experimental. The case-by-case method can be frustrating for patients and health care providers because they don't know what the insurance company will pay for and what it will not.

Surgical procedures that are considered **elective** or **diagnostic** may also be excluded from health insurance coverage policies. Elective surgical procedures are those that are not considered necessary from a medical perspective; instead, having them performed is the individual's choice. As an example, an athlete who has 20/25 vision and is able to read, write, and participate in sports without harmful risk might opt for a vision correction procedure that would improve her vision to 20/20. Although the procedure would clearly improve the person's visual sense, it might not be considered medically necessary. A diagnostic surgical procedure is performed when a diagnosis cannot be made from clinical findings and surgery would more accurately identify the diagnosis and enable the selection of the appropriate treatment. In the past, the use of arthroscopy as a less invasive surgical technique for exploring joint pathology was found to be beneficial as a diagnostic procedure. Recently, however, the prevalence of arthroscopic diagnostic procedures has decreased as a result of the surgical risks and liability associated with the lack of a specific diagnosis before performing surgery.

Usual, Customary, and Reasonable Fees

Another insurance concept that athletic trainers should understand is **usual, customary, and reasonable (UCR)** reimbursement for medical services. The UCR concept is a flexible-fee system originally developed by the federal government to reimburse health care providers through the Medicare system. Most insurance companies now use this system. A combination of the following factors determines the amount of money that insurance companies will pay to health care providers for a particular service under the UCR system:

- The usual fee charged by each health care provider for the particular service

- The customary fee for the geographic area (either the average fee or the **90th-percentile fee**, whichever is lowest)

- The reasonable fee (the lower of either the usual or customary fee)

To reduce the likelihood of having a claim denied, an athletic trainer should make sure that physicians and other health care providers the patient will be referred to will perform only nonexperimental procedures and that they will accept the UCR fee as payment in full for services rendered. If the planned procedure could potentially be considered experimental, the athletic trainer should consult a representative of the insurance company before referral.

Even the most circumspect athletic trainer will have claims denied from time to time for reasons that might not seem fair. Lawsuits to recover the costs of denied claims should be the last option. The following suggestions might help resolve claims denied because of experimental treatment or UCR clauses:

- Find out the exact reasons the claim was denied. The law requires insurance companies to provide this information.

- Obtain a statement from the physician or other health care provider explaining why the treatment was implemented and justifying the fee.

- If the self-insurance fund of a parent's employer covers a patient, correspond with the employer directly. The employer, not the insurance administrator, has final legal authority to reverse the denial.

- Provide evidence from clinical studies to support your claim that the treatment should not be considered experimental.

- Try to convince the physician or other health care provider to waive the portion of the fee above the UCR amount.

- Contact the state insurance commissioner and request assistance in challenging the denial.

Types of Athletic Insurance

Academic institutions that sponsor athletic programs have the option of choosing from three types of medical insurance for their student-athletes: self-insurance, primary coverage, and secondary coverage. As with any management option, each system offers advantages and disadvantages, including cost.

Self-Insurance

Institutions that choose to self-insure are speculating that the amount they pay out for medical expenses will be less than the amount they will pay for insurance premiums. The institution typically purchases no medical or accident insurance except for catastrophic coverage and pays medical bills incurred by student-athletes. Many national governing organizations such as the NCAA have rules that prevent educational institutions from paying for medical expenses not directly related to participation in intercollegiate or interscholastic athletics. Institutions that self-insure must be particularly careful to create and monitor procedures used to ensure compliance with these rules. Compliance and clearly disseminated policies are of particular importance as they relate to off-season conditioning programs and other directed activities performed absent the supervision of official personnel.

Self-insuring offers several advantages. Saving money is possible because the institution retains the potential profit that an insurance company normally earns. Processing claims is also simplified because there are no insurance claim forms to complete. Institutions have the flexibility to pay for procedures that a normal insurance policy might exclude.

Although cost can be an advantage with self-insurance, it can be a significant disadvantage as well. A large claim can deplete an institution's

<table>
<tr><td>

Advantages and Disadvantages of Self-Insurance

Advantages
- Potential savings
- Simplified claims process
- Greater flexibility

Disadvantages
- High risk for large claims
- Risk of bankrupting fund
- Institutional dollars tied up

</td><td>

Reasons for Purchasing Primary Insurance Coverage

- Sense of responsibility for paying all medical expenses
- Large percentage of uninsured student-athletes
- Simplified and accelerated claims processing

</td></tr>
</table>

insurance fund, making it difficult or impossible to pay other, less costly claims. For that reason, it is typically large, financially healthy university athletic programs that employ self-insurance. One method of providing for the possibility of a large claim is to set aside leftover insurance funds in an endowment account that will eventually provide a cushion against large claims. The disadvantage of this method is that it ties up a substantial amount of money that the institution could use for more productive purposes. Institutions that self-insure can decrease their annual expenses by using a student-athlete's personal insurance as the primary source of coverage wherever possible. In this case, the institution becomes a secondary payer. The following sections discuss primary and secondary coverage.

Primary Coverage

Primary coverage is medical or accident insurance that begins to pay for covered medical expenses as soon as the institution pays the deductible. The athlete's (or the athlete's parents') personal medical insurance is not a source for payment of medical bills arising out of athletic participation. Institutions adopt primary insurance plans for a variety of reasons. Some feel a moral obligation to pay for all athletic medical expenses without involving families or their insurance companies. Others have a student population that is substantially uninsured anyway, so it is logical to choose primary coverage. Finally, primary coverage simplifies and accelerates claims processing because the family does not need to be involved.

The disadvantage of primary coverage is the expense. Because the insurance company takes on all the risk for an institution's student-athletes, as opposed to sharing the risk with personal medical insurance, it must charge a substantially higher premium for the coverage.

Secondary Coverage

Secondary coverage, also known as *excess insurance,* is a policy that pays for covered medical expenses only after all other insurance policies, including the athlete's personal medical insurance, have reached their limit. The most obvious benefit of this approach is that institutions can lower their costs by spreading the risk associated with athletic injuries to other potential payers. Because personal insurance companies share the risk, the cost of secondary coverage can be as much as 60% lower than the cost of primary coverage. Another, less tangible benefit is that this approach, if used properly, can help develop a sense of shared responsibility for safety in an athletic program. Most parents want to provide a safe environment for their children. Presumably, their interest rises when they have a financial interest as well. An additional advantage of the secondary approach is that it encourages athletic administrators to find ways to reduce and control medical costs. A section on reducing insurance costs is presented later in the chapter.

The disadvantages of secondary coverage relate to claims processing. Because personal insurance serves as a primary layer of coverage, an institution must spend substantial time and energy communicating with parents and their insurance carriers to move claims along. This process can delay settling insurance claims, which can frustrate the medical vendors that the institution wants to keep happy. Another potential problem is that the secondary system requires more communication and understanding of the shared responsibility for paying medical costs. Ethical dilemmas may also arise

Advantages and Disadvantages of Secondary Insurance Coverage

Advantages

- Less costly
- Shared responsibility
- Promotes cost controls

Disadvantages

- Longer claims process
- Requires more communication
- Labor-intensive claims process

when organizations institute secondary insurance policies. Parents of student-athletes who use their own insurance as primary insurance will realize that their claims may rise and thus their future deductibles may also increase. In contrast, if they do not include their son or daughter as a dependent on their insurance plan, then the student-athlete would have no primary coverage, leaving the school to absorb all medical costs associated with claims. In this case, the parents will have recognized that they would not be responsible under their own insurance plan for athletically related medical bills.

Reducing Insurance Costs

Premiums for medical or accident insurance are closely linked to an institution's past claims history, enhancing the incentives for institutions to establish risk management programs and decrease medical costs. Insurance companies track the cost of claims made by an institution and compare those costs to the premium that the institution pays. Because all insurance companies must make a profit to stay in business, they will adjust the premium to help ensure that it will cover the likely cost of the claims, the administration of those claims, and the desired profit margin. Some insurance companies adjust premiums every year in an effort to balance this equation. Others make adjustments less frequently so that over the long term, say five years, they meet their financial goals.

In any case, athletic trainers and other members of the sports medicine team can help their institutions keep insurance premiums to a minimum by instituting the following measures. Keep in mind that institutional philosophy will govern which, if any, of these suggestions the institution will adopt.

- Spread the risk among all concerned parties. The best way to do this is to buy secondary coverage so that the personal insurance of athletes or their parents becomes the primary source of payment for athletic injuries.

- Adopt and communicate policies that limit the institution's financial obligations to those injuries that the school's insurance policy covers. For example, some athletic accident policies exclude certain kinds of conditions (for example, stress fractures). The institution can limit its financial risk if it also refuses to pay for those kinds of injuries. To do otherwise results in institutional expenditures far in excess of the annual insurance premium. Despite clear communication regarding such policies, one should always expect to exercise diplomatic skills with parents and caregivers when such noncovered injuries and illnesses arise. It is common for people to pay insufficient attention to the details of documents, policies, and procedures prior to the occurrence of an injury or illness. If they have not acknowledged agreement to guidelines and instead learn of the guidelines only after the occurrence of adverse events, there may be disagreement regarding the policy and who should be responsible for payment.

- Insist that athletes buy their own personal insurance. Remember, even if the institution has secondary coverage, it will end up paying from the first dollar of the claim for injured athletes without their own personal insurance. Some institutions will not allow students to participate in athletic programs without their own personal insurance. Other institutions provide their students with the opportunity to buy university-sponsored health insurance; however, most of these policies have relatively low coverage caps and will not pay for injuries associated with intercollegiate athletics. When working at the collegiate level for a program that offers scholarships to student-athletes, an athletic trainer should be prepared to hear the expressed concerns of coaches who feel that requiring an incoming student-athlete to have a primary insurance coverage plan is an obstacle to their recruiting efforts.

- Pass the cost—or some fraction of the cost—of the athletic accident insurance along to the athletes by requiring them to pay a modest sum for the insurance.

- Limit the institution's financial obligation for costs associated with athletic injuries to those medical services that an institutional representative, usually the athletic trainer or team physician, has preapproved. In effect, you will be creating your own health maintenance organization, because all injured athletes will have to pass through a gatekeeper to have the school or its insurance company cover the cost of their injuries. Injured athletes could still receive medical care from the provider of their choice, but they would have to pay for it if they had not use the services of the athletic trainer, team physician, or some other approved provider (Ray 1996). Establishing precedent and extremely clear guidelines for exceptions to this model is critical to the success of an internal gatekeeper-type model.

- Encourage medical providers to treat athletes from your institution on an insurance-only basis. If the physician is willing to accept whatever the athlete's personal insurance will pay as payment in full, little or no cost will be passed on to the institution or its insurance company.

- Require injured athletes covered by managed care plans to use medical providers approved by the plan. Many managed care plans, especially health maintenance organizations, will not pay for medical services provided by out-of-plan physicians. These costs are usually passed on to the institution.

- Conduct annual risk assessment audits to help reduce the incidence of athletic injuries.

Third-Party Reimbursement

Third-party reimbursement is the process by which health care practitioners receive reimbursement from a policyholder's insurance company for services they perform. A **third party** is defined as a person, in this case a medical vendor, who has no binding interest in a particular contract (the insurance policy). Third-party reimbursement is the primary mechanism for paying for medical services in the United States. Hospitals and private practice health professionals rely heavily on third-party reimbursement to generate the income that keeps their practices in business.

Leaders within the profession have launched proactive educational efforts for the past two decades, yet third-party reimbursement remains a growing practice for athletic trainers. Insurance companies, concerned about financial issues, have been slow to cover athletic trainers' services, even though the percentage of the population demanding those services is increasing. One of the main reasons for the lack of athletic training services reimbursement is the attainment of goals set forth with student-athletes by athletic trainers seeking remuneration for services. For example, in the general public sector, a patient may be discharged when he meets his activities of daily living (ADL) goals and is able to return to work. However, with athletes, simply returning to sport may be deemed a minimal-level goal. Treatment interventions may continue well beyond the return-to-play phase, and the services of the athletic trainer may extend daily throughout an athletic season. This can become costly to an insurance company, despite the fact that the athletic trainer may perceive the ongoing care as necessary for a higher level of performance as compared to the performance level of a nonathletic patient.

Access to payment for athletic training services through insurance companies is becoming more available now that more states credential athletic trainers. One outcome study conducted by the National Athletic Trainers' Association (NATA) demonstrated that athletic training services are cost efficient and effective in the treatment of injuries in physically active populations (Albohm and Wilkerson 1999). As more state athletic trainers' organizations lobby their insurance commissioners and legislators for access to third-party billing, the number of athletic trainers who receive payment for their services in this manner is likely to increase (Keeley et al. 2016; Manspeaker and Van Lunen 2011). In 2014, the state of Indiana added 98 payers for athletic training services, demonstrating progress for the profession (Grantham 2017).

KEY POINT

Athletic trainers who work in hospitals and clinics might earn a portion of their income through third-party reimbursement. Reimbursement through this system requires knowledge of diagnostic and procedural coding and strict adherence to certain legal requirements on the part of the athletic trainer.

Although athletic trainers have historically lacked direct access to third-party reimbursement, they have been responsible in some settings for generating significant amounts of reimbursable dollars for the clinics and hospitals that employ them; therefore, they must understand this aspect of insurance. Within interdisciplinary settings, many athletic trainers perform similar tasks as other allied health care professionals with whom they often work side by side. Athletic trainers working in high school outreach programs are often responsible for bringing in referrals to the clinics that employ them. Many of these patients will pay for the services they receive by submitting a claim to their medical insurance carriers. **Carriers** are charge-based providers contracted by the federal government to review Medicare claims made by physicians or other health care providers. While the athletic trainer who better understands third-party reimbursement in the private sector will be valuable to the clinical and business operations, she will also become a more valuable commodity and potentially establish the rationale for earning a higher-than-average wage for a clinical athletic trainer.

Some athletic trainers in university sports medicine programs seek third-party reimbursement from their student-athletes' personal insurance companies. This is not common in a large number of settings for a variety of reasons, although there seems to be an upward trend recently in an attempt to offset rising costs of overall athletic training and athletic department costs. Many athletic trainers lack the necessary knowledge to successfully complete the steps required for successful reimbursement. Support staff is needed to assist with much of the paperwork, and athletic training departments find themselves lacking personnel to perform the necessary billing submission procedures. In out-patient medical practices, you may note the increasing size of support staff in the billing departments. The process is labor intensive, adding work to individuals who already carry a large workload.

National Provider Identifier Number

Every athletic trainer should possess a **National Provider Identifier (NPI) number**. An NPI is a unique 10-digit identification number used in standard health care transactions. It is issued by the Centers for Medicare and Medicaid Services (CMS) to health care professionals and covered entities in the United States that transmit standard HIPAA electronic transactions. The NPI fulfills a requirement of the Health Insurance Portability and Accountability Act of 1996 (HIPAA). It also replaces all provider identifier numbers assigned by payers and is used by health care professionals.

All individual HIPAA-covered health care providers (e.g., physicians, pharmacists, physician assistants, midwives, nurse practitioners, nurse anesthetists, dentists, denturists, chiropractors, clinical social workers, professional counselors, physical therapists, occupational therapists, pharmacy technicians, athletic trainers) or organizations (e.g., hospitals, home health care agencies, nursing homes, residential treatment centers, group practices, laboratories, pharmacies, medical equipment companies) must obtain an NPI for use in all HIPAA standard transactions, even if a billing agency prepares the transaction. Once assigned, a provider's NPI is permanent and remains with the provider regardless of job or location changes. Other health industry workers, such as admissions and medical billing personnel, housekeeping staff, and orderlies, who provide support services but not health care, are not required to obtain the NPI. Although some athletic trainers are not employed in settings that seek and obtain third-party reimbursement for their services, the profession highly encourages all athletic trainers to obtain an NPI number in an effort to enhance professional recognition as a health care provider. Athletic training students are eligible to obtain an NPI number and are also highly encouraged to do so. Commonly available websites can be used to locate a provider's or organization's unique NPI number.

KEY POINT

Applying for an NPI number is relatively simple, and no cost is associated with the process. Step-by-step instructions for applying for an NPI number can be found online at the NATA website or by accessing the CMS website.

Types of Third-Party Payers

Several models of third-party payment exist, and many health plans offer several models to their enrollees. Some companies even develop hybrid plans that mix the characteristics of the following models:

- Private medical insurance companies provide group and individual coverage for employees and their dependents. The medical insurance that these companies provide is typically the traditional **fee-for-service plan**. This insurance model is also known as an *indemnity plan* (DeCarlo 1997). Patients are free to go to the medical provider of their choice. The plan reimburses a portion of the cost of covered services, and the patient is responsible for the copayment or deductible. The managed care models described next are rapidly replacing fee-for-service plans.

- **Health maintenance organizations (HMOs)** provide participating health care practitioners with a fixed fee for services rendered to members. A **capitation** (per person) system usually, but not always, determines fees. HMOs that do not use a capitation system usually reimburse providers based on a fixed-fee schedule. Patients insured by an HMO must use a primary care provider that participates in the HMO. A modest copayment is usually charged. Some HMOs provide services at medical facilities, whereas others provide care through a network of individual medical practitioners (**individual practice associations**, or **IPAs**).

- **Preferred provider organizations (PPOs)** operate similarly to HMOs but usually allow greater choice of health care providers and pay medical vendors on a fee-for-service rather than a capitated basis. PPOs allow policyholders to choose any health care provider they wish, but offer financial incentives for policyholders to use providers identified by the PPO. When patients choose to see a medical provider who does not belong to the PPO, they can expect to pay for a greater percentage of the cost of the services. One variant of the PPO is the **exclusive provider organization (EPO)**, a hybrid health insurance plan whereby a primary care provider is not necessary, although health care providers must be seen within a predetermined network. Out-of-network care is not provided, and visits require preauthorization.

- A **point-of-service plan (POS)** is similar to a PPO. The primary difference between the two is that POS plans assign primary care physicians, who act as gatekeepers by coordinating patient care. Most PPO plans do not.

- Government-sponsored programs provide coverage for the elderly (Medicare), the needy (Medicaid), and members of the armed forces and their dependents (TRICARE).

KEY POINT

For an excellent summary of the current state of health care insurance options available to consumers, visit the Health Insurance Association of America's website.

Legal Requirements

Among the many legal considerations in third-party reimbursement, one of the most important is the requirement that health care practitioners obtain signed authorization from a patient for release of medical records. Unless the patient authorizes such a release, the patient–practitioner relationship requires the medical vendor to keep information confidential. Third-party payers, however, will not process claims unless they have access to the information to substantiate them.

Another legal issue related to confidentiality of the medical record involves answering an insurance company's questions about a patient's case over the telephone. Athletic trainers should always verify the identity of the caller and be sure that the patient has signed an authorization for release of medical records before answering questions over the phone. If the patient is a minor, it is required to have a parent or guardian signature on file for the release of information. Several steps can be taken to assist in assuring appropriate confidentiality:

- Ask the caller to read a portion of the claim information so that you can verify the legitimacy of the caller and agency.

- If you remain unsure as to the legitimacy of the caller, ask the caller to submit the questions in writing on company letterhead and mail it to you.

- If you prefer, you can ask the caller for the insurance company's telephone number. Call the person back through the company switchboard to verify identity.

- Never answer questions from attorneys until the authorization for release of information is in hand, even if the attorney claims to have it. The best practice is to correspond by mail with attorneys regarding insurance reimbursement cases. It is also wise to consult with your own organization's legal counsel before responding to a legal inquiry.

- Any medical information requested by a recruiter, scout, coach, agent, or other member affiliated with a college or professional team should be disseminated only after receipt of written permission on a case-by-case basis from the student-athlete, or the parent or guardian of the student-athlete in the case of a minor.

Fraud is another legal pitfall athletic trainers must avoid in the third-party reimbursement process. Fraud is a significant problem in the insurance industry. An athletic trainer must never change the date of an injury, treatment, or assessment, or fail to record payments from an insurance company on a patient's bill. Other fraudulent acts committed by unscrupulous health care providers include claiming reimbursement for treatments that were not provided and increasing the charges for treatments for patients with insurance. The penalties for medical fraud are substantial and can include fines and possibly imprisonment. Additionally, athletic trainers run the risk of losing certification and state licensure, which damages their professional career and affects the reputation of the athletic training profession overall.

Diagnostic and Procedural Coding

Reimbursement for sports medicine and all other medical services is based on the coding system used when submitting claims to third-party payers. Two kinds of codes must be submitted: diagnostic and procedural.

Diagnostic coding is required for all forms of third-party billing. The International Classification of Diseases (ICD-10-CM) 10th Revision is a book specifying the code that should be applied to every injury or condition that athletic trainers or other health professionals treat. It consists of three volumes. Volume 1 is a numerical listing of all diagnoses using a five-digit code. Volume 2 is an alphabetical listing of the diagnoses using the same five-digit codes. Volume 3 is a listing of inpatient or in-hospital procedure codes. The system defines each condition as a five-digit code that must be entered on all claim forms. Table 8.1 is an example of the diagnostic code for acute sprains and strains of the ankle and foot.

The Current Procedural Terminology (CPT) is a list of codes published by the American Medical Asso-

Table 8.1 ICD-10-CM Codes for the Foot and Ankle

Code	Subcode 1	Subcode 2	Condition
845			Sprains and strains of the foot and ankle
	845.0		Ankle
		845.00	Unspecified site
		845.01	Deltoid (ligament), ankle
		845.02	Calcaneofibular (ligament)
		845.03	Tibiofibular (ligament), distal
		845.09	Other
	845.1		Foot
		845.10	Unspecified site
		845.11	Tarsometatarsal (joint) (ligament)
		845.12	Metatarsophalangeal (joint)
		845.13	Interphalangeal (joint)
		845.19	Other

Reprinted from Center for Disease Control and Prevention. *International classification of diseases (ICD-10-CM)*, 10th Edition.

ciation that represents the vast majority of medical procedures. The person completing a claim form for sports medicine services selects the most appropriate code for each of the services rendered. On January 1, 2017, new codes and guidelines were revised and implemented for athletic trainers that will directly affect those involved with billing for services.

KEY POINT

Information pertaining to the Current Procedural Terminology can be found in the American Medical Association's CPT Code Manual.

The January 1, 2017, changes will most affect the CPT evaluation codes. For example, what used to be CPT evaluation code 97005 is now three different codes (low, moderate, high) in an effort to better describe the severity of a patient's condition, comorbidities identified in the medical history, and the complexity associated with the clinical decision making. Additionally, what had been CPT reevaluation code 97006, now has a new number designation and includes a time element associated with face-to-face contact. Again, athletic trainers who seek reimbursement from third-party payers should be intimately familiar with the most current codes, definitions, and related terminology.

CPT Evaluation Codes

97169 Athletic Training Evaluation (low complexity)

- A medical history and physical activity profile with no comorbidities that affect physical activity.
- An examination addressing 1-2 elements from: body structures, physical activity, and/or performance deficiencies.
- Clinical decision making of low complexity using standardized assessment instruments and/or functional outcomes.

97170 Athletic Training Evaluation (moderate complexity)

- A medical history and physical activity profile with 1-2 comorbidities that affect physical performance.
- An examination addressing 3 or more elements from: body structures, physical activity, and/or participation deficiencies.
- Clinical decision making of moderate complexity using standardized assessment instruments and/or functional outcomes.

97171 Athletic Training Evaluation (high complexity)

- A medical history and physical activity profile with 3 or more comorbidities that affect physical activity.
- A comprehensive examination addressing 4 or more elements from: body structures, physical activity, and/or performance deficiencies.
- Clinical presentation with unstable and unpredictable characteristics.
- Clinical decision making of high complexity using standardized assessment instruments and/or functional outcomes.

97172 Re-Evaluation of Athletic Training Established Plan of Care

- Assessment of patient's current functional status when there is a documented change. A revised plan of care with an update in management options.

Physical Medicine and Rehabilitation Codes

The application of a modality that does not require direct (one-on-one) patient contact.

- 97022 Whirlpool therapy

(continued)

(continued)

The application of a modality that requires (one-on-one) patient contact.

- 97032 Electrical stimulation, manual, each 15 minutes
- 97035 Ultrasound therapy, each 15 minutes

Neuro-Cognitive Assessments/Tests

- 96119 Neuropsychological testing (e.g., Halstead-Reitan Neuropsychological Battery, Wechsler Memory Scales and Wisconsin Card Scoring Test), with qualified health care professional interpretation and report, administered by technician, per hour of technician time, face-to-face
- 96120 Neuropsychological testing (e.g., Wisconsin Card Sorting Test), administered by a computer, with qualified health care professional interpretation and report

Application of Casts and Strapping

- 29280 Strapping; hand or finger
- 29540 Strapping; ankle and/or foot

Health Care Common Procedure Coding System (HCPCS) Level II Codes

The HCPCS coding system is divided into two levels. Level I of the HCPCS is comprised of CPT codes. Level II of the HCPCS is a standardized coding system that is used primarily to identify products, suppliers, and services not included in the CPT code set jurisdiction. For more information on the HCPCS coding system, please refer to Centers for Medicare & Medicaid Services page.

- E0110-E0118 Crutches
- L1500-L2999 Orthotic devices

Reprinted by permission from National Athlete Association. Available: www.nata.org/practice-patient-care/revenue-reimbursement/general-revenue-reimbursement/commonly-used-cpt-codes

The importance of carefully checking the accuracy of the diagnostic and procedural codes listed on the claim form cannot be overstated. Using improper codes will significantly increase the time required by the insurance company to process the claim and might result in denial of the claim.

KEY POINT

A thorough description of various revenue resources can be found on the NATA website.

Claims Processing

Filing claims quickly and properly is one of an athletic trainer's most important insurance functions. The claims process for athletic trainers in educational settings is distinctly different from that of athletic trainers in private or hospital-based sports medicine clinics. Athletic trainers in educational settings file all (or nearly all) claims with a single insurance company to pay other medical vendors for services rendered to the institution's student-athletes, whereas athletic trainers in sports medicine clinics file claims with a wide range of insurance companies for reimbursement for services they provide. Some universities operate their athletic training programs like sports medicine clinics by routinely seeking third-party reimbursement. The two settings will be discussed separately, however, because the claims process is usually different in each.

KEY POINT

Claims processing is the act of formally communicating with an insurance company or other third-party payer to seek payment for services rendered to an injured patient. The process is different for athletic trainers working in educational settings than it is for those working in sports medicine clinics.

Claims Processing in Educational Settings

An athletic trainer can take preliminary steps to make claims processing easier. Collecting accurate and current insurance information for every student-athlete in the program should be completed well in advance of a season. For participants who are not identified until the beginning of the season, the preseason physical exam offers an excellent opportunity to collect the information. Personal insurance information forms should be updated annually. Another preparatory step that will save time and prevent confusion after an injury occurs is to communicate by letter with the parents of all student-athletes, informing them of the limits of the school's accident insurance policy and the steps they will need to take to process an insurance claim (see figure 8.1). If the school has a secondary policy, be sure to explain to parents that they must submit all medical bills to their insurance company before submitting the balance to the school.

When the athletic trainer receives a bill for processing, she should create an insurance file for the student-athlete. Many programs now use a software system to store such data. However, for those that do not, a useful approach is to use adhesive labels to color code each file according to its status. As the status of the claim changes, a different-colored label can be applied over the old one. Consider the following system:

- Red label—bills and other information being collected, claim not yet submitted
- Yellow label—full claim submitted but not yet paid
- Green label—claim paid in full and case closed

Dear Student-Athlete and Parents:

At the beginning of every sports season, the athletic department sends the parents of each student-athlete information regarding our insurance coverage. We hope all participants will be injury free; however, if an athlete is accidentally injured, the following information should be useful.

If a student-athlete is accidentally injured and generates medical expenses associated with the accident, all claims must be filed first with the student's or parents' personal insurance company. If a balance remains after the personal insurance company has paid its maximum, that balance will be submitted to the school's athletic accident insurance company. If covered, the school's insurance company will pay the balance of the eligible medical expenses not covered by the personal insurance company up to the maximum of the policy. This excess insurance program is being used at many of the nation's high schools and colleges.

The school's insurance policy covers only new accidents that are sustained during competition or supervised practice. Any bills related to injuries that fall into the category above should be mailed to the athletic department only after first being submitted to the personal insurance company. Preexisting injuries, off-season injuries, injuries incurred during the season that are not directly related to in-season competition or supervised practice (physical education injuries, intramural injuries, and so on) or routine medical care (eye care, dental care, care for illnesses) are NOT COVERED. Also not covered are injuries or "conditions" caused by overuse, such as tendinitis and stress fracture. We strongly recommend that a personal health and accident insurance policy be maintained for all student-athletes.

If you have questions regarding the accident insurance program, please feel free to contact us at your convenience. We look forward to serving you again this year and hope that your experience will be enjoyable and accident free.

Sincerely,

Athletic Director   Athletic Trainer

Figure 8.1 Sample letter to parents and student-athletes explaining the athletic accident insurance plan.

Besides creating an individual insurance folder, the athletic trainer should enter each claim on an **insurance claim tracking form** (see figure 8.2). This document provides the athletic trainer with a quick reference for determining which claims are paid and which are outstanding. For individuals using electronic medical records, these forms can be synced with the software to submit the claims online.

The athletic trainer should not submit a claim to the school's secondary insurance company before receiving an **explanation of benefits form (EOB)** from the athlete's personal insurance company. The EOB describes how the insurance company paid benefits for the claim. The EOB is proof of which bills the insurance company paid and to whom, either medical vendors or parents, the company wrote the checks (see figure 8.3).

HMOs, part of a larger concept in the medical insurance industry known as **managed care**, remain the predominant form of health insurance available, particularly with the implementation of the Affordable Care Act previously discussed (see figure 8.4). If a student's personal insurance carrier is an HMO, the student will be required to seek treatment from a physician designated as her **primary care provider** except in life-threatening emergencies. This requirement frequently poses problems for athletic trainers because student-athletes must seek medical treatment from physicians not associated with the school's sports medicine program. Most HMOs refuse to pay for treatment performed by a nonparticipating physician or other health care provider without prior approval. When the athlete is a high school student living in the same town as her HMO physician, the problem is merely an inconvenience. When the athlete is a college student living hundreds of miles from home, however, the problem can become more serious. Most

INSURANCE CLAIM TRACKING FORM

Patient's name	Social security number	Insurance company	Date claim filed	Amount due	Amount of payment received

Figure 8.2 Sample insurance claim tracking form.

GOOD Insurance Company

Date:

EXPLANATION OF BENEFITS

EMPLOYEE:	SSN:
GROUP:	CLAIM #:
GROUP ID:	DATE INCURRED:
PROCESSED BY:	PATIENT:

TREATMENT DATES	CHARGE AMOUNT	PATIENT COPAY	NOT COVERED	REASON CODE	PPO DISCOUNT	ELIGIBLE CHARGES	DEDUCTIBLE AMOUNT	PCT	PAYMENT AMOUNT

TOTAL INDIVIDUAL DEDUCTIBLE MET	$	
TOTAL FAMILY DEDUCTIBLE MET	$	
OUT-OF-POCKET YTD	$	

TOTAL CHARGES	$
LESS DEDUCTIBLE	$
PATIENT RESPONSIBILITY	$
TOTAL PAYMENT	$
OTHER INSURANCE/ADJUSTMENTS	$

PAYMENT DISTRIBUTION

CODE	PAYEE	AMOUNT	CHECK NUMBER

SERVICE CODE	REASON CODE

MESSAGES

IF THE PARTICIPANT BELIEVES THE CLAIM HAS BEEN IMPROPERLY DENIED, HE OR SHE HAS THE RIGHT TO HAVE IT RE-VIEWED. THE APPEAL MUST BE FILED IN WRITING WITHIN SIXTY (60) DAYS OF RECEIPT OF THIS WORKSHEET. ADDITIONAL INFORMATION ABOUT WHERE THE CLAIM SHOULD BE SENT IS CONTAINED IN THE EMPLOYEE BENEFIT HANDBOOK.

Figure 8.3 Sample explanation of benefits form.

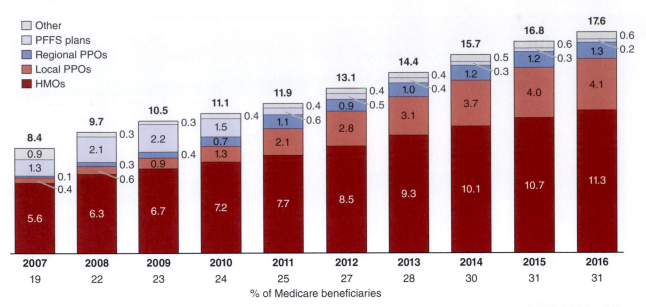

Figure 8.4 Top Medicare Advantage enrollment (in millions), by plan type, 2007-2016. *Other* includes MSA, cost plans, and demonstrations. Includes special needs plans as well as other Medicare Advantage plans. Excludes beneficiaries with unknown county addresses and beneficiaries in territories other than Puerto Rico.

The Henry J. Kaiser Family Foundation. Authors' analysis of CMS Medicare Advantage enrollment files, 2008-2016, and MPR, "Tracking Medicare Health and Prescription Drug Plans Monthly Report," 2007; enrollment numbers from March of the respective year.

secondary carriers will not pay the full cost of an athletic accident if the student's HMO denies the claim because the student sought treatment from a physician outside the plan. Although some large university athletic programs might be able to absorb the costs incurred by avoiding the inconvenience of using a student-athlete's HMO-approved physician, most school- and college-based programs lack the financial resources to become, in effect, primary coverage providers for these students.

An athletic trainer can take several steps with students who are insured through an HMO:

- Contact the HMO in writing and request information about the procedure to be followed in the event of an athletic accident (see figure 8.5). Do this for all the managed care plans that operate in your area so that you can learn the limitations and rules for each of the policies.
- Place an "HMO ALERT" label on the athlete's medical record as a reminder to contact the HMO in the event of an injury that requires outside medical care.
- If the student is in college and lives a great distance from the HMO service area, determine whether the HMO will assign a physician in the local college community as the student's

primary care provider during the time the student is in school.

- If the school's secondary insurance policy will not honor claims rejected by an HMO for noncompliance with the HMO plan, be sure to remind parents of that fact. This reminder should be part of a larger effort to educate parents and student-athletes about the institution's athletic accident insurance. Among the many ways to educate parents and student-athletes are brochures, letters, team meetings, and parent meetings. This educational effort will help prevent confusion and anger later if a claim is denied.

PEARLS OF MANAGEMENT

Keep in mind that athletic trainers who have converted to electronic medical systems may be able to flag HMO alerts within the program.

Insurance claim forms must be complete and accurate to be processed quickly. Athletic accident insurance claim forms include at least the following elements:

- Student's name and address (home and local when appropriate)
- Student's date of birth, sex, and year in school
- Sport in which the student was injured
- Date, time, and place of the accident

- Description of how the accident occurred
- Nature of the injuries suffered, including specific body parts
- Names and titles of witnesses to the accident
- Parent's medical insurance information

HMO OR PPO AUTHORIZATION FORM

Name of student-athlete: _____

Name of covered person: _____

(Parent or Guardian)

Name of employer: _____ HMO or PPO certificate #: _____

Dear _____:

_____ is a student-athlete at _____ College and has indicated that he/she is covered under your plan for health and accident coverage while he/she is a student here.

_____ is participating in our intercollegiate sports program and there is a possibility that he/she may suffer an accidental injury while competing. The athletic accident coverage purchased by _____ College is an excess policy that requires all medical bills be first submitted to the student's primary health plan for payment before it assumes any liability. It also requires that all student-athletes must follow any procedures required by their HMO or PPO, should they be covered by such a plan.

As the head athletic trainer, it is my responsibility to process any insurance claims that are made by our student-athletes. I am requesting your assistance in properly administering your plan for _____ _____.

If you have any printed material that would assist in this matter, please send it to me as soon as possible. If there is a phone number that should be called prior to _____ receiving any medical treatment, I request that you send it to me as well. It is most important that I be informed of all medical vendors in the immediate area of _____ College that qualify under your plan to treat _____.

At various times our athletic teams will be several hundred miles from our campus, and I need to know the proper procedures for handling any emergency that might take place. I also need to know whether your coverage has a particular definition of "emergency" and whether there are different procedures for treating a life-threatening emergency and a less serious problem such as a fractured leg or dislocated shoulder that requires the immediate attention of a physician.

Thanks in advance for your help. I look forward to your early reply.

Sincerely,

Director of Sports Medicine

Figure 8.5 Sample HMO or PPO authorization form.

Adapted by permission from First Agency, Inc. HMO/PPO authorization (Kalamazoo, MI).

Finally, First Agency, one of the oldest and largest athletic accident insurers, recommends that athletic trainers avoid the following claims-processing pitfalls:

- Do not wait until an injury occurs to obtain the parent's insurance information from the student-athlete.

- Do not convey the impression that the institution will pay all expenses involving athletic injuries. One of the ways athletic departments can avoid this problem is to appoint a sole spokesperson who is responsible for managing the insurance program. All questions related to the insurance program should be directed to this person.

- Do not take primary responsibility for filing claims with the student's personal insurance company. Either the parents or the medical vendor should file such claims.

- Do not prepay medical vendors from the athletic budget. Prepaying can result in duplicate payments and arouse animosity between physicians and parents.

- Do not delay filing claims with either the primary or secondary insurers. Many policies have time limits beyond which they will not pay.

- Do not assume that medical bills have been filed with the parent's insurance company. Athletic trainers should contact parents soon after an injury occurs to remind them of the process for settling claims. In many cases, parents receive a bill and assume that the institution is taking care of it, causing delays in claim processing that lead to past-due accounts.

- Do not submit incomplete claims. Make sure that bills are itemized and accompanied by the parents' insurance information.

Claims Processing in Sports Medicine Clinics

The claims process in sports medicine clinics is fundamentally different from the process in educational institutions for two reasons. First, the athletic trainer or clinic administrator must integrate claims processing within the context of a larger patient billing system. Because of this arrangement, the livelihood of the sports medicine clinic depends on the ability to secure a steady flow of referrals from primary care physicians and specialists and to obtain reimbursement from third-party payers for patient bills. The second fundamental difference is that sports medicine clinics receive direct payments from third-party payers, whereas in the educational setting the money generally does not pass through the hands of an athletic trainer but goes directly to the medical vendor. This distinction is important, because it means that athletic trainers working in sports medicine clinics face a greater accounting burden than those working in educational institutions do.

One of the most important steps that athletic trainers in sports medicine clinics can take to ensure a smooth claims process is to seek prior authorization from a patient's insurance company before providing treatment. Some third-party payers, such as HMOs and PPOs, require this action; they usually will not provide reimbursement without preapproval by the primary care physician. Some Blue Cross plans will reimburse for rehabilitation and other sports medicine services, whereas other plans might not. The prudent clinic administrator should use the toll-free number provided by Blue Cross to determine in advance the limitations of the patient's policy.

Several steps can be followed when filing insurance claims with third-party payers, although one should always verify what is required from each individual payer and use systems and forms that are required for successful reimbursement (Albohm, Campbell, and Konin 2001):

- Use the required electronic forms for each specific provider policy and procedures.

- Submit the required patient information such as the patient's name, date of service, type of service, and balance due.

- Convert all the procedures performed to CPT codes and list prices.

- Identify all procedures, charges, and payments in a timely and accurate manner.

- Complete the claim form. Most third-party payers will accept the CMS 1500 claim form from private practice clinics (see figure 8.6). The UB-04, also known as the CMS 1450, is the appropriate form for hospitals (see figure 8.7).

- Obtain the authorized signature on the claim form.

- Place a copy of the insurance claim form in the patient's record.

- Enter the claim on the insurance claim tracking form.

- Mail (or transmit electronically) the claim form to the insurance company.

HEALTH INSURANCE CLAIM FORM

APPROVED BY NATIONAL UNIFORM CLAIM COMMITTEE (NUCC) 02/12

CARRIER

▢▢ PICA   PICA ▢▢

1. MEDICARE ▢ (Medicare#)   MEDICAID ▢ (Medicaid#)   TRICARE ▢ (ID#/DoD#)   CHAMPVA ▢ (Member ID#)   GROUP HEALTH PLAN ▢ (ID#)   FECA BLK LUNG ▢ (ID#)   OTHER ▢ (ID#) | 1a. INSURED'S I.D. NUMBER   (For Program in Item 1)

2. PATIENT'S NAME (Last Name, First Name, Middle Initial) | 3. PATIENT'S BIRTH DATE MM DD YY   SEX M ▢ F ▢ | 4. INSURED'S NAME (Last Name, First Name, Middle Initial)

5. PATIENT'S ADDRESS (No., Street) | 6. PATIENT RELATIONSHIP TO INSURED Self ▢ Spouse ▢ Child ▢ Other ▢ | 7. INSURED'S ADDRESS (No., Street)

CITY   STATE | 8. RESERVED FOR NUCC USE | CITY   STATE

ZIP CODE   TELEPHONE (Include Area Code) ( ) | | ZIP CODE   TELEPHONE (Include Area Code) ( )

9. OTHER INSURED'S NAME (Last Name, First Name, Middle Initial) | 10. IS PATIENT'S CONDITION RELATED TO: | 11. INSURED'S POLICY GROUP OR FECA NUMBER

a. OTHER INSURED'S POLICY OR GROUP NUMBER | a. EMPLOYMENT? (Current or Previous) YES ▢ NO ▢ | a. INSURED'S DATE OF BIRTH MM DD YY SEX M ▢ F ▢

b. RESERVED FOR NUCC USE | b. AUTO ACCIDENT? YES ▢ NO ▢ PLACE (State) | b. OTHER CLAIM ID (Designated by NUCC)

c. RESERVED FOR NUCC USE | c. OTHER ACCIDENT? YES ▢ NO ▢ | c. INSURANCE PLAN NAME OR PROGRAM NAME

d. INSURANCE PLAN NAME OR PROGRAM NAME | 10d. CLAIM CODES (Designated by NUCC) | d. IS THERE ANOTHER HEALTH BENEFIT PLAN? YES ▢ NO ▢ If yes, complete items 9, 9a, and 9d.

READ BACK OF FORM BEFORE COMPLETING & SIGNING THIS FORM.
12. PATIENT'S OR AUTHORIZED PERSON'S SIGNATURE I authorize the release of any medical or other information necessary to process this claim. I also request payment of government benefits either to myself or to the party who accepts assignment below.

SIGNED _____ DATE _____ | 13. INSURED'S OR AUTHORIZED PERSON'S SIGNATURE I authorize payment of medical benefits to the undersigned physician or supplier for services described below.

SIGNED _____

PATIENT AND INSURED INFORMATION

14. DATE OF CURRENT ILLNESS, INJURY, or PREGNANCY (LMP) MM DD YY QUAL. | 15. OTHER DATE QUAL. MM DD YY | 16. DATES PATIENT UNABLE TO WORK IN CURRENT OCCUPATION FROM MM DD YY TO MM DD YY

17. NAME OF REFERRING PROVIDER OR OTHER SOURCE 17a. 17b. NPI | 18. HOSPITALIZATION DATES RELATED TO CURRENT SERVICES FROM MM DD YY TO MM DD YY

19. ADDITIONAL CLAIM INFORMATION (Designated by NUCC) | 20. OUTSIDE LAB? YES ▢ NO ▢ $ CHARGES

21. DIAGNOSIS OR NATURE OF ILLNESS OR INJURY Relate A-L to service line below (24E)   ICD Ind. |
A. ___ B. ___ C. ___ D. ___
E. ___ F. ___ G. ___ H. ___
I. ___ J. ___ K. ___ L. ___ | 22. RESUBMISSION CODE   ORIGINAL REF. NO.
23. PRIOR AUTHORIZATION NUMBER

24. A. DATE(S) OF SERVICE From MM DD YY To MM DD YY	B. PLACE OF SERVICE	C. EMG	D. PROCEDURES, SERVICES, OR SUPPLIES (Explain Unusual Circumstances) CPT/HCPCS	MODIFIER	E. DIAGNOSIS POINTER	F. $ CHARGES	G. DAYS OR UNITS	H. EPSDT Family Plan	I. ID. QUAL.	J. RENDERING PROVIDER ID. #
1										NPI
2										NPI
3										NPI
4										NPI
5										NPI
6										NPI

25. FEDERAL TAX I.D. NUMBER SSN ▢ EIN ▢ | 26. PATIENT'S ACCOUNT NO. | 27. ACCEPT ASSIGNMENT? (For govt. claims, see back) YES ▢ NO ▢ | 28. TOTAL CHARGE $ | 29. AMOUNT PAID $ | 30. Rsvd for NUCC Use

31. SIGNATURE OF PHYSICIAN OR SUPPLIER INCLUDING DEGREES OR CREDENTIALS (I certify that the statements on the reverse apply to this bill and are made a part thereof.)

SIGNED _____ DATE _____ | 32. SERVICE FACILITY LOCATION INFORMATION a. NPI b. | 33. BILLING PROVIDER INFO & PH # ( ) a. NPI b.

PHYSICIAN OR SUPPLIER INFORMATION

NUCC Instruction Manual available at: www.nucc.org | **PLEASE PRINT OR TYPE** | APPROVED OMB-0938-1197 FORM 1500 (02-12)

Figure 8.6 CMS 1500.

Reprinted from Centers for Medicare and Medicaid Services. Available: www.cms.gov/medicare/cms-forms/cms-forms/cms-forms-items/cms1188854.html

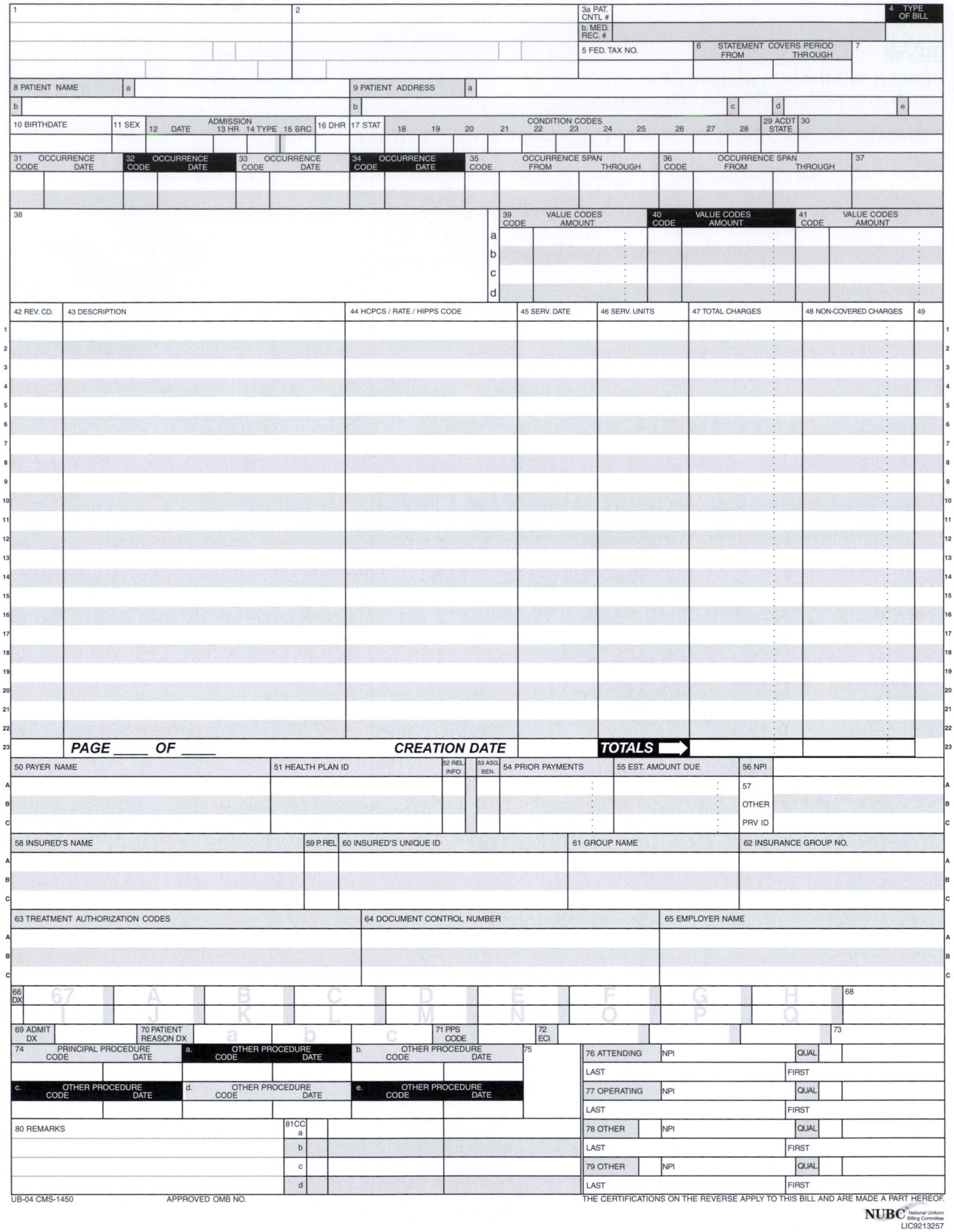
1
2
3a PAT. CNTL #
b. MED. REC. #
4 TYPE OF BILL
5 FED. TAX NO.
6 STATEMENT COVERS PERIOD FROM THROUGH
7
8 PATIENT NAME a b
9 PATIENT ADDRESS a b c d e
10 BIRTHDATE
11 SEX
ADMISSION 12 DATE 13 HR 14 TYPE 15 SRC
16 DHR
17 STAT
CONDITION CODES 18 19 20 21 22 23 24 25 26 27 28
29 ACDT STATE
30
31 OCCURRENCE CODE DATE
32 OCCURRENCE CODE DATE
33 OCCURRENCE CODE DATE
34 OCCURRENCE CODE DATE
35 OCCURRENCE SPAN CODE FROM THROUGH
36 OCCURRENCE SPAN CODE FROM THROUGH
37
38
39 VALUE CODES CODE AMOUNT
40 VALUE CODES CODE AMOUNT
41 VALUE CODES CODE AMOUNT
a b c d
42 REV. CD.
43 DESCRIPTION
44 HCPCS / RATE / HIPPS CODE
45 SERV. DATE
46 SERV. UNITS
47 TOTAL CHARGES
48 NON-COVERED CHARGES
49
PAGE ____ OF ____
CREATION DATE
TOTALS
50 PAYER NAME
51 HEALTH PLAN ID
52 REL. INFO
53 ASG. BEN.
54 PRIOR PAYMENTS
55 EST. AMOUNT DUE
56 NPI
57 OTHER PRV ID
58 INSURED'S NAME
59 P. REL
60 INSURED'S UNIQUE ID
61 GROUP NAME
62 INSURANCE GROUP NO.
63 TREATMENT AUTHORIZATION CODES
64 DOCUMENT CONTROL NUMBER
65 EMPLOYER NAME
66 DX
67 A B C D E F G H
I J K L M N O P Q
68
69 ADMIT DX
70 PATIENT REASON DX a b c
71 PPS CODE
72 ECI
73
74 PRINCIPAL PROCEDURE CODE DATE
a. OTHER PROCEDURE CODE DATE
b. OTHER PROCEDURE CODE DATE
c. OTHER PROCEDURE CODE DATE
d. OTHER PROCEDURE CODE DATE
e. OTHER PROCEDURE CODE DATE
75
76 ATTENDING NPI QUAL
LAST FIRST
77 OPERATING NPI QUAL
LAST FIRST
78 OTHER NPI QUAL
LAST FIRST
79 OTHER NPI QUAL
LAST FIRST
80 REMARKS
81CC a b c d
UB-04 CMS-1450
APPROVED OMB NO.
THE CERTIFICATIONS ON THE REVERSE APPLY TO THIS BILL AND ARE MADE A PART HEREOF.
NUBC National Uniform Billing Committee
LIC9213257

Figure 8.7 UB-04 (also CMS 1450).

Reprinted from Centers for Medicare and Medicaid Services. Available: www.cms.gov/Regulations-and-Guidance/Legislation/PaperworkReductionActof1995/PRA-Listing-Items/CMS-1450.html

The CMS 1500 and the UB-04, also known as the CMS 1450, are both available in electronic format at the Centers for Medicare and Medicaid Services website.

The Committee on Practice Advancement of the National Athletic Trainers' Association offers members an excellent guide to help athletic trainers who wish to charge for their services. Information specific to current resource documents can be found on the NATA website.

Medical practice software packages that help automate many of the steps for filing insurance claims are available. In addition, some insurance companies allow medical vendors to submit their claims either in the traditional manner, as just described, or in a scannable format. Preparing the scannable claim form (according to insurance company specifications) allows for quicker claims processing because a scanner automatically enters it into the insurance company's computer system. Claims that require a written explanation, however, will usually be held for review by a processing clerk.

It is not uncommon for submitted claims to be returned with payment denied. This can occur for a variety of reasons; these include incomplete or unsigned forms, services rendered by an ineligible provider, lack of medical necessity, services considered to be maintenance without expectations for improvement, invoices not submitted within a specific time period, no physician prescription, or a difference in diagnosis from that of the referring physician's office (Konin and Frederick 2018). Providers may take up to 90 days to pay an invoice even without an initial denial. If a claim is denied, it can be resubmitted as an appeal after corrections are noted by the payer.

Purchasing Insurance Services

An athletic trainer might be responsible for evaluating and buying an athletic accident policy for a school sports medicine program. A variety of people, including athletic directors, business office personnel, and risk managers, often share this function. Even if athletic trainers are not directly involved in evaluating and selecting insurance, they should not hesitate to offer their input, especially if they will be responsible for implementing the system.

PEARLS OF MANAGEMENT

Athletic trainers should work with an insurance agent to purchase insurance services. Although athletic trainers can buy insurance directly or by bidding, those pursuing this option should always be sure to determine the layers and limits of the coverage, deductibles and copayments that might be required, and exclusions to the policy.

Like sports medicine supplies and equipment, athletic accident insurance can be purchased in a variety of ways. One method is simply to contact a local insurance agency and ask the agent to write a policy covering the elements that the institution desires. This method requires the least time and effort on the part of the athletic trainer, but it is without question the least desirable. Investigating the wide range of insurance products and their prices is the surest method of obtaining the best protection for the lowest cost.

Another method that educational institutions commonly use is a formal bidding process to purchase insurance services. The advantage to the bidding method is that it allows institutions to obtain athletic accident insurance at the lowest possible cost. This system has disadvantages too. First, every insurance plan has hidden costs, the most significant of which is usually the time the institution's employees spend learning the system and filing the claims. If an institution awards athletic accident contracts to the lowest bidder annually, employees will spend a great deal of time learning new insurance systems—time that they could spend on more productive work. Another disadvantage of the bidding system, especially for institutions that bid for multiyear contracts, is that the initial low price of the premium may rise as the institution establishes a claims history with the company, which may raise rates to ensure that it makes a profit.

Bidding for insurance coverage can be a stressful and often frustrating process. The inexperienced athletic trainer may be involved in making a decision that affects tens of thousands of dollars for an institution yet possess no formal training or experience regarding the process. One method of improving leverage during bidding and negotiations is to consider collaborating with institutions that may be in your conference, in your geographical region, or of like size in terms of the number of participating student-athletes. This can also help inexperienced athletic trainers. Regardless of how the process is managed, an athletic trainer should be prepared to provide the past three to five years of a claims history to present to potential insurance providers so that they can analyze the trends of the injury claims in an effort to provide a fair bid for services.

An alternative to both the bidding and direct purchasing systems just described is for the athletic trainer and other institutional representatives to interview several insurance companies and carefully evaluate their products and prices. This process allows for easy clarification of questions and provides an opportunity to determine the procedures for processing claims.

No matter which purchasing method is used, each proposal should be evaluated with the following points in mind:

- What are the monetary limits of the coverage? What are the time limits of the coverage? Does the policy offer **layered coverage**? If so, what are the limits for each layer of coverage? Is there a layer of catastrophic coverage?

- What specific exclusions to the coverage are listed? What riders are available to cover these exclusions?

- Does the policy provide primary coverage or secondary (excess) coverage? If secondary, how does it interface with personal insurance? How does it handle student-athletes whose parents are covered by HMOs or PPOs?

- What deductibles, if any, apply to the policy? Who will be responsible for paying the deductible?

- What **copayments**, if any, does the policy require? Who is responsible for the copayments?

- Whom does the policy cover? Does it cover ancillary and support personnel, such as athletic trainers, coaches, student managers, and cheerleaders?

- Under what circumstances are covered individuals protected? How does the policy handle out-of-season injury?

- What is the annual premium? If a multiyear contract, how and under what circumstances will the annual premium change?

- What specific steps must the institution take to file claims? How much staff time and effort will be required to do so?

Revenue Models

As discussed in this chapter, athletic trainers historically have not been deeply involved with the expenses and revenues generated via athletic training services. Now more than ever, athletic trainers serving in administrative roles need to understand the business models associated with the cost of operating athletic training health care services and the various means of generating potential revenue to offset such costs. NATA offers resources to assist the athletic trainer in the secondary school and college and university settings with what is referred to as value models. These models educate athletic trainers on the types of metrics that can be performed and measured, ways to minimize risk and keep costs down, budgetary skills, and fund-raising possibilities, among other helpful tools.

One emerging area of practice for athletic trainers involves direct fee for services, or what is referred to as a cash-based service (Matney and Husen n.d.). Cash-based services are typically contractual in nature and may be delivered one-on-one with a patient or client, or may be offered in other formats where the services rendered are paid in cash. This model is attractive because it bypasses the comprehensive and often complicated third-party reimbursement. Athletic trainers involved in cash-based practices are more involved in a self-started business plan and set their own fees based on their perceived value. The reputation of the athletic trainer, the clinical and business experience, the geographical location, and the potential for client growth are just a few of the many factors that will determine the success of a cash-based practice.

Summary

Reimbursement provides an opportunity to receive equitable remuneration for professionally delivered health care services. While reimbursement for services and involvement with various forms of insurance did not play a role in the early days of athletic training, they have become more commonplace in the practice of athletic training today. Various types of insurance exist, including (but not limited to) health, accident, medical, and liability. For student-athletes, medical, health, and accident insurance exist to support injuries and illnesses that occur as a result of sport participation. The athletic trainer is often involved with the data collection and claims processing associated with these types of insurance plans. A series of steps are taken to ensure proper filing of an insurance claim, and the types of services provided will often be dictated by the specific type of plan an individual or the individual's affiliation (or both) has contracted with. All policies and plans offer advantages and disadvantages, and each person should take the time to understand the specific type of insurance plan that he maintains. The entire process associated with insurance and reimbursement can be time sensitive and complicated, requiring the athletic trainer to be competent and remain current regarding industry standards. Athletic trainers should use the resources available to understand revenue models.

Learning Aids

Case Study 1

Rosita was beginning to have second thoughts about her decision four months earlier to sell her private sports medicine and physical therapy practice to Universal Health Care Services. She had thought that by selling the practice to Universal, a huge medical practice conglomerate operating in 47 states, she would be able to improve her bottom line while the parent company assumed the risk of adding the new, expensive equipment she desperately needed to remain competitive with the local hospital's sports medicine clinic. Unfortunately, she soon discovered that Universal put so much pressure on her to increase revenue that patient care was beginning to suffer. Still, she thought that she had to do something to meet Universal's expectations or she would have to leave the practice she had worked so long to establish.

Bob, Universal's manager of clinic operations for 10 northern states, visited Rosita's clinic and told her she would have to institute the following billing and insurance practices immediately:

- All new patients were to be discharged immediately when they met their insurance limits.
- No patients were to be discharged until their insurance expired.
- Every patient was to be billed for a minimum of 1 hour of therapy to cover expenses associated with overhead at the home office.
- Patients without insurance were not to be accepted.

Although Rosita was upset with the new regulations, she thought she had no choice but to conform to the standards established by the company. The day after Bob's visit, she implemented the new regulations.

Questions for Analysis

1. What potential legal pitfalls do the new billing and insurance regulations pose for Rosita and her staff? What ethical dilemmas, if any, do these regulations pose?
2. How could Rosita implement the regulations without violating the law? Would these actions serve her patients well? Why or why not?
3. What other revenue-enhancing procedures, besides those mandated by Universal, could Rosita implement? How would they serve her patients more efficiently and effectively than the procedures required by Universal?

Case Study 2

Libby, Northwest State University's head athletic trainer, was called into the athletic director's office and told that a new university policy required all service contracts to be awarded to the lowest bidder. The new rule was to take effect beginning with the next fiscal year, which was only two months away. Libby would have to put together a bidding package for the university's athletic accident insurance, the ambulance service, and the team physician's contract. The athletic director gave her one month to secure the bids. This schedule would give him enough time, he thought, to evaluate the bids, award the contracts, and have the services in place by the time the new fiscal year began.

Although Libby was not happy about having to put these services out for bid, she went to work right away. She knew that the insurance bid would be the most complicated, so she decided to tackle that part of the project first. She put together a bidding document that requested cost quotations based on the following requirements:

- Excess coverage for 500 student-athletes in 18 sports, including football and gymnastics
- Excess coverage for all ancillary and support personnel
- Coverage limits up to $50,000 with lifetime catastrophic coverage for amounts above $50,000

Libby included a copy of the university's claims history for the previous five years (an average of 75 claims per year) and sent the bidding package to three insurance companies that specialized in athletic accident insurance. Two weeks later she received the bids. She developed this table to help the athletic director understand the bids:

| | | Premium | | |
| | | Deductible per claim | | |
Company	Coverage	$0	$100	$250
Professional Underwriters	$50,000	$20,000	$17,500	$15,000
Best Insurance Company	$50,000	$18,000	$16,000	$14,000
Good Insurance Company	$25,000	$12,000	$10,000	$8,000

Questions for Analysis

1. What advantages and disadvantages are likely to accompany the university's new policy regarding the athletic accident insurance program?

2. If you were in Libby's position, would you have followed the same process in securing bids for insurance? Why or why not? What would you have done differently?

3. Based on the information in the table, which company's insurance policy represents the best value? Do you need any other information to reach this conclusion?

4. The Good Insurance Company will write a policy only with a maximum of $25,000 per claim. The university's catastrophic insurance coverage does not take effect until $50,000 in medical bills has been paid. If the university decided to purchase the Good Insurance Company's policy, what options should it investigate to decrease its risk between $25,000 and $50,000?

Key Concepts and Review

Understand the difference between medical, health, and accident insurance.

As the cost of medical care continues to rise and the quality of insurance (e.g., coverage, cost, time to pay claims) continues to fall, it is becoming increasingly important for athletic trainers to understand insurance systems. Insurance not only protects the assets of educational institutions that sponsor athletic programs, but also safeguards the income and livelihood of athletic trainers employed by sports medicine clinics. Most athletic accident policies cover only acute injuries with no connection to preexisting conditions and do not pay for illnesses or overuse conditions. Medical and health insurance policies are generally more comprehensive and are usually designed to help cover a percentage of an insured person's medical bills or to provide coverage for activities designed to maintain good health.

Understand the advantages and disadvantages of self-insurance, primary coverage, and secondary coverage.

The three choices available to most educational institutions when buying insurance services are self-insurance, primary coverage, and secondary (or excess) coverage. Secondary coverage is the most common type of insurance plan because it uses the patient's personal health insurance as a first layer of coverage. Primary insurance is expensive; it pays all covered expenses from the first dollar. Some institutions choose to self-insure, gambling that they will not incur large claims that would drain institutional coffers.

Define the types of injuries covered by most athletic accident policies.

Most athletic accident policies cover only acute injuries that occur in officially sanctioned practices or games. These policies usually do not cover chronic injuries, illnesses, or degenerative conditions.

Understand the basic legal responsibilities associated with third-party reimbursement.

Athletic trainers reimbursed for services through third-party insurance plans should maintain patient–practitioner confidentiality. They should never release medical records to third-party payers unless the patient has provided written authorization. Athletic trainers commit fraud when altering the date of an injury, treatment, or assessment or when failing to record payments from an insurance company on a patient's bill. Claiming reimbursement for services not provided is also illegal and is punishable by substantial fines.

Understand the role of procedural coding in the third-party reimbursement system.

CPT is a list of codes representing procedures and is used on insurance claim forms. Diagnostic coding provides third-party payers with a standardized system for determining the kinds of medical conditions that health care providers are treating when they seek reimbursement.

Organize a claims-processing system for a sports medicine program in an educational setting.

Claims processing in educational settings is different from claims processing in a sports medicine clinic. In each case, patients enrolled in some managed care plans must receive authorization from primary care providers before services are rendered. Athletic trainers in educational settings should communicate the limits of the school's athletic accident insurance policy to parents. Each athlete who submits an insurance claim needs a separate file, and bills should not be submitted to the school's insurance company until the athletic trainer has received an explanation of benefits report from the athlete's personal health insurance company.

Understand the steps required to file a claim for reimbursement from a third-party payer.

All diagnoses and procedures must be converted to coded form using the ICD-10-CM and the CPT list of codes. Claims can be submitted on the standard CMS 1500 form for private practice settings, the UB-04 (CMS 1450) form for hospitals, on a scannable form, or electronically using a computer. Athletic trainers responsible for this process must keep meticulous records of all procedures, charges, and payments.

Evaluate and purchase an athletic accident insurance policy for an educational institution.

Athletic trainers are frequently responsible for purchasing or recommending the purchase of athletic accident insurance. Price, policy exclusions, limits of coverage, deductibles, and claims-processing workload should all be considered when the policies offered by various insurance companies are being evaluated.

Ethics in Sports Medicine

Objectives

After reading this chapter, you should be able to do the following:

- Understand the definition and purpose of ethical standards and their relevance for the athletic trainer.

- Define what the term *professionalism* means as it relates to an athletic trainer.

- Identify the appropriate code of ethics that applies generally to the profession of athletic training, along with codes that might apply to specific settings within the profession.

- Identify the situations and circumstances in which ethical concerns are most frequent.

- Develop strategies for avoiding ethical problems and for dealing with them if they occur.

- Recognize the ethical challenges and overall issues associated with whistle-blowing.

- Recognize elements of cultural competence as they relate to athletic training.

Portions of this chapter are reprinted or adapted from R.R. Ray and D. Wiese-Bjornstal, *Ethical perspectives in counseling* (Champaign, IL: Human Kinetics, 1999), 161-175. By permission of Richard Ray.

Athletic training is a profession that places many pressures on its practitioners. Athletic trainers face pressure from coaches, whose security needs are met through winning games; from athletes and other physically active patients, who are often willing to sacrifice their health for short-term glory; and from a variety of other sources (Kroshus et al. 2015; Testoni et al. 2013). One common by-product of this pressure is the temptation to make decisions or perform acts that, although seemingly innocent, are not in the best interests of patients or of the profession.

As professionals, all athletic trainers have a responsibility to act in an ethical manner. Unfortunately, fulfilling this responsibility is not always easy. Ethical decision making requires both the knowledge of ethical responsibilities and the willpower to endure the inevitable hardships that accompany ethically correct decisions. This duty to report is endorsed by the strategic alliance composed of the Commission on Accreditation of Athletic Training Education (CAATE), the National Athletic Trainers' Association (NATA), the NATA Research and Education Foundation (NATA Foundation), and the Board of Certification (BOC) (Strategic Alliance n.d.). The purpose of this chapter is to introduce the topic of ethics as it applies to athletic trainers. We will identify some of the most common situations in which ethical breaches can occur, and we will consider steps that the athletic trainer can take to minimize their occurrence.

Ethical practice is not limited to the managerial roles assumed by athletic trainers; ethical dilemmas arise in other domains of the profession as well. An athletic trainer's injury management, rehabilitation, education, and counseling roles are particularly rich with potential ethical problems. Although not all ethical problems are related to the managerial role, many are. All require some degree of decision making. Decision making is the single most common element among all managerial functions, and the ability to make good decisions is one of an athletic trainer's most important managerial skills.

Defining Ethics

Ethics is the study of the rules, standards, and principles that dictate right conduct among members of a society. Such rules are based on moral values. Principles of ethics have developed from a long, rich history of philosophical debate. They are deeply embedded in our choices of how we govern and conduct ourselves as a civilized society and serve as the basis for many of our norms for social interaction. Ethics also reflect many of the tenets of a variety of religions and have been influenced by religious philosophies from around the world. All of these influences and history have led us to depend on the principles of ethics to form the moral backbone of the most important things that we do as contributors to a conscientious society. In athletic training, individual moral philosophies and ethical decision making has been studied for both athletic training students and athletic training educators looking at idealism and relativism scores (Caswell and Gould 2008). Whereas *idealism* reflects how the fundamental rightness of an action should ultimately determine one's behavior, *relativism* more closely identifies situations where individuals reject a universally accepted moral principle. Examples of relativism according to Caswell and Gould (2008) include "never lie or cheat" and "abide by the golden rule." In their findings, undergraduate students rated higher than educators in their idealism scores, with gender playing no significant difference in the results.

KEY POINT

Ethics help define acceptable behavior among members of a group. Professions establish codes of ethics to provide behavioral guidelines for their members and to help protect the public from the actions of unethical practitioners.

Why Professions Establish Ethical Standards

Professions are defined by a commitment to certain characteristics that set them apart from nonprofessional groups within our society. One of the most important of these characteristics is a commitment to high standards of ethical behavior by the members of the profession. The professional organization of each of the professions that provide health care services to athletes and other physically active patients writes a code of ethics to establish its ethical standards. The purpose of these codes is to provide a guide to appropriate conduct for members, to provide a reference by which to judge members when their conduct comes into question, and to provide assurance and protection to the public served by members of the profession.

PEARLS OF MANAGEMENT

Even though a code of ethics is not a formal legal document, violating an ethical code oftentimes can lead to a violation of the law.

Ethical Standards Relevant to Athletic Training

Sports health care professionals should comply with the code of ethics of the national professional organization for their primary profession. Athletic trainers must adhere to several sets of professional standards. The NATA Code of Ethics (National Athletic Trainers' Association 2016) is intended to guide the actions of every member of NATA in the practice of athletic training (see appendix C). The code consists of four general principles, each with its own substatements. Violation of the code may result in one or more of the following sanctions: denial of eligibility, cancellation, nonrenewal, and suspension of membership; public censure; or private reprimand.

Athletic trainers who hold dual credentialing as physical therapists must adhere to the American Physical Therapy Association Code of Ethics. Similarly, athletic trainers who hold other certifications or credentials, such as those for nurses, occupational therapists, physicians, physician assistants, or emergency medical technicians, are bound by the codes of ethics of the organizations that represent those professions. Code of ethics documents provide guidelines for ethical conduct within the respective professions and apply to the entire range of practice patterns and settings applicable to those professions. Their standards are enforceable for the members of each organization but should also be considered applicable to nonmembers within the profession as it relates to an overall standard of care and behavior of an athletic trainer.

Despite variations in how different professions view their own ethical conduct, the foundation for forming guidelines for each can be based on six underlying principles (Rubin 2002):

1. *Autonomy.* A patient's right to be fully informed, to make his or her own health care decisions, and to have his or her inherent dignity respected
2. *Beneficence.* Commitment to do good and to try to do the best for each patient
3. *Nonmaleficence.* Commitment to avoid doing bad things and to do no harm
4. *Fidelity.* Subordination of one's needs to those of the patient
5. *Veracity.* Truth telling and honesty
6. *Justice.* Concept that all patients should be treated fairly without regard to race, religion, and so on

Unfortunately, becoming informed about NATA's code of ethics is often not enough, even for athletic trainers without dual credentials. The various practice domains force athletic trainers to examine the ethical codes of other disciplines to make sure that they do not stray from accepted practice in those disciplines. For example, when providing counseling to student-athletes, athletic trainers should be sure to adhere to the *Code of Ethics* of the American Counseling Association or to the *Ethical Principles of Psychologists and Code of Conduct* of the American Psychological Association. Athletic trainers who are also teachers might be bound by the ethical codes of professional educators' societies, such as the American Association of University Professors. Finally, ethical standards exist that are specific to particular employment settings.

KEY POINT

Go online to find the code of ethics for the following organizations: American Counseling Association, American Psychological Association, American Association of University Professors *(Statement on Professional Ethics)*, the International Federation of Sports Medicine, and the American Physical Therapy Association.

Efforts to implore members of professions and professional associations to adhere to an ethical code of conduct are necessary to establish public trust that in the eyes of some has been waning in recent years (Cohen 2006). Public trust is based on altruism, respect, honesty, integrity, dutifulness, honor, excellence, and accountability. While the overwhelming majority of health care providers abide by their professional ethical guidelines, some are faced with a unique set of challenges related to these principles. This is seen in cases in which individuals hold dual certifications and credentials, such as a certified athletic trainer who is also a physical therapist, or a physical therapist who is also a chiropractor. In these circumstances, the professional who attempts to follow ethical principles of both professionally affiliated organizations may find that the organizations are at odds with one another. Position statements and other organizational initiatives may conflict between the two organizations, placing the health care professional in a difficult predicament. Professional organizations are focused on supporting, endorsing, and protecting their professional members; thus, they may not be sympathetic toward health care professionals who hold dual memberships. Core competencies for interprofessional collaborative practice is a standard that all health care providers should adhere to.

Medical Ethics

While professionals in different disciplines define their own set of ethical standards, those in health care typically follow a set of guidelines referred to as **medical ethics**. Campbell and colleagues (2005) defined medical ethics as a moral philosophy that helps practitioners and others discern whether and under what circumstances various health care practices are right or wrong. For physicians, the foundation for ethical practice has been established by the Hippocratic Oath:

I SWEAR TO FULFILL, TO THE BEST OF MY ABILITY AND JUDGMENT, THIS COVENANT:

I will respect the hard-won scientific gains of those physicians in whose steps I walk, and gladly share such knowledge as is mine with those who are to follow.

I will apply, for the benefit of the sick, all measures [that] are required, avoiding those twin traps of overtreatment and therapeutic nihilism.

I will remember that there is art to medicine as well as science, and that warmth, sympathy, and understanding may outweigh the surgeon's knife or the chemist's drug.

I will not be ashamed to say "I know not," nor will I fail to call on my colleagues when the skills of another are needed for a patient's recovery.

I will respect the privacy of my patients, for their problems are not disclosed to me that the world may know. Most especially must I tread with care in matters of life and death. If it is given me to save a life, all thanks. But it may also be within my power to take a life; this awesome responsibility must be faced with great humbleness and awareness of my own frailty. Above all, I must not play at God.

I will remember that I do not treat a fever chart, or a cancerous growth, but a sick human being, whose illness may affect the person's family and economic stability. My responsibility includes these related problems, if I am to care adequately for the sick.

I will prevent disease whenever I can, for prevention is preferable to cure.

I will remember that I remain a member of society, with special obligations to all my fellow human beings, those sound of mind and body as well as the infirm.

If I do not violate this oath, may I enjoy life and art, respected while I live and remembered with affection thereafter. May I always act so as to preserve the finest traditions of my calling and may I long experience the joy of healing those who seek my help.

KEY POINT

Medical ethics is a moral philosophy that helps practitioners and others discern whether and under what circumstances various health care practices are right or wrong.

The **Hippocratic Oath** is believed to have been written by Hippocrates, who is considered the father of Western medicine, around the late fifth century B.C. The oath is taken by new physicians and other new health care practitioners to swear in the presence of others that they will uphold their professional ethical standards. Today, the Hippocratic Oath has been translated from its original format to both classic and modern versions (the modern version is presented here).

Medical ethics goes beyond the relationship between a single practitioner and a patient. All health care professionals must work collaboratively despite their variance of training in an effort to offer maximum benefits for all patients involved in the health care system (Davidoff 2000; Gibson 2002). A group of interdisciplinary health care providers consisting of physicians, nurses, health care admin-istrators, academics, ethicists, lawyers, economists, and philosophers met to develop ethical principles that might be useful for all individuals involved in the health care delivery system. This group has since become known as the Tavistock (named after a square in London where the meeting took place) group, and the set of principles derived from their discussions is referred to as the Tavistock principles. The principles were all encompassing, designed to benefit those who are responsible for the health care system, those who work in it, and those who use it.

The following are the seven principles defined by the Tavistock group (Magee 2010):

1. *A human right.* Health care is a human right.

2. *Balance between patient centered and population sensitive.* The care of the individual is at the center of health care delivery, but must be viewed and practiced within the overall context of continuing work to generate the greatest possible health gains for groups and populations.

3. *Comprehensive management of disease burden and promotion of prevention.* The responsibilities of the health care delivery system include the prevention of illness and the alleviation of disability.

4. *Professional collaboration.* Cooperation with each other and those served is imperative for those working within the health care delivery system.

5. *Quality improvement.* All individuals and groups involved in health care, whether providing access or services, have the continuing responsibility to help improve its quality.

6. *Safety.* Initially there was anxiety over "do no harm" because it is so strongly associated with doctors. But this principle seemed important to include because there is increasing recognition of just how much harm health care systems produce and of how policies with benign intentions can create harm.

7. *Openness.* This last principle might be both the most banal and the most profound. Nobody could argue against being open, honest, and trustworthy; yet every day in every health care system, people fail on all three counts.

KEY POINT

Athletic trainers can usually act in an ethical manner by acting within the law. They can become involved in ethical dilemmas as either a primary party or a third party.

Relationship Between Legal and Ethical Considerations

Ethical considerations often overlap with, contradict, or otherwise interact with issues of **law**. In convenient circumstances, difficult ethical decisions are consistent with the law, but an athletic trainer must recognize that in some situations what is ethical might not be legal and what is legal might not be ethical. This issue is especially difficult for those in health care roles who must consider issues of confidentiality and protection of individual **rights** to privacy. The right of an athlete to privacy might well conflict with the law when the law dictates that a specific type of information be reported. The multiple roles served by athletic trainers make the issue even more difficult because of the many types of information for which they are responsible. The most recent large-scale issue of this kind is the reporting of human immunodeficiency virus (HIV) status required by some health departments. Ideas regarding how an athletic trainer might deal with such conflicts are included later in this chapter. What is clear is that professional codes of ethics usually dictate that it is unethical to engage in any practice activity that is illegal (Makarowski and Rickell 1993).

Defining Professionalism

As simple as the term may sound, *professionalism* is not clearly defined and agreed on among those in all health care disciplines (Craig 2006; Doherty and Purtilo 2016; Swick 2000). Concepts of professionalism have been reported to change according to age, experience level, educational rank, and gender (Nath, Schmidt, and Gunel 2006). Nath and colleagues found that younger health care professionals in training were more likely than their older peers or faculty to view certain behaviors as unprofessional. Isear (1997) originally defined three elements of professionalism:

1. Clinician–patient relationship (trust, confidence)
2. Collegial relationships (with other health care professionals, including professional growth)
3. Attire and hygiene (personal intangibles, such as punctuality, adhering to commitments, understanding role limitations)

Isear's elements are similar to those of Chambers (2004), who incorporates more of a community-based approach toward the characteristics of a professional:

1. Form a community of practitioners who simultaneously work for themselves, customers, and peers.
2. Help patients and clients who are individuals making their own personal choices.
3. Serve private and personal needs of customers seeking wholeness.
4. Work as agents on behalf of customers instead of transacting services.
5. Function in a relationship of trust.

Implementing these elements does not appear to be an overwhelming task to request of a health care professional. Why, then, are they not adhered to regularly by all? Even though most health care professionals place a high value on the components of professionalism, not all believe that they are easy to incorporate into daily practice. The three most common barriers to professionalism as reported by medical residents are time constraints (51.5%), high workloads (21.9%), and having to work with challenging or difficult patients (16%) (Ratanawongsa et al. 2006).

Professionalism is not an expectation only for practicing clinicians, educators, and administrators. The process of developing skills and characteristics to become a competent professional must also be nurtured while students engage in their formal academic preparation (Cruess and Cruess 2012). Professionalism is one of the six core competencies of both the Accreditation Council for Graduate Medical Education (ACGME) and the American Board of Medical Specialties (ABMS) (DeRosa 2006). Professionalism is taught at the medical school level and in residency programs, as well as in all athletic training education programs. A fact that merits discussion is that after one completes all academic requirements and becomes further removed from formal education, less emphasis is placed on grade point average and more attention is paid to interpersonal skills and professional behaviors. Physical therapy educators have also attempted to define professionalism in an effort to promote such behavior as a part of student preparation (Jette and Portney 2003). Similar to what Isear (1997) suggested for athletic trainers, surveys of physical therapy students identified the following attributes associated with professionalism: self-presentation, accountability, integrity, and values.

The Athletic Trainer as a Primary Party

An athletic trainer may face ethical issues in many different forms. The most menacing will be those in which the athletic trainer is a **primary party** to the ethical concern. To be a primary party means that the athletic trainer is directly involved in the situation as a person who has behaved in an ethically questionable manner or who is the victim of an unethical act committed by another person. Of primary concern in this chapter is the first situation, in which the athletic trainer is the **perpetrator** of an unethical act.

The next few paragraphs address three types of situations in which an athletic trainer might become entangled as a primary party in an ethical dilemma. Although this set of situations is not exhaustive, these are the scenarios that occur most often or that have the greatest potential to harm the individuals involved. By adhering to codes of ethics, the athletic trainer will do much to protect both the patient and himself.

Breach of Confidentiality

One of the most frequently recurring ethical situations faced by athletic trainers involves **breach of confidentiality**. This situation is especially difficult for several reasons. First, an athletic trainer often serves in many roles that relate to an athlete. The athletic trainer often needs to share information with the team organization, with coaches, or with colleagues who are also responsible for some aspect of the athlete's care. Those needs, legitimate or not, sometimes conflict with what is in the best interest of athletes and with the responsibilities that the athletic trainer has for their health care.

Confidential information obtained as part of the professional relationship that an athletic trainer has with an athlete or other physically active patient might be personal, private, and sensitive. The athletic trainer should handle such information carefully to avoid ethical as well as legal breaches

Types of Unethical Conduct

The following are the most common or serious situations in which an athletic trainer might become a primary party:

- Breach of confidentiality
- Conflict of interest
- Exploitation

of confidentiality. In some situations, the most appropriate ethical behavior might even jeopardize an athletic trainer's job.

The second reason it might be difficult for an athletic trainer to maintain confidentiality is that often many people are involved in the care of an athlete or other physically active patient. This situation is especially common when student and intern practitioners who might not be fully cognizant of concerns for confidentiality are involved. When an athletic trainer is responsible for the supervision of students and interns, she will also be held responsible for student or intern actions. The athletic trainer can become a primary party in a breach of confidentiality even if she was not the immediate perpetrator of the breach.

The final concern relative to confidentiality is the high profile of athletes and of the athletic industry in our society. The pressures of the press and the public's desire to know everything possible about a high-profile athlete can pose significant threats to an athlete's right to privacy and to the confidentiality of information that an athletic trainer is privy to. To avoid breaches of confidentiality, athletic trainers should take proactive and diligent measures to protect information and communications. Several suggestions for such measures are offered in the following sidebar.

The codes of ethics note three exceptions to the rule of confidentiality:

1. When the client is in clear and imminent danger
2. When other persons are in clear and imminent danger
3. When legal requirements demand the release of confidential information

No reason for a breach of confidentiality other than those listed serves as an excuse for its occurrence. A professional should recognize the difference between a **reason** and an **excuse** and should accept a reason as an excuse only when it is both unavoidable and justifiable. These reasons would be considered excusable; any other reason would be inexcusable.

Conflict of Interest

Athletic trainers are also susceptible to ethical breaches based on **conflicts of interest**. Here again, the particular threat to ethical practice is a result of the multiple roles that an athletic trainer might fill. The responsibilities that an athletic trainer has to a team organization, to the coaching staff, and to himself will often conflict with his responsibilities

Measures to Protect the Confidentiality of Information and Communications

- Publish established policies regarding communication with coaches, administrators, media, and so on.
- Establish and follow responsible procedures for documentation, and store records in a secure environment.
- Allow access to the records only to persons with a legitimate role in providing health care to the patient.
- Release information only with written permission of the patient involved.
- Designate a specific person to handle all requests for health-related information; train all people in the organization and remind them regularly to refer all inquiries to that person.
- Never discuss the health status of an athlete or other physically active patient in public, and never in private, unless all persons present have a legitimate need and have authorization to access the information.

to an athlete or other physically active patient. The temptation to act or to advise an athlete or other patient in a manner that serves the team or protects the job or other interests of the athletic trainer might go unrecognized. Return-to-play decision making can often place an athletic trainer in a conflicted situation because of external pressures surrounding the individual circumstances (Kroshus et al. 2015).

A nearly universal component in most codes of ethics for health care professionals is the responsibility to place the best interests of the patient above all other concerns. This standard applies to every role assumed by an athletic trainer. Athletic trainers who receive payment to use a particular product might face a conflict of interest when treating patients with that product. An athletic trainer's role is particularly sensitive because the athletic trainer and the patient must develop a high degree of trust in one another. If the athletic trainer breaches this trust through a conflict of interest, rebuilding it might be impossible and the relationship might disintegrate. For that reason, among others, athletes with sensitive counseling or psychological concerns might be better off if they are referred to a counselor not affiliated with the institution or the team. The athletic trainer's role as administrator is also subject to conflicts of interest. When decisions regarding allocation of resources, including time, money, and personnel, clash with the health care needs of the athletic patient population, a conflict of interest might be present that could lead to an ethical breach.

Avoiding conflicts of interest is not enough. Athletic trainers should be careful to avoid even the appearance of a conflict. People interpret ethical standards in different ways. Sometimes a well-considered action will appear unethical to those who don't know why the decision was made or why the action was taken. Unfortunately, if the action appears to involve a conflict of interest and is therefore considered unethical, the trust required to maintain a reputation of high integrity will be damaged.

Exploitation

Exploitation of an athlete or other physically active patient by an athletic trainer is a particularly manipulative and self-interested form of conflict of interest. Exploitation involves the intentional use of another person or group of persons to achieve a selfish objective. When patients confide in an athletic trainer, they become particularly vulnerable to exploitation because they might reveal things about themselves that would otherwise be unknown. Under such circumstances, patients are vulnerable to exploitation for money, information, sex, self-endangerment (for example, manipulating an athlete to play while injured), goods, or any number of other reasons. For an athletic trainer to perpetrate such a situation would be clearly unethical.

The Athletic Trainer as a Third Party

An athletic trainer might also be involved in ethical dilemmas as a **third party**. To be a third party means that the athletic trainer is not personally involved in the dilemma but has professional responsibilities because of her knowledge of the situation. An athletic trainer has the responsibility not only to intervene in the best interest of the client, but also to protect others from harm whenever there is apparent risk of harm occurring.

One of the primary differences between being involved in a situation of ethical concern as a third party and being involved as a primary participant is that as a third party, an athletic trainer can act more appropriately to help find a resolution. When an athletic trainer's involvement is as a primary participant, especially in the presence of a conflict of interest or exploitation, he must often remove himself from the situation and request that someone else intervene to help resolve it. If he is involved in an ethical concern as a third party, the circumstance is much different. In this case the athletic trainer is often in a position to orchestrate a solution. The solution will often entail providing information and perspectives to the patient or managing other people and information to resolve the ethical dilemma.

An athletic trainer can become a third party to an ethical dilemma because of what she learns directly from a patient or because knowledge comes to her attention from other sources. Such knowledge can create difficult circumstances, because conflicts often occur between the professional's responsibility to maintain confidentiality, her responsibility to protect the patient from harm, her responsibility to protect others from harm, and other loyalties she might have that affect the patient.

Five categories of knowledge are most likely to render an athletic trainer a third party to an ethical dilemma.

Breach of Confidentiality, Conflict of Interest, and Exploitation of a Patient

As in situations when the athletic trainer is directly involved, breach of confidentiality, conflict of interest, and exploitation of a patient by a third party can be harmful to patients. Knowledge of such situations makes it incumbent upon the athletic trainer to intervene on behalf of the patient. Intervention usually does not mean that the athletic trainer has responsibility for correcting the situation. Bringing the situation to the patient's attention is usually sufficient because the patient can then take responsibility for the circumstance from a fully informed perspective. In the case of patients who are **minors** or who might otherwise be unable to protect themselves in such a situation, the athletic trainer should inform the parents or **guardians**, refer the situation to the appropriate authorities (particularly when there are legal concerns), or intervene directly.

Imagine, for example, that a college softball player goes to her athletic trainer for advice because she is frustrated about not getting enough playing time. She states that she thinks the woman playing ahead of her is getting all the playing time not because she is a better player but because she has a romantic relationship with the coach. The athletic trainer, as a third party having knowledge of this exploitation, would be ethically bound to intervene on behalf of both athletes.

Forbidden Knowledge

Forbidden knowledge is information about a situation that an athletic trainer is forbidden to act on. Such information might come from athletes or other physically active patients (about themselves or others), or it might come from another person. Typically, the person prefaces the sharing of information with a phrase such as "If I tell you this, you must promise not to share it with anyone" (Makarowski and Rickell 1993).

An athletic trainer should be wary of anyone who wants to share information but refuses to allow it to be acted on. To agree to such terms might preclude the athletic trainer from taking necessary actions that would otherwise supersede the promise, including the reasons cited earlier. An athletic trainer who receives forbidden information should insist that the patient offering it trust him to act in the patient's best interests. The patient should be assured that the athletic trainer will maintain the confidentiality of the information (provided that there is no threat of harm to the patient or to other persons affected by the information, and provided that the athletic trainer is not legally required to release the information). If a patient is unable to agree to those terms, the athletic trainer should offer him a referral to someone with whom he can trust the information, and the athletic trainer should strongly encourage the patient to follow through with it.

Categories of Knowledge That Make an Athletic Trainer a Third Party to an Ethical Dilemma

1. Knowledge of the occurrence of a breach of confidentiality, conflict of interest, or exploitation involving a patient
2. Forbidden knowledge
3. Knowledge of high-risk behaviors
4. Knowledge of illegal activities
5. Knowledge of situations in which the welfare of the patient conflicts with the welfare of another individual or group of individuals

When someone other than the patient involved offers forbidden information, an athletic trainer must clarify that she is obligated to act in the best interest of the patients under her care. Offering to use the information in an anonymous fashion might be appropriate, but an athletic trainer must not forfeit the right to use it when necessary.

A word of caution regarding the use of knowledge is in order, particularly in the context of forbidden knowledge. To take action on knowledge that is inaccurate or untrue can be harmful to athletic trainers, to the athletes or other physically active patients they are responsible for, or to others. The offer of forbidden knowledge by a patient or by others is a common avenue by which an athletic trainer is at risk for being **manipulated**. The athletic trainer should use information cautiously, particularly when the accuracy of the information is in doubt. In some circumstances, delaying action on a piece of information until it can be verified might be appropriate.

Knowledge of High-Risk Behaviors

Knowledge of **high-risk behaviors** is another area of potential ethical concern for an athletic trainer. This knowledge might come to you from your own observation, from a report from an athlete or other physically active patient under your care, or from others. This particular concern extends to situations in which a patient is at risk for harm because of his high-risk behaviors or the high-risk behaviors of others. It also includes situations in which the high-risk behavior of the patient puts others at risk.

When an athletic trainer has knowledge that a patient is engaging in potentially harmful high-risk behaviors that put only the patient at risk, the ethical responsibility is not to prevent the behaviors as much as it is to be sure that the individual involved is aware of the associated risks. The athletic trainer may also wish to help the person find alternatives to the high-risk behaviors. The athletic trainer's responsibilities in a case like this, therefore, are to provide the patient with information, education, and counseling so that she can make an informed choice regarding her participation in the behaviors.

When the high-risk behavior of an athlete puts others at risk, the athletic trainer has the responsibility to intervene, if only to make the other individuals aware of the risk so that they can protect themselves. For example, if an athletic trainer becomes aware that one of the athletes in her care is engaging in unprotected sexual activity with multiple partners, she might have an ethical duty to confront the athlete in a private setting and warn him of the consequences of such behavior. Another example is often seen in a college or university setting when a student-athlete tests positive following a drug screen. While established guidelines of confidentiality may exist regarding which individuals within an organization need to know of the positive test results, these guidelines may cover only the communication methods with administrators and coaches. However, others, such as strength and conditioning coaches, may have a justified need to be informed because they are working with student-athletes in a potentially risky environment—one in which a lack of judgment in thought processes could certainly lead to serious injury.

Knowledge of Illegal Activities

Knowledge of illegal activities related to an athlete or other physically active patient can also create a difficult ethical situation. An athlete might admit to illegal activities as part of an advising session, or the information might come to the attention of the athletic trainer from an outside source.

One of the difficulties of having knowledge of illegal activities is that legal authorities might be aware of those activities and seek information from the athletic trainer. The other difficulty occurs when legal authorities are unaware of the illegal activities. Both of these circumstances demand that the athletic trainer be familiar with her legal obligations as a professional and also demand careful consideration of the specific situation. Legal concerns become entangled with issues of confidentiality, responsibility to the client, privileged communication status, legal reporting requirements, and many others. Athletic trainers who have knowledge of a patient's illegal activities should consider seeking legal counsel to protect their own status and that of the patient.

Knowledge of Conflicting Interests

Self-determination is the freedom to judge for oneself, to determine one's own course of action, and to manage one's own affairs. This right, however, can come into conflict with the rights and welfare of other individuals or groups in society. For example, suppose an athletic trainer knows that a wrestler has a contagious skin disease that is difficult to see. In this example, the right of a capable and otherwise healthy athlete to compete would conflict with the right of other athletes to be protected from the skin disease.

Knowledge of situations in which the welfare of a patient conflicts with the welfare of another individual or group of individuals can present challenging ethical questions for the athletic trainer. Social conventions or law governs many of these types of situations, but some areas are not clearly defined. The athletic trainer might have the opportunity to remediate some of these difficult ethical situations. It is possible to resolve many of them by seeking permission to take action or disclose information, or by bringing the involved parties together to develop a mutually acceptable solution to the problem. Indeed, most situations in which the rights and welfare of individuals conflict can be resolved by providing an opportunity for the affected parties to become familiar with the perspectives of the other parties. Most people are reasonable and willing to compromise when they understand the concerns of others who might be affected by their actions.

The Act of Whistle-Blowing

A professional athletic trainer who feels obligated to abide by established policies might view the initial actions of informing a basketball coach of his player's misconduct as completely appropriate; others may think such a matter could be handled in a softer way, intending no formal inquiry beyond a friendly discussion between the coach and the player.

Even though reporting people who are perceived to have violated rules follows a set of rules in an attempt to do the right thing, it is often referred to as **whistle-blowing**. Whistle-blowers may report what they see or hear through proper reporting channels or to someone that they feel will be able to act on their information. Although the reporting in some cases can be done anonymously, the act is still considered whistle-blowing. Individuals may initiate or participate in whistle-blowing for a variety of reasons. It is believed that the typical whistle-blower is motivated by a sense of altruism and egoism while possessing strong moral convictions and a sense of responsibility to act appropriately. Whistle-blowers often think that the consequences of failing to bring the truth to light may be too great to bear and therefore they must act (Alford 2001). Some whistle-blowers feel that double standards exist within their employment setting and are uncomfortable not bringing issues to superiors; they may even feel ashamed of their work setting for allowing wrongdoing to go on.

The reporting of possible wrongdoing would appear on the surface to be the appropriate form of action in any workplace. As previously discussed in this chapter, this is an ethical decision that people must make on their own because there may be significant adverse consequences for the whistle-blower. However, the duty to report developed by the strategic alliance is something that all athletic trainers should become familiar with and take seriously. As Bok (2004) said of the whistle-blower's situation:

"The whistle blower hopes to stop the game; but since he is neither the referee nor the coach, and since he blows the whistle on his own team, his act is seen as a violation of loyalty."

Laws designed to protect the whistle-blower have not worked very well. Even if the whistle-blower has disclosed an obvious wrongdoing, there are a host of procedural and technical legalities that can fail to protect him (Alford 2001). All health care organizations should establish procedures for employees to report wrongdoing without fear of reprisal. These should include a range of actions such as anonymous reporting. In 2001, the corporate world faced a financial scandal in which numerous employees of the company known as Enron sensed a betrayal of financial responsibility on the part of their superiors, when their initial actions were not responded to. The result was federal criminal charges against the leaders of the organization and a significant amount of lost life earnings for the employees. This outcome led to the passing of the Sarbanes-Oxley Act, written to prohibit retaliation against whistle-blowers in publicly traded companies. This act also encouraged a standard for other industries to follow, including for-profit and not-for-profit health care organizations (Griffin 2005). Laws that have been enacted have not completely addressed the repercussions seen with whistle-blowing. Alford (2001) reported that two-thirds of whistle-blowers he had worked with ended up losing their jobs. Most never got their jobs back or even ended up working in the same field again. Some lost significant wages leading to bankruptcy, loss of their homes, and even loss of their families. Many of these individuals at the time of their reporting felt strongly that they were doing the correct thing. However, after dealing with the consequences, they regretted their actions and would advise others against whistle-blowing.

At the time of decision making, judgment as to whether or not one should report another person for a possible wrongdoing is not always clear. Why is judgment unclear in the heat of the moment, with the right decision becoming more apparent to a whistle-blower only as time passes? This thought process and learning from a particular situation are not unique to whistle-blowing. Many decisions in life are confusing and difficult to make at the most critical time. However, after time has passed and we have the opportunity to assess the outcomes, we learn from our experiences and apply the knowledge toward future situations.

Athletic trainers are not immune to negative outcomes, even when they believe whistle-blowing is a viable solution. For example, Weuve and colleagues (2014) demonstrated the prevalence of workplace bullying among athletic trainers in collegiate settings and how such behaviors can lead to stress and anxiety for the employee. They stated that proper workplace training and administrators who create a culture of respect are critical to minimizing bullying behaviors and incidents. However, absent these interventions, coworkers and others who witness such inappropriate behavior must decide whether or not to report these observations to proper authorities.

The act of whistle-blowing requires making a difficult decision that could have adverse ramifications, despite believing you are doing the right thing. Perhaps asking a series of questions first can help you decide whether or not to move forward with the act:

- How certain are you factually that wrongdoing has occurred? Did you witness firsthand, or are you relying on hearsay?

- Do you have anything in writing, audio, or video to support your claim?

- Can anyone else support your claim, or will you be the only one who has such knowledge or the only one willing to speak up?

- Should your whistle-blowing act result in adverse ramifications, have you thoroughly considered how you could be affected?

- Have you practiced your responses through role-playing exercises with close family members, close friends, or other trusted individuals?

- Are you prepared for a potentially lengthy and unpleasant period during the inquiry of the wrongdoing?

- If you are retaliated against and find yourself in a legal dilemma, do you have legal protection?

Practicing Ethically as an Athletic Trainer

The following recommendations are intended to serve as a functional guide to ethical practice in athletic training. The guidelines in this list should minimize the occurrence of ethical conflicts and facilitate the resolution of those that do occur.

PEARLS OF MANAGEMENT

Most athletic trainers are committed to practicing ethically, but they are not interested in becoming ethicists to do so. Fortunately, ethical practice doesn't require becoming an ethicist, but it does require an understanding of the meaning and intent of the relevant codes of ethics, reflection on the situations and actions that occur in practice, and the development of professional habits and awareness that are consistent with ethical practice.

- *Study the relevant professional codes of ethics.* Begin with the code of ethics of NATA and then review the codes of ethics of organizations that apply to your specific employment setting and the roles you play in that setting.

- *Learn to recognize situations in which ethical concerns are present or might appear to be present.* This undertaking requires careful consideration of how all your personal and professional relationships might affect the athletes or other physically active patients whom you treat.

- *Increase your sensitivity to situations in which ethical concerns are present.* Remember that ethics are relative and that the athletic trainer needs to be aware of how a situation may appear to persons viewing it from their own social or cultural perspective. Sensitivity requires that you be able to appreciate a situation from the point of view of others who are affected, particularly the patients under your care. Beyond that, you should treat every ethical concern seriously, or you will be perceived as insensitive and uncaring—and there is no better formula for professional trouble than that.

- *Consult with others whenever there are questions, especially when the answers are not clear or when they are not clearly defensible.* Good consultation serves to protect the athletic trainer as well as the patient because it provides an outside, objective perspective on the situation of concern. In addition, a small group often has more wisdom than an individual does.

- *Refer when the concern is beyond your legal scope of practice or your competence.* Everyone's best interests are served when athletic trainers make prudent use of referrals in critical, complicated, and difficult cases. To do this, however, athletic trainers must be acutely aware of their own limitations and must be sure to follow prescribed protocols for referral.

- *Refer when you become a primary party in an ethical dilemma or when you might be perceived by a patient or outside observers to be a primary party.* When an athletic trainer becomes a primary party in a situation of ethical concern, both the professional and the patient are at risk and the situation might become worse. In addition, even the perception of such a situation can be destructive. Referral to a health care professional not involved in the conflict is generally considered necessary and prudent in such situations.

• *Document carefully and often.* As in all areas of practice, careful, accurate documentation is essential. This includes documentation of all policies and procedures that have been read and agreed to by all those that the guidelines pertain to.

• *Follow your conscience.* A clear conscience requires knowledge and awareness. For the athletic trainer, good conscience requires knowledge of the moral and ethical standards applicable to the profession, and it requires awareness of the individual circumstances that each patient faces. Athletic trainers most often fail to be conscientious not so much because they lack knowledge but because they lack awareness. To be aware, they must be reflective and considerate, which takes time and effort. As athletic trainers, we must guard against becoming too busy or too routinized to allow ourselves the time and energy to be reflective and considerate. Otherwise we risk failing to be conscientious.

• *Fully disclose to a patient all your roles.* More than anything else, disclosure is an ethically critical component for informed consent in an athletic trainer's relationship with an athlete or other physically active patient. Identify all the roles you assume that might involve the athlete directly or indirectly. Avoid circumstances in which you are responsible for roles that present conflicting interests regarding the patient (Riendeau et al. 2015). Examples of the types of situations that warrant disclosure include, but are not limited to, the following:

- You should be sure that athletes understand that you also have responsibility for other athletes on a team and that you might be obligated to use or act on information that affects their health or safety.

- The organization that an athlete plays for often employs the athletic trainer. The athlete needs to understand this potential conflict of interest, because the practitioner might be required or might have strong incentives to act in the best interest of the organization rather than of the athlete.

- Athletic trainers often make available services, referrals, or goods in which they have a financial interest. The athletic trainer should disclose this conflict of interest to the athlete or other physically active patient and provide alternatives.

- Patients should be informed that an athletic trainer also has social and legal obligations that might require her to divulge information that could be in conflict with the patient's own best interest. If a patient tells her about certain illegal activities, the law might require her to report that information. Furthermore, the patient should be informed that information might be divulged when it indicates that the patient or others are in imminent danger.

• *Consider possible courses of action carefully.* When confronting an ethical dilemma, (1) identify the greatest variety of choices possible, including those that might seem extreme; (2) investigate each of the possible choices identified; and (3) judge your choices from an other-centered perspective rather than from a self-centered or egocentric perspective.

• *Allow patients to make their own fully informed choices rather than imposing solutions on them.* An informed perspective requires exploration of the positive and negative implications of every conceivable choice. Having relevant information allows athletes or other physically active patients to judge which course of action is in their best interest and is a necessary prerequisite to self-determination. Allowing patients to make their own choices helps them take responsibility for their destiny.

These actions, when combined, dramatically reduce the occurrence of ethical conundrums.

Cultural Competence

Diversity is observed each day in all facets of life. Health care providers are diverse both as individuals and as practitioners. Similarly, athletes and patients are diverse. They are diverse in their thinking, in their values, and in their actions. The cultural background of individuals is recognized as a major contributor toward their actions and expressed beliefs.

It is not uncommon for health care providers to make decisions for patients taking into account their own values. While a provider may mean well, this approach may not be optimal if his values differ from those of the patient (Campbell, Gillett, and Jones 2015). What part of one's cultural background leads to the development of values and beliefs? There is no one simple component. Numerous elements integrate with one another to formulate cultural beliefs.

Campinha-Bacote (2003) and Spector (2016) have identified the following as indicators of one's cultural makeup:

- Race
- Ethnicity
- Religious affiliation
- Language
- Physical size
- Gender
- Sexual orientation
- Age
- Disability
- Political orientation
- Socioeconomic status
- Occupational status
- Geographic location

Despite whatever indicators compose one's makeup, all individuals should be provided health care services on an equitable basis (Campbell, Gillett, and Jones 2015). In athletics, such indicators may also include type of sport (revenue generating versus nonrevenue generating) and level of participation (varsity versus junior varsity, travel team versus recreation team, Division I versus Division III).

Cultural competence has taken on a greater role over the last three decades in the United States as the result of rapidly changing population demographics. The Census Bureau estimates that by 2050, diverse racial and ethnic groups will constitute approximately 48% of the U.S. population (Bigby 2003b; Callister 2005; Institute of Medicine 2002).

Defining Cultural Awareness and Cultural Competence

Schlabach and Peer (2008) define culture as the shared values, beliefs, traditions, and customs of a particular group. A group can be identified by similar race, religion, ethnicity, or any of the previously mentioned indicators. While there is no single acceptable definition of *culture*, it consists of a sum of social characteristics of a given group of people (Spector 2016). Coaches fall under this definition of culture; to a certain extent, subgroups of coaches exist who form cultural views related to their own sport and its idiosyncrasies. Athletic trainers have become accustomed to working with some coaches who truly believe that an athlete's health and well-being come first above all other aspects of sport and life, with equal health care afforded to all. Some coaches, however, seek preferential treatment for athletes who play more significant roles on the team. While this lends itself to an ethical dilemma, the example demonstrates the ongoing relationship between cultural competence and ethical decision making.

As a health care professional, the athletic trainer will cross the paths of individuals on a daily basis who represent different cultures. While it is unrealistic to assume that an athletic trainer can become aware of all of the potential cultural differences, cultural awareness in and of itself is a critical first step toward becoming a competent health care provider (Perrin 2015). As one becomes aware, one becomes more competent. **Cultural awareness** represents a set of behaviors that an individual or group of individuals (organizations, businesses) possesses and implements through consistent actions that demonstrate appropriate awareness of diverse cultures. As there are numerous versions of the definition for culture, there are also several components of cultural competence (Bigby 2003b). Within health care, being culturally competent equates to being sensitive to issues of culture, race, gender, sexual orientation, social class, language, and economic situation (Stuart, Cherry, and Stuart 2011). Callister (2005) explained cultural competence nicely by relating areas of culture to a particular domain:

- Cultural awareness and knowledge (cognitive domain)
- Cultural skills (behavioral domain)
- Cultural sensitivity (affective domain)
- Cultural encounter (environmental domain)

With the growing cultural shift in the United States, cultural competence has taken on an increasingly important role in an effort to eliminate health care disparities (Callister 2005; Spector 2016). However, cultural awareness and cultural competence are not simply talked about and learned in a meeting. Athletic trainers should strive to systematically incorporate culturally competent principles into policies, the administrative structure, and clinical service delivery models in their athletic training settings (Bigby 2003b; Taylor and Lurie 2004). To put it simply, cultural awareness reflects on the process of an individual self-reflecting, while **cultural competence** is the process of applying one's cultural awareness toward one's actions and the actions of others.

Athletic trainers interact daily with individuals from a broad spectrum of cultural backgrounds. When Marra and colleagues (2010) studied the levels of cultural competence in the athletic trainers' delivery of health care, they found that athletic trainers believed that they possessed a higher level of cultural competence than that indicated by their scores on cultural assessment tools. Furthermore, and of greater concern, their cultural behaviors did not equitably reflect their cultural awareness and sensitivity. Of interest in these findings were that female athletic trainers and athletic trainers of multiracial or African American background scored higher on cultural competence scores. And they found that one's experience had no significant impact on cultural competence levels. This suggests that perhaps one's upbringing plays a greater role in cultural awareness and competence than formal teachings and actual work experience. Volberding's work (2013) reflects similar findings in that students of color demonstrated higher levels of cultural competence compared to their Caucasian counterparts, believed in part to be related to personal history and experiences. Nynas (2015), using a small sample size, reported that athletic training students possessed a good sense of cultural awareness and sensitivity but were less likely to actually apply culturally competent care. Students surveyed suggested enhanced integration within clinical environments that reinforce didactic material and require the athletic training to incorporate and implement cultural awareness and sensitivity into decision-making situations.

Challenges Associated With Establishing Cultural Competence

Reading and learning about different cultures is helpful for any practitioner. Most athletic trainers are confronted with issues of race, class, sex, and cultural diversity on a daily basis (Geisler 2003). Equally important is understanding how certain cultures perceive how they are treated within the health care system. For example, blacks and Latinos perceive that they receive a lower quality of health care than whites do. Blacks, Hispanics, and Asian Americans are more likely to report difficulty in accessing health care, paying for medications, and identifying a regular physician than whites; they are also more likely to rate the quality of care they receive from health care providers and the health care system in general more negatively (Bigby 2003a; Johnson et al. 2004). How does knowing this type of information help an athletic trainer become more culturally competent? This is part of becoming culturally sensitive, a component of the affective domain as defined by Callister (2005).

Culturally sensitive challenges may also be prevalent and may be exacerbated by the behaviors of health care practitioners who knowingly or unknowingly provide differential treatment, lack a sense of awareness of cultural issues, and perhaps even choose to spend less time with certain patients (Bigby 2003a). Ethnocentrism, the conviction that one's own culture is superior, can also hinder effective cross-cultural care (Juckett 2005).

National Standards for Cultural Competence

The profession of athletic training does not have set guidelines related to cultural competence. While the guidelines for accreditation for entry-level athletic training education programs refer to ethical behaviors, learning styles, and other related indicators, the words *cultural* and *diversity* do not appear in the guidelines administered by the Commission on Accreditation of Athletic Training Education (CAATE). However, NATA established the Ethnic Diversity Advisory Committee, defining its purposes as follows: "Identify and address issues relevant to American Indian/Alaskan Natives, Asian/Pacific Islanders, Black, non-Hispanic and Hispanic members. Additionally, address health care concerns affecting physically active individuals in these ethnic groups. Advocate sensitivity and understanding toward ethnic and cultural diversity throughout the profession and the association." The profession of athletic training would benefit from strategies designed to incorporate cultural awareness and competence into the formal didactic and clinical curriculums (Geisler 2003). NATA educational competencies that do refer to cultural competence state that cultural competence should be incorporated into all aspects of professional practice as a foundational behavior.

The Office of Minority Health of the U.S. government published the *National Standards on Culturally and Linguistically Appropriate Services in Health Care (CLAS Standards)*. These standards (presented in the following sidebar) provide a framework for building the cultural and linguistic competence of home health care agencies and can be integrated into athletic training practice settings (U.S. Department of Health and Human Services n.d.).

Cultural awareness and competence can be as simple as respecting others' beliefs and interest in receiving alternative or complementary therapies. Nontraditional athletic training treatment interventions, such as aromatherapy, reflexology, or hypnotherapy, may be the treatment of choice for some patients. While disagreeing with such forms of care and perhaps even being able to cite a lack of evidence to support such treatments, an athletic trainer should respectfully acknowledge the wishes of a patient and perhaps take the time to learn more about why the patient prefers a particular form of care (Spector 2016).

Athletic training curriculums and clinical education experiences teach us formal and informal methods of what we perceive to be appropriate health care delivery services. However, some elements of our health care delivery approach may seem strange to people from different cultures. For example, preventive medicine is not practiced in all cultures, and in some countries patients must wait months just to see a physician regardless of the severity of

National Culturally and Linguistically Appropriate Services Standards

The National CLAS Standards are intended to advance health equity, improve quality, and help eliminate health care disparities by establishing a blueprint for health and health care organizations.

Principal Standard

- Provide effective, equitable, understandable, and respectful quality care and services that are responsive to diverse cultural health beliefs and practices, preferred languages, health literacy, and other communication needs.

Governance, Leadership, and Workforce

- Advance and sustain organizational governance and leadership that promotes CLAS and health equity through policy, practices, and allocated resources.
- Recruit, promote, and support a culturally and linguistically diverse governance, leadership, and workforce that are responsive to the population in the service area.
- Educate and train governance, leadership, and workforce in culturally and linguistically appropriate policies and practices on an ongoing basis.

Communication and Language Assistance

- Offer language assistance to individuals who have limited English proficiency and/or other communication needs, at no cost to them, to facilitate timely access to all health care and services.
- Inform all individuals of the availability of language assistance services clearly and in their preferred language, verbally and in writing.
- Ensure the competence of individuals providing language assistance, recognizing that the use of untrained individuals and/or minors as interpreters should be avoided.
- Provide easy-to-understand print and multimedia materials and signage in the languages commonly used by the populations in the service area.

Engagement, Continuous Improvement, and Accountability

- Establish culturally and linguistically appropriate goals, policies, and management accountability, and infuse them throughout the organization's planning and operations.
- Conduct ongoing assessments of the organization's CLAS-related activities and integrate CLAS-related measures into measurement and continuous quality improvement activities.
- Collect and maintain accurate and reliable demographic data to monitor and evaluate the impact of CLAS on health equity and outcomes and to inform service delivery.
- Conduct regular assessments of community health assets and needs and use the results to plan and implement services that respond to the cultural and linguistic diversity of populations in the service area.
- Partner with the community to design, implement, and evaluate policies, practices, and services to ensure cultural and linguistic appropriateness.
- Create conflict and grievance resolution processes that are culturally and linguistically appropriate to identify, prevent, and resolve conflicts or complaints.
- Communicate the organization's progress in implementing and sustaining CLAS to all stakeholders, constituents, and the general public.

Reprinted from U.S. Department of Health & Human Services. Available: www.thinkculturalhealth.hhs.gov/clas/standards

the symptoms. Additionally, we have been taught to expose the body part that needs to be examined for proper skin inspection. Some cultures find it offensive to remove portions of clothing even for medical purposes (Padela and del Pozo 2010). As an athletic trainer, being aware of such concerns prior to performing an assessment or treatment intervention will likely lead to an improved patient–practitioner interaction.

Cultural awareness and competence can also take the form of recognizing certain medical conditions that are associated with a specific race, gender, or ethnicity. For example, the sickling of red blood cells is a genetically inherited trait that occurs only in blacks and causes normally shaped red blood cells to assume a sickle shape. This can result in hemolysis and thrombosis of the red blood cells because the abnormally shaped cells do not move easily through the blood vessels. Proper screening and recognition of individuals who carry the sickle cell trait and who are involved with competitive and contact or collision types of sports are essential. This demonstrates not only competent health care delivery but also cultural competence.

The process of becoming culturally competent must be differentiated from what can be referred to as stereotyping. Salimbene (2015) offers the following tips for avoiding a stereotypical approach to patients:

- Find out where the patient is on the continuum of health beliefs and practices often associated with his or her population group.
- Refrain from judging any of the beliefs or practices the patient reveals during the interview.

- Honor the patient's decision-making process.
- Negotiate, don't dictate, your treatment plans.
- Modify both your personal and your medical approach according to where the patient is on the continuum of health beliefs and practices.

Summary

Being a professional is part of being an athletic trainer. Professionalism has been defined in many ways, although it encompasses one's level of trust, appearance, communication, and interpersonal relationships with colleagues and patients, among other characteristics. Being a professional also involves following a set of ethical principles. NATA has established a code of ethics, and states that enforce regulatory status also abide by a set of ethics. Athletic trainers should follow a strategic process designed to avoid unethical behaviors and also be familiar with the steps they should take when making ethical decisions. Whistle-blowing is a process whereby an employee reports a colleague for unethical behavior, and the individual who makes the report or complaint sometimes faces retaliation. Despite an effort to do the right thing, the whistle-blower must decide whether the act of reporting is worth the potential consequences. As the population of the world around us changes, we become more aware of other cultures and how that affects our communities, our professions, the sporting world, and the health care delivery system. Becoming culturally aware of one's own values and beliefs is a component of becoming culturally competent overall.

Learning Aids

Case Study 1

Julio is an athletic trainer at a large university with a successful athletic program. One morning, Julio made a routine trip to the student health service to pick up lab reports and X rays. As he gathered his materials, an administrative assistant asked him whether Sean (a star basketball player) had been dating a student named Mary (a nonathlete on campus). When Julio responded that Sean had dated Mary a few months ago, the administrative assistant proceeded to say how unfortunate it was that Mary had recently tested positive for HIV. Julio was startled to hear this news. Although Mary wasn't under the care of the athletic training staff and Julio didn't really know her, he was concerned about how this circumstance might affect Sean, who was under the care of the athletic training staff.

Questions for Analysis

1. What are the major ethical issues Julio should be concerned about following this exchange? Should Julio pursue additional details and information from the administrative assistant? If so, what?

2. To whom is Julio primarily responsible in this situation? What responsibilities does Julio have toward Sean, and what responsibilities does Julio have toward Mary? What other people might be involved and warrant consideration?

3. What should Julio do with the information about Mary's HIV status? Should Julio use the information as a basis for counseling Sean? Under what conditions should Julio use the information? What alternatives should Julio be investigating?

4. What is the worst mistake Julio could make in trying to fulfill the responsibilities of an athletic trainer to an athlete in this situation? What would be the ideal resolution to this ethical situation? What alternatives fall between the two extremes? How should Julio proceed?

5. If it is determined at some time that Sean is HIV positive, how should the athletic training staff handle that outcome? Who needs to know? What permission is necessary for the staff to relay the information? Who is responsible for the safety of other athletes, for coaches, for the athletic training staff, and for officials with regard to their risk of exposure?

6. What risks does Julio face because he has this information? What steps should Julio take to avoid becoming another victim in this ethical dilemma?

7. What elements of professionalism are involved in Julio's decision-making process?

Case Study 2

Shawna, an athletic training student at Big Hills University, was assigned to work with the cross country team this fall. As was their custom, the team always spent the first week of the season at a mountain lodge to facilitate both intense training and a sense of team unity. During the first day at the lodge, a runner approached Shawna complaining of pain in his left great toe. Shawna examined the toe and noted that it was red, warm, and tender around the margin of the nail. "You're probably just developing a small blister from all the running you've been doing," Shawna informed the athlete. "Let's try padding and lubrication and see whether that makes it feel better." Shawna applied a felt doughnut and lubricant, and the runner told her that the toe felt better. Shawna didn't see the athlete for this or any other injuries the rest of the week.

A few days after the team returned from their trip, the same runner who had seen Shawna nearly 10 days earlier limped into the athletic training room and told Maria, the staff certified athletic trainer, that he had pulled his left groin. When Maria asked him when this happened, the athlete shrugged his shoulders and told her that it had started hurting a little the day before but that it was much worse today. When Maria examined the athlete, she observed several cracked calluses and blisters on his left foot. The left great toe was swollen, red, and warm. A faint red streak ran from the ankle to the posterior aspect of the knee. The left inguinal lymph nodes were swollen to golf-ball size. Maria told the runner that he had a serious infection in his left leg and made an immediate appointment for him to be seen by the team physician.

When Maria returned from taking the cross country runner to the hospital for IV antibiotic therapy, she checked his file and found the note that Shawna had entered describing her physical exam and treatment for the runner's "blister." Maria immediately picked up the phone and dialed Shawna's room.

Questions for Analysis

1. What are Maria's ethical responsibilities in this case? What ethical responsibilities does Shawna have? Are they the same? Are they different? Why or why not?

2. Should Maria tell the athlete that Shawna might have mishandled his toe injury? Does the athlete have a right to know this? Why or why not?

3. Which, if any, of the five principles of the NATA Code of Ethics apply (applies) to this case?

4. How do ethics and the law interface in this case? Where do the athletic trainer's ethical responsibilities end and the athlete's legal rights begin?

5. Does the concept of whistle-blowing come into play in this case? If so, how?

Key Concepts and Review

Understand the definition and purpose of ethical standards and their relevance for the athletic trainer.

Ethics is the study of the rules, standards, and principles that dictate right conduct among members of a society. Ethical standards are useful for athletic trainers because they provide a framework for decision making that helps the athletic trainer place the needs of the patient above all other considerations. Athletic trainers who practice unethically are at risk of failing to meet the needs of their patients.

Define what the term *professionalism* means as it relates to an athletic trainer.

Professionalism is not clearly defined and agreed on among those in all health care disciplines. However, most agree that certain elements compose professional behaviors. These include, but are not limited to, trust, confidence, professional growth, punctuality, and service-oriented behaviors.

Identify the appropriate code of ethics that applies generally to the profession of athletic training, along with codes that might apply to specific settings within the profession.

Athletic trainers are often called on to serve in many roles while working with athletes and other physically active patients. To carry out each role well, it is essential that they be familiar with the ethical standards that are customarily applied to these roles. Athletic trainers should review the code of ethics of NATA as well as those of other professional groups that might credential them.

Identify the situations and circumstances in which ethical concerns are most frequent.

The most common types of ethical problems that directly involve an athletic trainer are breach of confidentiality, conflict of interest, and exploitation. Athletic trainers might also have ethical responsibilities when they have knowledge of such situations; when they are privy to forbidden knowledge; or when they have knowledge of high-risk behaviors, illegal activities, or conflicts between the welfare of different parties involved in a situation.

Develop strategies for avoiding ethical problems and for dealing with them if they occur.

Athletic trainers can reduce the occurrence of ethical dilemmas by studying the appropriate codes of ethics and learning to recognize and be sensitive to situations in which ethical concerns are present. Prudent practice includes obtaining consultation with an uninvolved professional whenever there are questions about an ethical situation and referring patients when their problems are beyond the legal scope of practice or competence of the athletic trainer. Athletic trainers should present patients seeking their services with the conditions of the activity, including disclosure of potential conflicts between roles, and the circumstances that affect the confidentiality of information transmitted in their professional relationship. They should document all professional activities prudently and make referrals whenever they become involved as a primary party in an ethical dilemma. Whenever possible, athletic trainers should encourage athletes and other physically active patients to make their own fully informed choices regarding their care.

Recognize the ethical challenges and overall issues associated with whistle-blowing.

Whistle-blowing poses ethical challenges for how an individual chooses to report perceived or known wrongdoing within one's own organization. Formal versus informal reporting mechanisms are considered, and challenges such as retaliation and workplace humiliation may result following a whistle-blowing episode.

Recognize elements of cultural competence as they relate to athletic training.

Cultural competence is the ability to act with sensitivity to issues of culture, race, gender, sexual orientation, social class, language, and economic situations.

10

Legal Considerations in Sports Medicine

Objectives

After reading this chapter, you should be able to do the following:

- Define and discuss the legal principles most applicable to athletic training settings.

- Identify the types of situations most likely to hold liability concerns for athletic trainers.

- Understand the different types of credentialing laws that affect the practice of athletic training.

- Differentiate between Board of Certification (BOC) certification and state regulation for athletic trainers.

- Understand the elements required to prove negligence on the part of an athletic trainer.

- Be aware of the various legal defenses available to athletic trainers against charges of malpractice.

- Identify the most important elements of providing effective legal testimony.

- Identify and put into practice methods that avoid legal liability while improving the quality of athletic training care.

Many athletic trainers face similar pressures: too many athletes to care for and not enough time to provide that care. Yet the expectations faced from coaches, physicians, parents, and administrators are substantial. They expect athletic trainers to be caring, thorough, tireless, and wise every day (and night and weekend) of work. If a mistake is made, it is typically overlooked. However, if the wrong mistake with the wrong person is made, one's professional standing, personal assets, and self-respect could be seriously jeopardized.

Athletic trainers have been aware for more than three decades that they need a general understanding of certain legal principles to protect themselves and the institutions that employ them from the risk of lawsuits (Gieck, Lowe, and Kenna 1984). Wise athletic trainers, however, also realize that basic knowledge of legal principles, when applied thoughtfully and consistently, helps inform and improve their professional practice. In general, legal standards enacted by state and federal jurisdictions set minimal expectations of practice guidelines that oftentimes influence one's decision-making process.

Of course, this chapter cannot provide definitive, comprehensive coverage of all the laws related to the practice of athletic training. However, it does present the legal issues that athletic trainers are likely to encounter in their professional practice. If an athletic trainer confronts a specific legal issue or problem, the best source of information is an attorney who is experienced in handling similar cases. Effective policies and procedures, formed by consultation with both attorneys and insurance companies, also help guide athletic trainers through the minefield of legal perils they face daily.

KEY POINT

Laws are the rules and regulations governing the affairs of a community or society.

Legal Principles

The common threat that confronts all athletic trainers who provide sports medicine services to patients is **malpractice** (Root 2009). In health care, malpractice is related to one's responsible conduct that results in an adverse outcome of an intervention. Liability may be based on

- negligent patient care,
- failure to obtain informed consent,
- intentional conduct,
- breach of a contract,
- use or transfer of a defective product, or
- abnormally dangerous treatment.

KEY POINT

Athletic trainers can be subject to judicial claims based on a variety of legal theories, and professionals in different settings must be aware of the legal concepts specific to their setting.

Torts

Although athletic trainers may enter patient–practitioner relationships that are implied contracts, unhappy patients are less likely to bring a legal action based on **breach of contract** than on an accusation that the athletic trainer committed a **tort** (Sanders et al. 2005). A tort is a legal wrong other than breach of contract for which a remedy will be provided by the courts, usually in the form of monetary damages. Actions based on tort law are pressed by plaintiffs in civil legal proceedings, whereas criminal cases are initiated by the government. All the legal grounds for malpractice, other than breach of contract, are based on tort law. Of the three types of tort—intentional tort, negligent tort, and strict liability tort—negligence, which

focuses on the conduct of the practitioner, is the most common basis for most malpractice actions.

Negligence

Negligence is a type of tort in which an athletic trainer fails to act as a reasonably prudent athletic trainer would under the circumstances (Pearsall, Kovaleski, and Madanagopal 2005). Athletic trainers can demonstrate that their actions have been both reasonable and prudent by adhering to certain standards in the performance of their duties. Standards emerge from several sources and include all legal guidelines such as state practice acts, ethical codes of professional conduct, and other expected behaviors of one in a similar profession and circumstance. Standards derived from individual and societal values are often implicit (for example, patients should be treated with respect). Standards derived from institutional and professional values are typically more explicit. Policies and procedures usually codify these standards. Position statements of professional associations also include standards. For example, the joint position statement on exercise and type 2 diabetes published by the American College of Sports Medicine and the American Diabetes Association (Colberg et al. 2010) creates a professional standard that athletic trainers and others involved in the health care of physically active patients should adhere to. Similarly, the National Collegiate Athletic Association (NCAA) has established a comprehensive set of standards to which athletic trainers in college athletics should adhere (see the *NCAA Sports Medicine Handbook*).

Athletic trainers can be negligent through either omission or commission. **Omission** is the failure to do something that one should have done under the circumstances. **Commission** occurs when an athletic trainer performs an act that she should not have performed. The three basic forms of negligence include **malfeasance** (performed an improper act), **misfeasance** (improperly performed an act), and **nonfeasance** (did not perform an act). To prove that an athletic trainer was negligent, a complainant must be able to substantiate each of the following (Pozgar 2016):

- Conduct by the athletic trainer
- Existence of duty
- Breach of duty
- Causation
- Damage

Conduct

To substantiate a charge of negligence, the plaintiff must be able to prove that the athletic trainer's **conduct**, by either commission or omission, is behavior that links her to the case. Nonactions, such as thoughts, attitudes, or intentions, cannot render the athletic trainer negligent. Only when athletic trainers take an action (or fail to take an action) can the plaintiff successfully accuse them of negligence.

Duty

When does an athletic trainer owe a **duty** to an injured athlete or other physically active patient? Generally, athletic trainers employed by educational institutions have a duty to provide athletic training services to student-athletes actively engaged in those institutions' athletic programs. Athletic trainers employed by professional sports teams have the same duty toward team members. This duty has its legal origin in the athletic trainer's contract, in which he or she agrees to provide these services in return for payment. Whether a high school or university athletic trainer owes a duty to the student who is injured in an intramural basketball game or a physical education class is less clear—it depends on the responsibilities defined by the employment contract. In many athletic training settings, coaches, coaches' families, athletic department staff, and other personnel often ask the athletic trainer for a consult and assume that such interaction is a courtesy. While this courtesy is often extended without question, it remains unclear from contract to contract whether or not it is considered an appropriate part of the job description of the athletic trainer. For that reason, athletic trainers should have an employment contract with a clearly written position description delineating their specific responsibilities.

Athletic trainers employed by sports medicine clinics have greater leeway in deciding whom they will accept as patients. Consequently, the injured athletes and other physically active patients they owe a duty to should, in theory, be only those patients they choose to treat in their clinics. Enough exceptions to this general rule exist, however, that sports medicine clinic owners should consult with their attorneys to find out whom they might owe a duty to and under what circumstances. For example, sports medicine clinics that have a contract to provide services to a health maintenance organization might have a duty to provide services to the HMO's subscribers.

Abandonment is another issue related to duty that affects athletic trainers. Once an athletic trainer chooses to provide services to an injured athlete or other physically active patient, whether a duty originally existed or not, the athletic trainer does not have the legal freedom simply to walk away from the case except under certain circumstances. Athletic trainers cannot forsake patients who do not cooperate or who fail to pay their bills—unless they provide adequate warning and enough time for the patient to find alternative care.

If the physically active patient recovers and the athletic trainer and the patient agree that further treatment is no longer necessary, they can jointly terminate the relationship. If the patient has been referred, the athletic trainer has a duty to inform the referring agent, usually a physician, that treatment is being discontinued.

An athletic trainer can also discontinue services without fear of being charged with abandonment if the patient voluntarily terminates the relationship. The athletic trainer should make sure (and should be able to prove), however, that the patient understands the consequences of discontinuing the therapy. If the patient simply stops coming for treatment, the athletic trainer should be sure to document his attempts to make contact. If the athletic trainer is away from the sports medicine center and leaves the patient's care in the hands of another practitioner, abandonment might also be charged. If the practitioner substituting for the athletic trainer commits a negligent act, the athletic trainer might be found negligent as well. Athletic trainers can avoid this problem by informing patients when they plan to be gone and making sure that patients agree to be treated by the substitute practitioner. The athletic trainer owes a duty to the patient to make sure that the substitute is competent and is capable of providing the same standard of care.

In general, the duties owed by an athletic trainer to athletes and other physically active patients are those described in the Board of Certification's *Role Delineation Study*. The courts have identified several specific duties:

- Provide or obtain reasonable medical assistance for injured patients as soon as possible under the circumstances in such a way as to avoid aggravation of the injury. This implies having an effective emergency action plan, complete with necessary first aid supplies and communications with ambulance services.

- Maintain the confidentiality of the patient's medical records.
- Provide adequate and proper supervision and instruction.
- Provide safe facilities and equipment.
- Fully disclose information about the patient's medical condition to the patient.

KEY POINT

You can go online to find the Board of Certification's most recent *Role Delineation Study/ Practice Analysis* for athletic training.

Breach of Duty

After a duty has been established, the next step in proving negligence against an athletic trainer requires the aggrieved athlete or other physically active patient to establish by a preponderance of the evidence that the athletic trainer actually **breached a duty** owed the patient. The issue here is whether the athletic trainer exercised the **standard of care** that other reasonably prudent athletic trainers would have exercised under the circumstances. The athletic trainer can consult the standards of practice of various medical and athletic professional organizations to determine a standard of care if questions arise. Note that the standard of care does not require an athletic trainer to be the *most* knowledgeable or competent athletic trainer in the profession. If this were the case, nobody could meet the standard. Instead, the standard requires athletic trainers to perform their duties as other competent athletic trainers would under similar circumstances. In determining whether athletic trainers have met the standard of care, the laws of various states require that their actions be compared with those of other athletic trainers This includes not only athletic trainers in similar general circumstances, but may also include similar types of practice and geographic settings.

Causation

After an aggrieved athlete or other physically active patient has demonstrated that an athletic trainer breached a duty to exercise reasonable care, the patient must prove that the breach was in fact the legal cause of the injury (or made the original injury worse). The courts use two tests to determine causation. First, the plaintiff must prove **actual cause**. Actual cause is established if the patient can demonstrate that the athletic trainer's actions were a considerable determining factor in the damage claimed. The athletic trainer might be found only partially responsible for causing or aggravating the injury. Team physicians, coaches, and institutions might be named as codefendants in negligence cases, because all of them might have contributed to the injury. If more than one defendant was responsible for causing or aggravating the injury, those defendants will be found jointly and severally liable for the negligence, which means that each might end up paying a portion of the damages, consistent with her percentage of fault as determined by the court.

The second causation test is the requirement to demonstrate the existence of **proximate (legal) cause**. Proximate cause exists when an athletic trainer acts in a way that leads to harm or injury to another or to an event that injures another. Inherent in the notion of proximate cause is the **foreseeability** of the harm allegedly precipitated by the athletic trainer. The requirement that harm must be foreseeable is positive for athletic trainers—it doesn't penalize them for results that were improbable or unlikely.

Damage

The final element in establishing negligence is to determine whether the aggrieved patient actually suffered **damages**. If an athletic trainer breached a duty without causing any harm or injury, no negligence occurred. The athletic trainer who oversteps his level of training by injecting a medication directly into someone's inflamed knee joint, for example, cannot be found negligent unless it can be proved that the plaintiff suffered harm as a result (but a charge of practicing medicine without a license would probably have merit). Although physical damage is the most common and easily proved, the law recognizes other forms of damage as well. Emotional distress and a loss of income or reputation are considered examples of damage that one can claim as the result of harm.

Federal Laws and Athletic Training

From a legal perspective, athletic trainers should also be familiar with two federal laws, both in place to prevent inappropriate self-referral for profit: the **Stark Law** and the **federal Anti-Kickback Statute**. Both of these laws prevent health care practitioners from referring patients to entities with whom they or their family members have a financial relationship with. The Stark Law, also referred to as the physician self-referral law, applies primarily to physicians and those entities that present bills to governmental health care programs. The federal Anti-Kickback Statute is inclusive of all health care providers, including athletic trainers. Athletic trainers employed in settings where patient referrals generate revenue should be sure to review employment contracts prior to signing and agreeing to all terms. Not abiding by these federal laws may result in severe penalties to include monetary fines or professional licensure and business operation ramifications or both.

Reducing the Risk of Legal Liability

In addition to the certification requirements of the BOC, most states regulate the practice of athletic trainers, which requires a state credentialing process. This state credentialing is important for the protection of the public and the advancement of the profession.

Credentialing

Athletic trainers must become familiar with the practice acts that regulate the profession. Both practicing athletic trainers and students should have this understanding because the law is likely to define different roles and responsibilities for these two groups. Athletic training practice acts vary a great deal among states. The acts define *athlete* and *athletic trainer* differently. Some limit the scope and setting in which an athletic trainer may practice. Some limit the types of therapeutic modalities athletic trainers can use. Most impose specific educational requirements that might or might not correspond to those required for certification by the BOC. Most state laws require direction by a physician, which is not the same as supervision. Direction means that the athletic trainer has established a relationship with a physician and follows the physician's treatment plans and protocols. Some states also allow other health professionals, such as physical therapists, chiropractors, and dentists, to direct an athletic trainer under certain circumstances. In states without specific credentialing for athletic training, an athletic trainer should obtain a copy of the state's **medical practice act** to determine the scope and setting of practice that the law permits athletic trainers and other health care providers.

Four types of credentialing laws regulate the practice of athletic training: **licensure**, **certification**, **registration**, and **exemption**. Athletic trainers practicing in states with athletic training practice acts should review the state law to determine what type of credentialing they require—each type has different implications. In addition, the definitions and level of restrictiveness of each type of credentialing vary from state to state.

- *Licensure.* Licensure is the most restrictive form of governmental credentialing. The intent of licensure is to protect the public by limiting the practice of athletic training to those who have met the requirements of a licensing board established under the law. Licensure laws generally prohibit unlicensed individuals from calling themselves athletic trainers. More important, they prohibit unlicensed persons from performing the tasks reserved for athletic trainers under the law. States that license athletic trainers usually require a specific educational background that comprises both course work and experience, in addition to passing the Board of Certification exam. Some states, such as Washington, also require athletic trainers to pass a small exam on the licensing law or bloodborne pathogens or both. Texas is the only state that has its own licensing exam, but athletic trainers who are certified by the BOC are exempt from the exam. The Texas licensing exam is for athletic trainers who attend state-approved (not accredited by the Commission on Accreditation of Athletic Training Education [CAATE]) athletic training programs. This license is only recognized in Texas, so these individuals must complete a CAATE-accredited athletic training program and pass the BOC exam before they are eligible to practice in other states. Licensing boards are powerful legal entities because they are usually authorized to set the rules, in accordance with the law, that govern who may practice and who may not. They also set the fee required for license applications and renewals. Because licensure is the most restrictive form of state credentialing, athletic trainers commonly view it as the most desirable of the four regulatory options. Athletic trainers should be aware that some states offer a grace period and others do not. For example, in some states, an athletic trainer who is in the process of becoming certified by the BOC may be allowed to practice under direct supervision of a licensed AT with a temporary license or permit while waiting for final approval of the licensure application. In almost every state with licensure, athletic trainers cannot practice independently until their license has been fully approved.

- *Certification.* Certification is a less stringent form of professional regulation than licensure. A person who is certified is generally recognized to have the basic knowledge and skills required of practitioners in the profession. Both states and professional associations can certify health care practitioners. The Board of Certification, for example, is the recognized certifying agency for ensuring that athletic trainers have the basic knowledge and skills to carry out their duties as defined by the *Practice Analysis* (formerly referred to as the *Role Delineation Study*). Athletic trainers who meet the requirements for BOC certification and maintain their certification are entitled to use the board's credential: ATC. Some states also certify athletic trainers. As of 2016, New York and South Carolina required state certification, although neither state required a certification exam, beyond the BOC exam. States get the authority to certify athletic trainers from a credentialing law passed by the state legislature and signed by the governor, the same process that gives them the authority for licensure. Unlike licensure, however, state certification usually protects only an athletic trainer's title, not the specific tasks that she performs. Noncertified people could not call themselves athletic trainers, but they could perform the duties of an athletic trainer.

- *Registration.* Registration is another form of professional regulation that is less restrictive than licensure. In states that have registration laws, athletic trainers are required to register with the state before practicing. Some states allow a grace period during which athletic trainers may practice without being registered as long as they begin their application for registration within the period established by the state's board. Because the registration law prohibits unregistered persons from practicing, it becomes a form of title protection for an athletic trainer. States that require registration might or might not require screening devices such as examinations, although most prescribe the educational requirements necessary to register as an athletic trainer.

- *Exemption.* Some states previously provided the legal basis for athletic trainers to practice by exempting them from complying with the practice acts of other professions, typically the physical therapy, physician assistant, medical, and massage therapy practice acts. Although exemption is often viewed as the least restrictive form of professional regulation, athletic trainers might still be required to meet a variety of standards, usually related to educational background or certification by the BOC, to qualify. In addition, athletic trainers are required to act according to the standards of the profession and the boundaries of their training. Currently, no states regulate athletic trainers under the exemption status.

Currently, athletic trainers are regulated in 49 states as well as the District of Columbia. California remains the only state with no regulation. Of the 49 regulated states (plus the District of Columbia), 43 regulate through licensure, five through registration, and two through certification.

One might wonder why athletic trainers would want to be regulated, because a fee is involved and it can restrict an AT's scope of practice. The main reason to do so is for public protection. Some feel that the national BOC certification should be more than adequate, but unless a law in the state requires someone to be BOC certified, it is optional. You might even think that employers wouldn't hire someone who isn't a certified athletic trainer, yet many employers have done so over the years to save money when their state laws did not require the certification. State regulation of athletic trainers requires that all ATs practicing in that state have earned the ATC credential through the Board of Certification.

Having a state regulatory body gives the BOC someone at the state level to communicate with if there are disciplinary issues. For example, if an athletic trainer violates the BOC Standards of Professional Practice, the BOC could suspend or revoke the AT's certification. However, without a state regulatory body, there is no mechanism for the BOC to let the state know that the AT should no longer be practicing and treating patients. The BOC also has no authority in the state to pull the AT from practice. The only mechanism for this would be for the BOC to contact the state regulatory board, which could then suspend or revoke the AT's license in that state. Many athletic trainer state regulatory boards also have the authority to issue "cease and desist" orders, which means that the AT cannot practice as an AT until the board lifts that order.

State regulation of athletic trainers also provides legitimacy to the profession because it is an important form of recognition. Not only does this make it easier for ATs to receive third-party reimbursement for services they provide (see chapter 8), but it also often provides protections for ATs. For example, many states have laws that protect health care providers from liability if they volunteer their services or assist in an emergency. However, if ATs are not recognized in the state's legal code as "health care providers," then this law will not protect the ATs from this type of liability. It is common for ATs to provide care outside of their direct job responsibilities such as when they attend a youth sporting event to watch a child participate or care for a spectator at an event.

KEY POINT

For the most current list of state regulation information, visit the Board of Certification's website and view the map of state regulatory agencies. When you click on a state, it provides the contact information for the regulatory agency in that state as well as links to the agency's website, the practice act, and rules and regulations. Appendix D lists state regulation information that was accurate at the time of this book's printing.

Athletic Training: State Regulations

States That License Athletic Trainers

Alabama
Alaska
Arizona
Arkansas
Connecticut
Delaware
Florida
Georgia
Idaho
Illinois
Indiana
Iowa
Kansas
Kentucky
Louisiana
Maine
Maryland
Massachusetts
Michigan
Mississippi
Missouri
Montana
Nebraska
Nevada
New Hampshire
New Jersey
New Mexico
North Carolina
North Dakota
Ohio
Oklahoma
Pennsylvania
Rhode Island
South Dakota
Tennessee
Texas
Utah
Vermont
Virginia
Washington
Wisconsin
Wyoming

States That Certify Athletic Trainers

South Carolina
New York

States That Register Athletic Trainers

Colorado
Hawaii
Minnesota
Oregon
West Virginia

States That Exempt Athletic Trainers From Other Health Professions' Practice Acts

None

States That Have No Regulation for Certified Athletic Trainers

California

Risk Management

Athletic trainers have been concerned with issues of legal liability for many years. As larger numbers of athletic trainers moved into management positions or took on management responsibilities along with their clinical duties, the broader construct of **risk management** became more important. Although athletic trainers are still concerned with the basics of avoiding legal liability in their clinical practices, they are increasingly called on to help their schools, professional teams, clinics, and companies manage the risks that form the foundation for this liability.

What Is Risk Management?

Simply put, risk management is a process intended to prevent financial loss for an organization. The goal of risk management is to prevent losses of all kinds (financial, physical, property, activity, time) for everyone associated with an organization, including its directors, administrators, employees, and clients. This broader application is warranted, because losses experienced at one level of an organization are usually felt at other levels, especially if formal legal action is taken.

As van der Smissen (2001) appropriately points out, risk management is more than the act of developing safety checklists. A comprehensive risk management program involves careful analysis of the risks facing the program or organization and development of a plan for addressing those risks. She recommends using four general strategies for managing risk:

1. *Avoidance.* When an activity, procedure, or event is so risky that dire consequences are likely, the organization may simply choose to avoid the activity. Avoidance is an especially appropriate risk management approach when the negative consequences of a particular activity have high costs.

2. *Transference.* When activities are associated with high financial risk but low frequency (for example, catastrophic sport injury) or lower financial risk but high frequency (for example, fractures, joint injuries requiring surgery), a common method to reduce the risk of these activities is to transfer all or part of the risk to another entity. The organization usually accomplishes this by purchasing insurance designed to cover the financial loss associated with certain well-defined risks. Exculpatory clauses in waivers signed by athletes and their parents are another example of a method to transfer the risk associated with sport participation to the participants and away from the organization, although this method has many flaws.

3. *Retention.* Every organization—including organizations in which athletic trainers work—hosts activities or sponsors programs that face a level of risk deemed acceptable in light of the organization's mission. These risks are viewed as part of the cost of doing business. To eliminate the activities associated with these risks would fundamentally change the nature of the organization. The organization accepts and retains risks like these. These risks are still associated with a predictable level of financial cost, however, and the organization must account for it in the organization or program budget. Ideally, the organization should establish a reserve fund to cover costs that rise above predicted levels.

4. *Reduction.* Careful development, implementation, monitoring, and evaluation of policies and procedures can reduce risks. Ideally, every risk that an organization knowingly retains should be accompanied by at least one policy and procedure designed to reduce the frequency and financial effect of that risk. For guidance on reducing risk in athletic programs, see the later section Specific Risk Reduction Strategies.

PEARLS OF MANAGEMENT

Athletic trainers can help prevent losses (physical and financial) for their employers and patients by instituting a risk management plan. Both real-world observations and controlled experiments can identify risks. Preparing properly for activity, conducting safe activities, managing injuries properly, and maintaining appropriate records are all part of a risk management plan.

How Are Risks Identified?

Risk identification is rarely as easy as it seems. Some risks are obvious to anyone. For example, if you begin to administer an ultrasound treatment to an athlete or other physically active patient and notice that the power cord is frayed and the wire is exposed, you have identified a rather obvious risk factor. You could even quantify the risk in this case, because you could safely assume that 100% of the people who contact the exposed wire will receive an injury ranging from a minor burn to an electrical shock that induces cardiac arrest. Most risks in athletics, however, are more difficult to identify and quantify. For example, how would you answer an athletic director who wanted to know whether the rubberized gym floor was the cause of the high rate of anterior cruciate ligament (ACL) injuries among your school's female basketball players? What evidence could you provide to support your answer? Could you calculate the risk of ACL injury with any accuracy? Assessing this risk is obviously difficult, because not every female basketball player at your school will suffer an ACL injury. Of those who do, not all will suffer the injury while playing in the gym at school. Two ways to identify and assess risk in athletics are real-world observation and inference from controlled experiments (Graham and Rhomberg 1996).

PEARLS OF MANAGEMENT

NATA members can link to the following page to access the "Liability Tool Kit," which serves as a guide to self-assess one's own professional as well as one's employer's risk of potential liability: https://www.nata.org/practice-patient-care/risk-liability#liability

Real-World Observation   Observation of real-world events is the most rudimentary form of risk assessment. This method involves making inferences regarding the risk of certain activities based on clinical practice and experience. Real-world observation is usually the first step in the discovery of cause-and-effect relationships between hazardous practices and their results.

For example, athletic trainers in the 1960s observed many cases of heat illness among athletes who had been denied access to fluids during heavy exercise in hot weather. The athletic trainers surmised that this practice led to dehydration and all its negative side effects. Their observations led to an accurate assessment of a risk that was later validated in laboratory studies. Unfortunately, however, real-world observation can often lead to spurious conclusions. In the case of the gym floor previously mentioned, all the women's sport coaches who used that gym were so convinced that the floor was the cause of the high incidence of ACL injuries that they

lobbied the administration to tear out the rubberized floor and replace it with a wooden floor. The project cost more than $1 million. Two years later, the rate of ACL injuries was just as high on the new wooden floor as it had been on the rubberized floor. In this case, factors other than the playing surface must have caused the high incidence of ACL injuries. The coaches' observations were incorrect and led to an expensive "solution" that solved nothing.

Controlled Experiments   Another way to identify and assess risks is to engage in data-driven controlled studies. This method is more difficult to implement because it is time intensive, costly, and frequently impractical. Using the preceding example, the people involved would probably have received better information regarding the effect of playing surfaces on ACL injuries if they had replaced one court with wood and left another with the original rubberized surface. If they had then randomly assigned players to practice on each of the courts and tracked the incidence of ACL injury as a function of player exposures, they would have gotten a much better answer (but not a perfect one) to the question of whether they should replace the rubberized floor.

This type of controlled study—the kind used to establish the safety and efficacy of prescription drugs—is rarely practical for athletic or physical activity settings. One method that is practical, however, involves using an epidemiological approach to identifying risks. Epidemiology can help athletic trainers draw inferences regarding potential risks by tracking the incidence of injuries and all their associated factors, including athlete characteristics, playing surface, weather, and type of activity. Most commercially available injury-tracking database software programs allow athletic trainers to do this.

When the school administration asked the athletic trainer in the gym floor case for an opinion regarding the advisability of switching to a wooden floor, he did an analysis of knee injuries in women's basketball and volleyball using 10 years of data from the school's injury-tracking database and the NCAA Injury Surveillance Study, in which his school was a participating member. The results indicated that the rate of injury was the same for wooden and rubberized gym floors. In addition, twice as many knee injuries occurred during away contests (where the teams usually played on wood surfaces) as occurred on the rubberized floor during home games. His conclusion was that there was no basis to recommend the commitment of $1 million to switch to a wooden floor. The money was spent anyway. Knee injury rates continued as before.

Planning for Risk

Even the most prepared and conscientious organizations will, despite their best efforts, experience unwanted events from time to time—including life-threatening emergencies. One of the most important roles that athletic trainers can play in helping the organization prepare for these events is by taking the lead in developing emergency action plans. An **emergency action plan (EAP)** is a blueprint for handling emergencies that helps establish accountability for their management (Andersen et al. 2002). Emergency action plans are discussed in detail in chapter 15.

Specific Risk Reduction Strategies

Besides considering van der Smissen's (2001) general risk reduction strategies, outlined earlier, athletic trainers should think about implementing Rankin and Ingersoll's (2001) four-part strategy to help control risk in athletic programs:

1. Preparation for the activity:
   - Administer preparticipation physical exams.
   - Monitor fitness levels.
   - Assess activity areas.
   - Monitor environmental conditions.
2. Conduct of the activity:
   - Maintain equipment.
   - Use proper instructional techniques.
   - Provide adequate work–rest intervals.
3. Injury management:
   - Have a physician supervise all medical aspects of the program.
   - Unchallengeable authority for the physician and athletic trainer, whereby coaches should not have medical decision-making authority over the physician and athletic trainer (NATA 2016).
   - Evaluate and treat injuries correctly and promptly.
   - Supervise student athletic trainers.
4. Records management:
   - Document physician orders.
   - Document the treatment plan.
   - Document the treatment record.
   - Document the patient's progress.

Mulder (2003) recommends implementing a computer-aided planned maintenance system for medical equipment monitoring because it is a relatively simple and straightforward task for most settings. The main purpose of such a system is to monitor and administer preventive maintenance activities. Although the cost of these systems may be more expensive in larger settings, such as hospitals, these types of settings often require a more formal tracking system to ensure compliance.

Medications, Legal Liability, and Athletic Trainers

The medical management of athletes' health with pharmaceutical agents is one of the areas of sports medicine that has great potential for legal liability for the athletic trainer. A growing concern is how college and university athletic programs, among other settings, improperly—and illegally—administer and dispense both prescription and nonprescription medications. Most do so in an effort to provide injured or ill athletes with a comprehensive regimen of therapeutic tools to encourage their full and speedy recovery. Providing medications in the athletic training facility is generally thought to improve physician and athlete convenience. However, poorly organized and delivered pharmaceutical management of athletic injuries and illnesses can both compromise an athlete's health and subject the athletic trainer and her employer to significant legal liability. More detailed information regarding pharmaceuticals in an athletic training setting is discussed in chapter 14.

Product Liability

Injured athletes and other physically active patients can sue equipment manufacturers based on any of three legal theories.

1. The manufacturer can be sued for negligence. If the risk of injury from the use of its product was foreseeable and the company did not exercise due care in reducing or eliminating the risk, the company may be found negligent.
2. The manufacturer can be sued for breach of an implied warranty. If a product is found by the court to be unfit for the purpose for which it was intended, then the plaintiff might be able

to collect damages because the equipment includes an implied warranty that it works the way it is supposed to work.

3. An injured patient might be able to argue that an equipment manufacturer is strictly liable. Under this legal theory, a company can be found liable if a patient using its product is injured, regardless of the foreseeability of risk or the care the manufacturer took to prevent an injury.

Athletic trainers must understand that the improper design, manufacture, or use of products can result in legal liability for the company that made the equipment and, in some cases, for the athletic trainer who issued or used the equipment. A product can be found defective in several ways (Feinman 2006):

- *Design defect.* Equipment that may have good intent may also have unplanned side effects that could result in injury or harm to a patient.

- *Manufacturing defect.* Sometimes something as simple as elastic bands may in fact contain a defect, leading to the band tearing with applied resistance and resulting in harm to the patient or others in the near vicinity.

- *Failure to warn.* Equipment and products may lead to harm if not properly used. Labels and instructions should always accompany a product or equipment device to clarify proper usage.

- *Breach of warranty.* Using products that have not been regularly calibrated or have passed their suggested dates of disuse poses great risk to patient safety.

Athletic trainers can help prevent lawsuits that have components of product liability by instituting the following practices:

- Read the warning labels and instruction manuals for every piece of equipment you use.

- Insist that athletes read the warning labels on all equipment they use.

- Make sure that athletes understand the information in the warning label. Ask them whether they have questions (this is especially important if their primary language is different from the language used on the label). Ask them to sign a statement indicating that they have read and understand the warning label.

- Never modify, alter, or otherwise reconfigure a piece of equipment. Doing so might invalidate its express warranty and might shift a sizable percentage of the legal liability away from the manufacturer and toward the athletic trainer.

- Inspect, fit, and maintain equipment according to the schedule recommended by the manufacturer. Keep records of all such maintenance.

- Require training for all products and equipment. Document the date for verification purposes. Establish a policy for retraining as appropriate.

KEY POINT

Athletic trainers can protect themselves against the threat of legal liability in many ways. Wise athletic trainers take care to implement each of these strategies in their practice.

Additional Strategies

At the beginning of this chapter, it was suggested that knowledge of legal liability would help improve the quality of care offered by an athletic trainer. To place that sweeping statement into context, consider the following suggestions as part of a strategy for avoiding the threat of legal liability (Graham 1985; Salyanarayana Rho 2008).

PEARLS OF MANAGEMENT

A common saying is "People don't care how much you know until they know how much you care." Demonstrating sincere patient concern is an interpersonal skill that can minimize legal liability.

- *Build relationships.* Develop and maintain good relations with athletes and other physically active patients, parents, coworkers, subordinates, and other health care professionals with whom you work or to whom you commonly refer patients. You should build trust relationships and promote a constant flow of two-way communication with these groups.

- *Insist on a written contract.* Have a written contract supported by a detailed position description that clearly delineates the athletic trainer's job functions. This document is one of the most important defenses you can offer against a charge of negligence because it helps establish those to whom you might owe a legal duty.

• *Obtain informed consent for the services you perform.* In the case of minors, obtain informed consent from their parents. Warn athletes and parents of the dangers, including permanent disability and death, inherent in their particular sport. Repeat such warnings annually.

• *Provide preparticipation physical examinations.* Be certain that every athlete undergoes a physical examination by a state-licensed medical practitioner. Make certain that the content of the physical examination is consistent with nationally recognized standards in terms of both content and frequency.

• *Know the profession and its standards.* Develop and maintain a database of information about injuries and illnesses that are most common to each sport you work with. This documentation will enhance your qualifications as an expert in your field. Practice your profession unafraid, but keep in mind the standards of practice embraced by the profession. Regularly refer to professional position and consensus statements for current acceptable approaches to the standard of care.

• *Document hazards.* Make a documented attempt to reduce injuries by recommending or personally taking action to remove or modify potential hazards. Consider establishing a safety committee charged with conducting an ongoing program of risk assessment and reduction. Be aware, however, that a paper trail documenting safety hazards can also be used against you or your institution, especially if the hazards are not corrected or the corrections go undocumented.

• *Establish policies.* Adopt and scrupulously adhere to policies and procedures designed to reduce the incidence of injury and to guide the actions of sports medicine personnel when injuries do occur. Keep all emergency first aid equipment in working order and available to those who might need to use it.

• *Document activities.* Document the details of all injuries, treatments, and rehabilitative procedures so that a chronology of events can easily be determined after the fact. Maintain medical records until well after the statute of limitations for malpractice liability has expired (this will vary from state to state).

• *Maintain confidentiality.* The patient's medical record must remain confidential. When you wish to share the information with others, obtain written permission of the patient first.

• *Provide proper instruction.* When interacting with athletes and other physically active patients, be certain that the instruction you provide allows for safe participation. If you give instructions to a patient in a rehabilitation program, for example, make sure that the patient understands how to progress and knows the warning signs associated with reinjury. If you are instructing athletes in an off-season conditioning program, make sure that they can perform the exercises properly and that they use commonly accepted safety techniques such as spotting each other when using free weights.

• *Supervise your staff.* Insist that all staff members adhere to prescribed programmatic procedures. Make sure that supervisees understand your requests. Make sure that they are carrying out your requests as required by the procedures specified in the program's handbook. When deviations occur, correct the supervisee's behavior.

• *Participate in continuing education.* Take part in continuing athletic training education by attending seminars and symposia and reading sports medicine literature. Alter your techniques as technology and knowledge advance. Document your continuing education activities and the changes that result.

• *Recognize your qualifications.* Practice only within the limitations of the laws of your state and the boundaries of your training. Be consistent with the standard of care expected of other reasonably prudent athletic trainers. Be quick to refer injured athletes and other physically active patients to physicians and be sure to follow their instructions carefully. Avoid the distribution of prescription medications and be cautious in your use of over-the-counter medications.

• *Maintain insurance coverage.* All athletic trainers, certified and student alike, should have malpractice and liability insurance to safeguard their personal assets in the event of a legal action. Even if a malpractice suit is frivolous and eventually dismissed, the costs associated with defense are usually beyond the means of most athletic trainers. In some cases, the employer's general liability policy will adequately protect the athletic trainer. In many cases, however, institutional liability insurance policies specifically exclude health care activities. In addition, the maximum benefit of institutional policies might not cover the fantastic costs associated with medical litigation. Athletic trainers who do not have adequate protection through their employer's liability insurance policy should seriously consider buying their own policies. Athletic trainers must evaluate the limits of coverage of both their employer's malpractice insurance policies and their personal malpractice insurance policies. The limits of these policies often determine what kinds of activities the athletic trainer can engage in. Some policies, for example, cover job-related duties but exclude volunteer activities. Under these circumstances, an athletic trainer who provides medical services at summer sports camps would probably want to have her employer write these activities into her job description so that the policy would cover them. Activities that an athletic trainer undertakes with malicious intent or gross negligence are frequently not covered.

Strategies for Dealing With Legal Challenges

Despite the best efforts of athletic trainers to practice within the law, some will inevitably face legal challenges at some point in their careers. When facing a lawsuit or other legal challenge, well-informed athletic trainers should be aware of both the defenses available to them and the dos and don'ts of providing testimony. The first step is to possess and understand professional liability insurance.

Professional Liability Insurance Coverage

Purchasing one's own professional liability insurance is something all athletic trainers should consider. A handful of insurance companies offer specific types of professional liability insurance for athletic training based on part-time or full-time employment. When purchasing professional liability insurance, be sure you understand exactly what you are receiving for services. This includes the amount of coverage, length of time that coverage is active, time when coverage is active, and many other benefits. You should also understand the proper process for activating your policy in the case of a claim being made against you. Policies are primarily of two types: claims made and occurrence.

1. Claims-made policies protect the insured from liability for covered events even if a claim and lawsuit are presented after coverage lapses, so long as the coverage was in effect at the time of the incident giving rise to the claim and lawsuit.

2. Occurrence policies provide protection only if a policyholder maintains his professional liability insurance coverage until a claim and lawsuit ensue. To have coverage similar to that of a claims-made policy, the holder of an occurrence policy must purchase one of two types of coverage: tail (postemployment) or prior acts (covering events before current employment and follow-on insurance coverage).

The following items should also be considered and reviewed carefully when purchasing professional liability insurance:

- What is the policy's limit for payment per incident and overall?
- Are there exemptions, in other words, are claims pertaining to certain acts not covered (e.g., sexual offenses, substance abuse)?
- What is the jurisdiction of the coverage? Will it cover out-of-state travel or international travel?
- How does the policy identify attorneys?
- How does the policy identify experts?
- How are attorneys, expert witnesses, and other fees for things such as exhibits, postage, and copying paid?
- Does the policy cover expense for travel to court if out of state?
- If an athletic trainer also holds credentials in another area (e.g., physical therapy, massage therapy) does the policy cover the AT for those services?

Possessing an active professional liability insurance plan is a wise choice for all athletic trainers. While the likelihood of being sued may not be high, it does happen, it can happen, and one should always be protected when it happens.

The next important step in risk management is knowing what to do when you are named in a lawsuit as a defendant. The first thing is to resist the temptation to tell everyone, and certainly don't say anything through social media outlets. Initial knowledge of being named in a lawsuit is not a comfortable feeling. In fact, it can be scary and unnerving. Regardless, you must not panic. If there is ever a time to remain calm—similar to managing an on-field emergency—this is it. While you may be tempted to speak with family, close friends, coworkers, and even supervisors, it is best to keep your communications to a minimum.

You should immediately contact your professional liability insurance provider, who will assign you an attorney. Based on your attorney's advice, you can proceed to communicate as deemed appropriate. You should contact your provider regardless of whether a lawsuit is named against you directly or whether you are part of one against your employer. While your employer may also have liability insurance that covers you, it is important for you to also have your own legal counsel. It is possible that at some point your employer's attorneys could suggest that the actions that led to the lawsuit were caused by your failure to act within the roles and responsibilities of your employment contract and job description. If this is the case, the employer will move to refuse to represent or defend your actions, and will instead defend themselves independently.

If named in a lawsuit, the following actions are recommended:

- Keep communications to a minimum, mainly based on your counsel's advice.
- Never modify, alter, or change any documents.
- Take time to write notes that may jog your memory of the incident.
- Do not contact others with the intent to influence facts or their recollection of events.
- Do not let the lawsuit affect your current practice ability.

Legal Defenses

Athletic trainers accused of malpractice have several possible legal defenses. None of these, however, provides ironclad protection against a lawsuit; each defense has exceptions that could leave the athletic trainer liable even though the general principle might be valid. The best defense, of course, is to provide high-quality athletic training services consistent with the standard of care expected in the profession and by the statutory regulations of the state. The statute of limitations, sovereign immunity, assumption of risk, Good Samaritan immunity, and comparative negligence are legal defenses that might apply to claims of athletic trainer malpractice.

KEY POINT

Athletic trainers will usually try to defend themselves against malpractice using one of five defenses: statute of limitations, sovereign immunity, assumption of risk, Good Samaritan immunity, and comparative negligence.

- *Statutes of limitations.* **Statutes of limitations** are state laws that fix a certain length of time during which an aggrieved patient may sue a health care provider. The statute of limitations applies in most states to health care providers who have been statutorily recognized by the state. States that regulate athletic training practice, therefore, probably extend the statutes of limitations to cover athletic trainers, but other states might not. Athletic trainers who are employed by physicians, hospitals, or physical therapists in states that don't provide credentials might also be protected because their employers are regulated. Although the statute of limitations usually specifies the period, many exceptions can lengthen the period during which an athlete or other physically active patient can bring suit.

- *Sovereign immunity.* **Sovereign (governmental) immunity** is a legal doctrine that holds that neither governments nor their agents can be held liable for negligent torts (Suk 2012). In theory, athletic trainers employed in public schools, colleges, and universities are immune from legal liability because they are agents of governmental entities. Case law reveals no less than three situations in which athletic trainers avoided liability based on a claim of governmental immunity (*Garza v. Edinburg Consolidated Independent School District* 1979; *Lowe v. Texas Tech University* 1976; *Sorey v. Kellett* 1988). However, athletic trainers employed in public institutions should never assume that they are covered by sovereign immunity.

- *Assumption of risk.* One of the oldest and most common defenses that educational institutions and their employees have used against legal liability in athletic injury cases is **assumption of risk** (Killion and Dempski 2000; Pozgar 2016). In this defense, the athletic trainer asserts that the injured athlete or other physically active patient was aware of the risks involved and decided to proceed anyway, thereby absolving the institution and the athletic trainer from any liability for damages. For assumption of risk to be used as a defense, the athlete must "fully appreciate" the type and magnitude of the risk involved in participating in the activity. The athlete must also "knowingly, voluntarily, and unequivocally" choose to participate in the activity in the face of the inherent risks. Skillful attorneys usually have little trouble defeating this defense, especially when the injured party is a minor. To protect against legal liability and improve their chances of being able to use this defense should the need arise, many schools and colleges provide educational sessions, complete with videos and printed materials, that warn student-athletes and their parents of the specific dangers inherent in their sport. Following these sessions, participants are asked to sign a statement affirming that they have been warned of the dangers associated with the sport (including permanent disability and death), that they understand these risks, that they have been offered the opportunity to ask questions regarding the risks, and that they voluntarily choose to participate regardless of the risks.

- *Good Samaritan immunity.* A possible defense that athletic trainers can use in a limited number of settings is immunity by virtue of a **Good Samaritan law**. Good Samaritan laws enacted in some states protect health care providers who voluntarily come to the aid of injured persons. These statutes might or might not cover athletic trainers. Specific Good Samaritan laws in some states protect volunteer team physicians from legal liability (Benda 1991). If the physician receives compensation of any kind, the immunity from liability does not apply. Because athletic trainers are increasingly volunteering to serve at state games and charitable athletic events, this defense might become more popular. The injured person, of course, must consent to be treated. The statutes do not protect an athletic trainer from willful or wanton misconduct or from gross or intentional negligence. Regardless, athletic trainers should always be familiar with the state law where one is practicing to know whether or not Good Samaritan laws apply.

- *Comparative negligence.* Physically active patients sometimes ignore the prescriptions of their health care providers, a disregard that can lead to injury or aggravate an injury. The courts often use the doctrine of **comparative negligence** to determine whether the liability for these injuries should be divided between the plaintiff and the defendant. Comparative negligence determines the degree of fault an athletic trainer and a patient have for causing an injury. The athletic trainer's financial liability depends on the formula used in the state in which the case is tried. In most states, patients can collect damages only if their comparative culpability is less than half the total. In some states, however, plaintiffs can be awarded financial restitution equal to the athletic trainer's percentage of fault.

Providing Testimony at a Deposition or Trial

As a fact witness, the athletic trainer either had responsibility for treating an injured patient or has knowledge of the facts of the case. The athletic trainer has little choice in whether or not to appear in court under this circumstance because the court will probably issue a **subpoena** ordering appearance. A **deposition** is a process of discovery, in which facts regarding the case are formally gathered through questioning under oath. This happens in the presence of attorneys and can last for many hours. The athletic trainer's attorneys will prepare him for and counsel him through the process. The process entails providing factual answers to the plaintiff's attorney's questions. It is important to always be truthful, factual, and consistent. If the athletic trainer does not remember something, he should state that instead of making up what he thinks he might recall.

An attorney might retain an athletic trainer as an expert to testify on behalf of a client. Expert witnesses are paid to provide **testimony** that educates the judge and jury about the standard of care that should be applied in a particular case. Typically both the plaintiff and the defense will hire their own expert witness, who must qualify as an expert in accordance with required state credentials (e.g., terminal degree, actively practice, accepted by both parties) (Florida Statute 90.702 2016). Expert witnesses sign a written affidavit providing a rationale behind their professional opinion. As an expert witness, the athletic trainer should agree with the positions that the attorney will ask her to take at trial. She should also be sure the attorney who hired her has the facts to support the case. Otherwise, she will appear ignorant and foolish on the witness stand. In many cases, the expert opinion of an athletic trainer is considered during pretrial phases, and the case itself may be settled or dismissed without a trial. The opinion of the athletic trainer is deemed valuable during these times because it may sway a plaintiff's or defendant's case in one direction or another, possibly leaning toward the determination of an outcome if a trial were to occur.

Whether athletic trainers are subpoenaed or appear as expert witnesses, many helpful guidelines can be implemented to safeguard their credibility and provide for a positive experience (Brodsky 2012):

- Avoid memorizing the testimony.
- Prepare for your testimony by carefully studying the records of the case before entering the courtroom or deposition. If you need to refer to the medical records while on the stand, understand that the records will be considered evidence that the opposing attorney will be able to access.
- Discuss your testimony with your attorney or the attorney retaining you as a witness before giving it in the courtroom.
- Never guess. If you're unsure of the answer to a question, admit lack of knowledge on that point.
- Testify only on issues about which you are an expert. Do not testify beyond the boundaries of your experience.
- Use common language. Whenever you use medical language, attempt to interpret it for the judge and jury.
- Avoid responding to hypothetically posed questions. These are not based on facts and merely serve as speculation.
- Be sure that your testimony in court is consistent with any depositions you might have made before the beginning of the trial. Always review the deposition before taking the stand.
- Ask the judge for guidance if you feel the need to expand on a yes-or-no question posed by an attorney.
- Ask the judge for guidance if you think that answering a question would violate the athletic trainer–patient relationship.

- Use illustrations (charts, drawings, slides, photographs, and so on) to help make your point when appropriate.
- If you are charged with malpractice and your malpractice insurance company has provided a lawyer you feel uncomfortable with, hire your own attorney.
- Maintain a professional, dignified demeanor at all times. Dress neatly; answer in a normal tone of voice at an even rate; and be respectful of the judge, jury, and attorneys.
- Remain composed at all times.
- Be prepared to be subjected to hostile questioning.

Summary

Athletic trainers are challenged every day with legal considerations. It is expected that all athletic trainers will practice within a standard of care, performing duties that other reasonably prudent athletic trainers would have performed under similar circumstances. Negligence occurs when an athletic trainer fails to act as a reasonably prudent athletic trainer would act under such circumstances. Malpractice refers to liability-generating conduct associated with the adverse outcome of a patient's treatment. To provide protection to the public, athletic trainers are regulated on a statewide basis (licensure, registration, certification, exemption). In addition to adverse treatment outcomes, liability also rests with adverse conditions arising from poor facility management, faulty equipment, and improperly dispensing medication, to name a few examples. Risk management is the process intended to prevent losses of all kinds (financial, physical, property, activity, time) for everyone associated with an organization, including its directors, administrators, employees, and clients. Ongoing evaluation of one's practice and practice setting helps to reduce the risk of adverse outcomes.

Learning Aids

Case Study 1

Lamar was pleased when the management of the professional football team that employed him allowed him to hire an additional athletic training student for the preseason training camp. The preseason was a hectic time, and he was grateful for the help that students were able to provide. One of the students whom he had decided to hire this year, Rich, was only a sophomore. Lamar usually hired only students who had completed their junior year, but Rich had come highly recommended by his supervising athletic trainer, an old friend of Lamar's, so Lamar decided to take a chance on Rich.

James was a 10th-round draft choice trying to make the team that summer. James had played college football at the university that Rich was attending. Although James felt good about his performance in the first two weeks, a knee injury suffered in the first scrimmage had kept him out of practice since then. Fortunately, the knee was starting to feel better, and James hoped that he could return to limited practice within a couple of days.

One day the head coach surprised everybody by announcing that the team would have the next morning off. The athletic training students, knowing they wouldn't have to wake up at 5:30 a.m. as usual, decided to visit a local pub that night. The bar was the only one in the small college town where the team had its training camp, so most of the players went there as well.

Rich saw James at the pub and joined him. Three beers later, the topic of James' knee injury came up. When James told Rich that he was feeling better and would probably be back in a couple of days, Rich confided that while he was cleaning a whirlpool a couple of days earlier, he had heard Lamar, the team physician, and the head coach talking about James. When James asked what they had said, Rich told him they were simply discussing the details of James' knee injury and his prospects for full recovery. After two more beers, James had the whole story.

When the team released him the next week, James immediately contacted his agent, an attorney, who filed a lawsuit on his behalf alleging that the team had concealed the true nature of James' injury, which resulted in his termination and subsequent unemployment.

Questions for Analysis

1. What legal principles are involved in this case? How do they apply? Does James have a strong case? Why or why not?

2. How could this situation have been avoided? What policies and procedures should Lamar institute to prevent this kind of problem?

3. Who, if anyone, is at fault in this case? If more than one person is at fault, how is a judge or jury likely to determine the percentage of each person's liability?

4. What records could Lamar use to defend himself and the team?

Case Study 2

Christine, the assistant athletic trainer for Northwest State University, was off the bench like a shot when she saw the basketball team's star center fall to the floor holding her knee. After conducting an examination on the floor, Christine decided to take the player to the athletic training room for a complete examination by the team physician. She and the student manager, who were both at least 10 inches (25 cm) shorter than the player, helped her hobble off the court toward the athletic training room. As they were passing the locker room, the student manager slipped on a wet spot, causing the player to put her full weight on the injured knee. She cried out in pain and told Christine that she felt a "pop."

After the team physician, a general practitioner employed by the student health service, completed his examination, he informed the player that she had torn the anterior cruciate and medial collateral ligaments in her knee and would need surgery to correct the problem. He instructed Christine to do the following things, all of which he recorded in his postevaluation dictation for the athlete's medical record:

- Apply an elastic wrap from the toes to midthigh.
- Apply a knee immobilizer.
- Fit the athlete with crutches.
- Arrange an orthopedic consultation for the next day.
- Give enough 800-milligram ibuprofen for three days.

Later that night, a phone call from the athlete's roommate woke Christine, who found out that the athlete had become violently ill and had been rushed to the hospital by ambulance after suffering a reaction to the medication that Christine had given her.

Questions for Analysis

1. What legal principles are involved in this case? What liability concerns should be addressed? What policies and procedures should be implemented to address these concerns?

2. What would you have done differently, if anything, if you had been in Christine's position?

3. Who, if anyone, is at fault in this case? If more than one person is at fault, how should a judge or jury determine the degree to which each person is liable?

Case Study 3

Adisa was an athletic trainer who worked mornings in an out-patient rehabilitation clinic and afternoons at a local, rural high school. As the end of the continuing education unit (CEU) reporting period was approaching, he worked diligently to make sure that he had completed the required number of CEUs and reported them to the Board of Certification. He also completed the necessary forms to renew his license in Washington before the deadline at the end of the year. In January, he received notification from the BOC that his CEUs were accepted and that his status as a certified athletic trainer was in good shape for another two years. He also received his renewed license from the state of Washington.

Adisa submitted all of the paperwork to his boss, Chandra, who thanked him for getting everything submitted on time. She asked Adisa if he would assist Charles, who missed both deadlines and seemed to be having some difficulty completing the required forms. Charles is another AT the same clinic who also works at a local inner-city high school in the afternoons. Adisa met with Charles the next day and learned that he had not yet completed all of his required CEUs, but was planning to do so by the end of the month, which is when he would submit his renewal forms for both his certification and license.

Questions for Analysis

1. Is Charles allowed to continue to practice as an athletic trainer in Washington? Why or why not?

2. Is Adisa obligated to report Charles to the Board of Certification or the state licensing body? Should Adisa report this information to anyone else?

3. How should Adisa advise Charles on how to proceed?

4. What could be the negative ramifications of Charles continuing to practice with an expired certification and license?

Key Concepts and Review

Define and discuss the legal principles most applicable to athletic training settings.

Although the thought of legal action against an athletic trainer is unsettling, prudent athletic trainers will take advantage of their legal knowledge to improve the quality of the service they provide to their physically active patients. The best and most important source of legal advice, of course, is an attorney experienced in dealing with health care malpractice issues.

Identify the types of situations most likely to hold liability concerns for athletic trainers.

Risk management is a process designed to prevent losses of all types for everyone associated with an athletic program. The two ways to identify and assess risks are real-world observation and inference from controlled studies. The best risk management programs use both methods. The athletic trainer can reduce risk in four areas: preparation for the activity, conduct of the activity, management of injuries, and proper records management.

Understand the different types of credentialing laws that affect the practice of athletic training.

Credentialing laws, including licensure, certification, registration, and exemption, are designed to ensure basic competencies to protect the public. All athletic trainers should become familiar with the laws in their state to determine their legal basis for practice. Athletic trainers who practice in states without credentialing laws might be held to the standard of care of a physician in a malpractice case.

Differentiate between Board of Certification (BOC) certification and state regulation for athletic trainers.

The Board of Certification (BOC) administers the national certification exam that one must pass to be recognized as a certified athletic trainer. State regulation is a separate process of recognizing an athletic trainer within an individual state's legal process, which is referred to as a regulatory process. Athletic trainers must typically be certified by the BOC in most states and then meet the qualifications for regulation in the form of licensure or registration.

Understand the elements required to prove negligence on the part of an athletic trainer.

Torts are legal wrongs, other than breach of contract, for which a court will determine a remedy, usually in the form of monetary damages. Negligence is the kind of tort most commonly charged against athletic trainers. To prove negligence, the aggrieved person must demonstrate conduct by the athletic trainer, existence of duty, breach of duty, causation (including actual and proximate cause), and damage. Athletic trainers will be held to the same standard of care as other reasonably prudent athletic trainers in the same or similar circumstances.

Be aware of the various legal defenses available to athletic trainers against charges of malpractice.

Although several defenses against charges of malpractice exist, including statutes of limitations, sovereign immunity, assumption of risk, Good Samaritan immunity, and comparative negligence, the athletic trainer's best defense is to practice in a manner consistent with the standards of the profession.

Identify the most important elements of providing effective legal testimony.

Should an athletic trainer be called to provide testimony, either as a fact witness or as an expert witness, he should prepare by reviewing the records of the case, consulting with the attorney, and speaking only of the facts of the case within the limits of his experience and training.

Identify and put into practice methods that avoid legal liability while improving the quality of athletic training care.

Athletic trainers will improve their practice while simultaneously protecting themselves from liability if they build relationships with their patients, insist on written employment contracts, obtain informed consent, screen all athletes during a physical exam, and abide by the standards of the profession. They should also document hazards, establish and adhere to written policies, document patient care activities, maintain confidentiality, and provide proper instruction to injured patients. Finally, athletic trainers must also supervise their staffs, participate in continuing education, practice within the boundaries of their qualifications, and maintain a liability insurance policy.

Professional Advocacy

Objectives

After reading this chapter, you should be able to do the following:

- Explain how a bill is introduced and becomes law.

- Explain the value and importance of youth sport safety legislation.

- Identify your state and federal representatives and senators and explain how to contact them to advocate for the athletic training profession.

- Describe the need to advocate for the athletic training profession.

The practice of athletic training is regulated in every state except California. In addition, many states have passed additional legislation that affect athletic trainers, such as concussion laws and laws related to heat illness and sudden death of athletes. It is important for athletic trainers to understand all of the laws in their state that affect their practice as well as the laws in the states they may visit when traveling with teams. Every athletic trainer can have a positive impact on the way these laws are written by understanding the legislative process and appropriately advocating for the profession throughout the process.

How Laws Are Made

Every law begins as an idea for how to solve a problem. These ideas can come from any individual, such as the governor, a state senator, a lobbyist, or a private citizen. However, only members of the legislature can introduce bills, which may eventually become laws. States and the federal government pass many new laws each year and revise existing laws. Some bills are reintroduced year after year without ever becoming law and others become law in the first year they're introduced. While each state's legislature functions a little differently, there are many similarities in how ideas become bills and how bills become laws.

The process to create a new law is similar in both the state and federal governments. However, the process outlined here is related to state legislative processes because this is where athletic trainers are most likely to be directly involved in drafting bills and lobbying for legislation.

Step 1: Identify a Bill Sponsor

The first step is to identify a legislator who will sponsor a bill addressing an idea or a problem. State associations typically employ **lobbyists** to help identify a legislator who would be willing to sponsor a bill addressing a certain issue. Choosing the right legislator to sponsor the bill also involves consideration of the legislator's influence and committee assignments. For example, a group might choose a legislator because she serves on or chairs a committee where the bill will likely be reviewed. It is also advantageous to choose legislators who are more senior and influential because they are more likely to be able to garner support from other legislators. Sometimes, the political party is considered as well. If the state's legislature is made up primarily of one party, then the bill is likely to be more successful if sponsored by a legislator from that same party.

Step 2: Discuss the Issue

Once a potential bill sponsor has been identified, the lobbyist will arrange a meeting between the state association's leaders or the state association's governmental affairs committee members or both to discuss the issue. The legislator should be well educated on the topic so that he or she can answer questions as they arise along the way. It is also important to let the legislator know where the organization is willing to compromise so that the main goal of the legislation is maintained. In many states, athletic trainers have agreed to compromise by stating that "athletic trainers treat and care for athletes," but the definition of who is considered to be an athlete was left open enough to include people who exercise outside of an organized sports team. For example, the state practice acts for both Idaho (Athletic Trainers, Idaho, Title 54, Chapter 39) and Utah (Athletic Trainer Licensing Act, Utah, 58-40a) define *athlete* as

> "*a person who participates in exercises, sports, or games requiring physical strength, agility, flexibility, range of motion, speed or stamina and which exercises, sports or games are of the type generally conducted in association with an educational institution or professional, amateur or recreational sports club or organization.*"

However, this language can result in a perception that athletic trainers are only qualified to treat *athletes*, which can result in other issues affecting employment in out-patient rehabilitation clinics and third-party reimbursement.

Step 3: Draft the Bill

The next step is to draft the language of the bill and determine where it will fit into the existing state legislative code. Sometimes, just adding or deleting a few words, or even punctuation, can completely change the law. In other situations, such as concussion legislation, it is a completely new topic and becomes a new section in the state code. Once the group (organization leadership, lobbyist, and legislator) has developed a draft of the bill, it should be reviewed by the membership of the state organization as well as by a staff member in the state legislative research office. The bill must be written in statutory language (i.e., legal language). See figure 11.1 for an example of a bill that amended the licensure law for athletic trainers in Florida. It is also wise to get feedback on the language from the Board of Certification as well as the NATA Government Affairs Committee, who have experience with athletic training legislation. The reviews should confirm whether the language will achieve the desired goal as well as whether unintended consequences could result. The bill is then often run by members of the state association and other health care groups to seek support and to identify issues that might arise during the legislative session. Whenever possible, it is better to work through the issues before the legislative session so that the bill goes forth with less or no opposition. This process can take several months, but it is important to make sure that the new law will make a positive difference (National Athletic Trainers' Association n.d.-b).

Step 4: Introduce the Bill

Once the organization and legislator are satisfied with the language (wording) of the bill, the legislator will introduce the bill. This typically involves the legislator filing for a bill number and then having a first reading in their assembly, chamber, or house.

KEY POINT

Most states have a **bicameral legislature**, made up of two separate bodies, typically a House of Representatives and a Senate. In California, these are referred to as the Assembly and Senate instead. Nebraska is the only state that has a unicameral legislature, in which the legislative body is not separated, but remains a single body simply called the Nebraska Legislature, and all legislators are referred to as senators.

HB 541: ATHLETIC TRAINERS

(CH. 2015-116, LAWS OF FLORIDA)

Bill Sponsor: Representative Palsencia

Effective Date: January 1, 2016

DOE Contact: Tanya Cooper, Director Governmental Relations, (850) 245-0507

EXECUTIVE SUMMARY:

The bill revises the requirements to become licensed as an athletic trainer by removing the requirement that the applicant must be at least 21 years of age. An applicant who graduated college prior to 2004 must hold a current certification from the Board of Certification. The bill requires the college or university from which the applicant holds a degree to be accredited by the Commission on Accreditation of Athletic Training Education. The degree must be from a professional athletic training degree program. The bill requires an applicant, who applies on or after July 1, 2016, to undergo a criminal background check. Applicants must also be certified in both cardiopulmonary resuscitation and the use of an automated external defibrillator.

SECTION 1.

Amends s. 468.70, F.S., Legislative Intent, to:

- Revise the legislative intent to state that athletic trainers in this state meet minimum requirements for safe practice and that an athletic trainer who falls below minimum competency or who otherwise presents a danger to the public be prohibited from practicing in this state.

SECTION 2.

Amends s. 468.701, F.S., Definitions, to:

- Delete the following definitions and terms:
  - Athlete;
  - Athletic Activity;
  - Athletic injury;
  - Direct Supervision; and
  - Supervision.
- Redefine the term Athletic Trainer as a person who is licensed and has met the education requirements set forth by the Commission on Accreditation of Athletic Training Education or its successor and necessary credentials from the Board of Certification.
- Specify that an Athletic Trainer may not provide, offer to provide, or represent that they are qualified to provide any care or services that they are not qualified to provide.
- Redefine the term Athletic Training to mean service by an athletic trainer under the direction of a physician as specified in s. 468.713, F.S.

SECTION 3.

Amends s. 468.703, F.S., Board of Athletic Training, to:

- Remove staggered terms for members of the Board of Athletic Training. Instead each board member shall be appointed by the Governor for a 4 year term.

SECTION 4.

Amends s. 468.705, F.S., Rulemaking Authority, to:

- Authorize the Board of Athletic Trainers to adopt rules for mandatory requirements and guideline for communication between the athletic trainer and a physician.

(continued)

Figure 11.1 Florida House Bill 541: Athletic Trainers. This is a summary of a bill that was passed in Florida in 2015 that amended (updated) the law relating to licensure of athletic trainers in that state.

SECTION 5.

Amends s. 468.707, F.S., Licensure, to:

- Revise the requirements to become licensed as an athletic trainer by removing the requirement that the applicant must be at least 21 years of age.
- Specify that an applicant who graduated college prior to 2004 must hold a current certification from the Board of Certification.
- Require the college or university from which the applicant holds a degree to be accredited by the Commission on Accreditation of Athletic Training Education. The degree must be from a professional athletic training degree program.
- Require an applicant, who applies on or after July 1, 2016, to undergo a criminal background check.
- Require that applicants must also be certified in both cardiopulmonary resuscitation and the use of an automated external defibrillator.

SECTION 6.

Amends s. 468.709, F.S., Fees, to:

- Remove the requirement that the examination fee not exceed $200.00.

SECTION 7.

Amends s. 468.711, F.S., Renewal of License, to:

- Align statutory language with changes made by the bill.

SECTION 8.

Amends s. 468.713, F.S., Responsibilities of Athletic Trainers, to:

- Remove the requirement for athletic trainers to practice within the written protocol of a physician, as determined by the Board. Instead, the bill requires athletic trainers to practice under the direction of a physician.
- Authorizes the Board of Athletic Training to adopt rules for mandatory requirements and guidelines for communication between the athletic trainer and a physician.

SECTION 9.

Amends s. 468.715, F.S., Sexual Misconduct, to:

- Align the definition of sexual misconduct for athletic trainers to s. 456.063, F.S.

SECTION 10.

Amends s. 468.717, F.S., Violations and penalties.—Each of the following acts constitutes a misdemeanor of the first degree, punishable as provided in s. 775.082 or s.775.803, to:

- Provide that practicing athletic training, representing oneself as an athletic trainer, or providing athletic trainer services to a patient without being licensed constitutes a first degree misdemeanor.
- Add the following terms under this section of law:
  - Licensed athletic trainer;
  - Abbreviation "AT" or "LAT"; or
  - A similar title or abbreviation that suggests licensure as an athletic trainer.

SECTION 11.

Amends s. 468.719, F.S., Disciplinary actions, to:

- Delete failing to include the athletic trainer's name and license number on any certain types of advertising as an act that constitutes grounds for denial of a license.
- Add that an athletic trainer can be denied a license if they are unable to practice athletic training with reasonable safety and skill because of a mental or physical condition or because of a controlled substance that impairs [one's] ability to practice.

(continued)

Figure 11.1 *(continued)*

SECTION 12.

Amends s. 468.723, F.S., Exemptions.—This part does not prevent or restrict, to:

- Define "direct supervision" as it relates to this section of law as, the physical presences of an athletic trainer so that the athletic trainer is immediately available to the athletic training student and able to intervene on behalf of the athletic training student in accordance with the standards set forth by the Commission on Accreditation of Athletic Training Education or its successor.
- State that nothing in the athletic training practice act prevents or restricts third party payors from reimbursing employers of athletic trainers for covered services rendered by a licensed athletic trainer.

SECTION 13.

Amends s. 456.0135, F.S., General Background Screening provisions, to:

- Align statutory language with changes made by the bill.

GENERAL IMPLEMENTATION TIMELINE:

January 1, 2016 The act becomes effective.

Figure 11.1 *(continued)*

PEARLS OF MANAGEMENT

To identify the legislators who represent you in your district, visit your state legislature's website. Most have a link called something like Find My Representative or Senator, where you can enter your ZIP code to get the name and contact information for your legislators. In some states, you might have to instead find your address on a map to determine your district and then identify your representative or senator by district.

The introduction of the bill is also often referred to as a **first reading**, in which the name of the bill is read and an overview of its goal may be provided by the bill sponsor. In some states, the first reading might include only reading the title and receiving a bill number. At the first or sometimes the second reading, the bill will be assigned to a committee that will review its language and purpose in more detail. Each committee focuses on specific types of issues such as health care, commerce, education, or agriculture (see the following sidebar for examples of senate committees). The legislator will often suggest a particular committee, but this is not always granted and bills sometimes end up in committees that were not anticipated. It can take several weeks or longer to get the bill on the committee's agenda, depending on how many other bills it is reviewing and how time consuming each one is.

When the bill is formally reviewed by the committee, members of the organization, the public, and anyone who wants to speak to support or oppose the bill are typically allowed to testify before the committee. At this point, data and justifications are often provided to either support or oppose the passage of the bill. **Amendments** (edits) to the bill may also be suggested at this time, but these can be added later in the process as well. The committee members may also request to hear testimony from certain individuals or groups and request specific information to aid their deliberations. The committee will then vote on the bill and must approve it before it can move on in the process. Bills sometimes die in committee, which means either that the committee opted not to put the bill on any of its meeting agendas or that the bill was voted down after review. Should this happen, the bill can be introduced again in subsequent years or on rare occasions, reviewed by the committee a second time after new information is presented or significant amendments are made (Vote Smart n.d.).

If the bill is passed by the committee, it will then go back to the legislative body where it originated (the house, senate, or assembly) for another reading, usually with more detail than the initial introduction and with a report regarding the committee's vote and feedback. Typically, only legislators can speak about the bill at this time, although they may share information provided by others. Sometimes, the bill will be debated and questioned by other legislators, but sometimes it will go directly to a vote. If the bill is voted down (not approved), the bill must usually go through the full process again during the next legislative session the following year. If the bill

Senate Committees in New Jersey

Budget and Appropriations

Commerce

Community and Urban Affairs

Economic Growth

Environment and Energy

Health, Human Services, and Senior Citizens

Higher Education

Judiciary

Labor

Law and Public Safety

Legislative Oversight

Military and Veterans' Affairs

Rules and Order

State Government, Wagering, Tourism, and Historic Preservation

Transportation

is passed (approved), it will then move to the other legislative body for review using the same process. For example, if a bill was introduced in the senate, it would then have to be reviewed and approved by a committee of the senate, before coming back to the senate floor for a vote. Once the bill is approved by the senate, it is introduced in the house or assembly, then reviewed by a house or assembly committee, and then it can be voted on by the full house or assembly. If the bill is significantly amended (modified) along the way, it may have to return to the other legislative body for another review.

If the bill has been approved by both houses (house or assembly and senate) or by the unicameral legislature (as in Nebraska), it then is referred to the governor. The governor can sign the bill to approve it, veto the bill to block its passage, or take no action (see figure 11.2). If the governor takes no action, meaning he or she does not sign it or veto it, it may result in the bill automatically becoming law or automatically being vetoed depending on how close to the end of the session the bill was passed. This varies by state quite a bit, so it is important to become familiar with these laws and timelines in your state.

KEY POINT

The bill-signing deadline for each state can be found on the StateScape website, although it would be wise to confirm this information within your state's legislative code. This website has other helpful resources, such as legislative session schedules, budget timetables, and a list of governors for each state.

Athletic Training Legislation

Athletic trainers have been involved in several types of legislation. The first involves the regulation of the profession, which can take the form of exemption, certification, registration, or licensure. See chapter 10, Legal Considerations in Sports Medicine, for more details regarding the types of professional regulation.

In addition, ATs also support youth sport safety legislation, both at the state and national levels. As of 2016, 49 states and the District of Columbia have passed concussion laws requiring that individuals who suffer concussions receive appropriate treatment from qualified health care professionals, such as athletic trainers, physicians, school nurses, and others with appropriate levels of training. Many of these laws specifically mention ATs as one of the

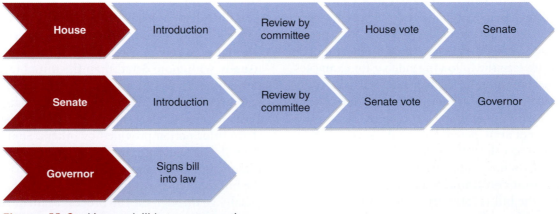

Figure 11.2 How a bill becomes a law.

health care providers who can evaluate concussions and make return-to-play decisions. Other states simply reference any licensed health care provider with appropriate training (Centers for Disease Control and Prevention n.d.). The state laws regulating athletic training also vary in their definition of *athlete* and who the law affects. In Utah, for example, the concussion law applies to anyone under the age of 18 who is involved in activities with sports teams, recreational sports (such as city leagues), sports camps, and public and private schools, which includes physical education classes (HB 204—Protection of Athletes with Head Injuries 2011). Some states have enacted similar youth sport safety laws addressing heat illness and sudden death.

At the federal level, NATA has supported bills that promote youth sport safety (National Athletic Trainers' Association n.d.-b). These bills received significant support in 2016, but as of 2017 have not yet been passed as laws. The Secondary School Student Athletes' Bill of Rights outlines 10 best practices that serve as recommendations for youth sport safety in secondary schools (see the following sidebar). It

> ### KEY POINT
>
> The Centers for Disease Control and Prevention's website on concussions is a resource for parents, coaches, schools, and health care providers. It provides basic information on traumatic brain injuries, handouts for various groups, and information on sports concussion policies and laws. It also includes training videos and a free app that contains concussion and helmet safety information.

encourages schools to adopt the recommendations, but is not a mandate to do so. The SAFE PLAY (Supporting Athletes, Families and Educators to Protect the Lives of Athletic Youth) Act also contains best practices, focusing on a multidisciplinary approach to research and policies related to concussions, heat illness, cardiomyopathy, and emergency action plans to protect young athletes (S.436—SAFE PLAY Act 2016). It also directs the Centers for Disease Control and Prevention to develop and disseminate educational materials to schools, parents, and health

Secondary School Student Athletes' Bill of Rights 10 Best Practices

Secondary school student athletes have the right to

1. be coached by individuals who are well-trained in sport-specific safety and to be monitored by athletic health care team members;

2. quality, regular pre-participation examinations and each athlete has the right to participate under a comprehensive concussion management plan;

3. participate in sporting activities on safe, clean playing surfaces, in both indoor and outdoor facilities;

4. utilize equipment and uniforms that are safe, fitted appropriately, and routinely maintained, and to appropriate personnel trained in proper removal of equipment in case of injury;

5. participate safely in all environmental conditions where play follows approved guidelines and medical policies and procedures, with a hydration plan in place;

6. a safe playing environment with venue-specific emergency action plans that are coordinated by the athletic health care team and regularly rehearsed with local emergency personnel;

7. privacy of health information and proper referral for medical, psychosocial, and nutritional counseling;

8. participate in a culture that finds "playing through pain" unacceptable unless there has been a medical assessment;

9. immediate, on-site injury assessments with decisions made by qualified sports medicine professionals; and

10. along with their parents, the latest information about the benefits and potential risks of participation in competitive sports, including access to statistics on fatalities and catastrophic injuries to youth athletes.

Reprinted from GovTrack, *114th Congress, 1st Session, H. Res. 112 – Supporting the goals and ideals of the Secondary School Student Athletes' Bill of Rights,* 2015.

care providers on these topics. The goal of both of these bills is to raise awareness of youth sport safety issues and ways in which we can make it safer for kids to play sports.

In 2009, NATA launched the Youth Sports Safety Alliance (YSSA) to advocate for youth sport safety through research, education, and legislation (Youth Sports Safety Alliance n.d.). As of 2016, the YSSA had 270 members including universities and other research groups, parent advocacy groups, youth sports leagues, and health care organizations. The YSSA has created a National Action Plan to identify and encourage best practices in youth sport safety. It also hosts a Youth Sports Safety Summit each year, presenting the latest research and current recommendations on topics such as concussions, cardiomyopathy, opiate abuse, and overuse injuries. The YSSA also publishes resources on these topics as well as a Youth Athlete in Memoriam, which tracks sports-related fatalities each year in youth participants.

KEY POINT

The Youth Sports Safety Alliance advocates for youth sport safety issues. More information can be found on their website.

Working with your state's high school activities and athletics associations is another way to advocate for youth sport safety. These organizations can establish rules for secondary school athletics that make playing sports safer. While each state has its own activities association, the National Federation of State High School Associations (NFHS) serves as a great resource for both interscholastic athletics and some recreational sports. Both state organizations and the NFHS establish rules and guidelines for sport participation; these often also apply to marching bands, debate teams, and theater activities. The Korey Stringer Institute also provides resources, including best practices for secondary school policies on topics such as automated external defibrillators, heat illness, and concussions.

Another bill that made significant progress in 2016 and 2017 is the Sports Medicine Licensure Clarity Act, which protects athletic trainers, physicians, and other health care providers who travel with teams across state lines (see figure 11.3). This requires their liability insurance to provide coverage even if the health care provider does not hold a license to practice in each state where she travels. As of November 2016, the bill had been passed by the U.S. House of Representatives and was headed to the U.S. Senate for consideration. Athletic trainers are not required

---

To provide protections for certain sports medicine professionals who provide certain medical services in a secondary State.

Be it enacted by the Senate and House of Representatives of the United States of America in Congress assembled,

SECTION 1. SHORT TITLE.

This Act may be cited as the "Sports Medicine Licensure Clarity Act of 2016."

SEC. 2. PROTECTIONS FOR COVERED SPORTS MEDICINE PROFESSIONALS.

(a) In General.—In the case of a covered sports medicine professional who has in effect medical professional liability insurance coverage and provides in a secondary State covered medical services that are within the scope of practice of such professional in the primary State to an athlete or an athletic team (or a staff member of such an athlete or athletic team) pursuant to an agreement described in subsection (b)(4) with respect to such athlete or athletic team—

> (1) such medical professional liability insurance coverage shall cover (subject to any related premium adjustments) such professional with respect to such covered medical services provided by the professional in the secondary State to such an individual or team as if such services were provided by such professional in the primary State to such an individual or team; and

> (2) to the extent such professional is licensed under the requirements of the primary State to provide such services to such an individual or team, the professional shall be treated as satisfying any licensure requirements of the secondary State to provide such services to such an individual or team.

(continued)

Figure 11.3 Sports Medicine Licensure Clarity Act

Reprinted from National Athletic Trainers' Association, *The sports medicine licensure clarity act.* (Carrollton, TX: NATA).

(b) Definitions.—In this Act, the following definitions apply:

(1) Athlete.—The term "athlete" means—

(A) an individual participating in a sporting event or activity for which the individual may be paid;

(B) an individual participating in a sporting event or activity sponsored or sanctioned by a national governing body; or

(C) an individual for whom a high school or institution of higher education provides a covered sports medicine professional.

(2) Athletic team.—The term "athletic team" means a sports team—

(A) composed of individuals who are paid to participate on the team;

(B) composed of individuals who are participating in a sporting event or activity sponsored or sanctioned by a national governing body; or

(C) for which a high school or an institution of higher education provides a covered sports medicine professional.

(3) Covered medical services.—The term "covered medical services" means general medical care, emergency medical care, athletic training, or physical therapy services. Such term does not include care provided by a covered sports medicine professional—

(A) at a health care facility; or

(B) while a health care provider licensed to practice in the secondary State is transporting the injured individual to a health care facility.

(4) Covered sports medicine professional.—The term "covered sports medicine professional" means a physician, athletic trainer, or other health care professional who—

(A) is licensed to practice in the primary State;

(B) provides covered medical services, pursuant to a written agreement with an athlete, an athletic team, a national governing body, a high school, or an institution of higher education; and

(C) prior to providing the covered medical services described in subparagraph (B), has disclosed the nature and extent of such services to the entity that provides the professional with liability insurance in the primary State.

(5) Health care facility.—The term "health care facility" means a facility in which medical care, diagnosis, or treatment is provided on an inpatient or outpatient basis. Such term does not include facilities at an arena, stadium, or practice facility, or temporary facilities existing for events where athletes or athletic teams may compete.

(6) Institution of higher education.—The term "institution of higher education" has the meaning given such term in section 101 of the Higher Education Act of 1965 (20 U.S.C. 1001).

(7) National governing body.—The term "national governing body" has the meaning given such term in section 220501 of title 36, United States Code.

(8) Primary state.—The term "primary State" means, with respect to a covered sports medicine professional, the State in which—

(A) the covered sports medicine professional is licensed to practice; and

(B) the majority of the covered sports medicine professional's practice is underwritten for medical professional liability insurance coverage.

(9) Secondary state.—The term "secondary State" means, with respect to a covered sports medicine professional, any State that is not the primary State.

(10) State.—The term "State" means each of the several States, the District of Columbia, and each commonwealth, territory, or possession of the United States.

Passed the House of Representatives September 12, 2016.

Attest: KAREN L. HAAS, *Clerk*.

Figure 11.3 *(continued)*

to be licensed in every state they travel to as long as they are appropriately credentialed in their home state and do not exceed a certain number of days in the state they are travelling to. The maximum number of allowable days varies from state to state. Athletic trainers with professional baseball teams who spend 3 to 6 months in Arizona or Florida for spring training typically have to be credentialed in those states because of the longer time period. It is important that athletic trainers remain up to date on the AT regulations in their own state as well as any states they travel to with teams to ensure that they remain in compliance with all regulations.

How to Become an Advocate for the Athletic Training Profession

One of the best ways that athletic trainers can serve the profession is to become an advocate. Serving in an advocacy role allows athletic trainers to let the public and legislators know why ATs are important members of the health care team. This can ensure that athletic trainers are allowed to use all their skills to provide high-quality health care to the patients they treat (National Athletic Trainers' Association n.d.-a). ATs can speak on behalf of youth athletes and other individuals who sustain injuries during sports, other activities, or while at work. They can work to convince insurance companies to reimburse for the services that ATs provide so that more individuals can benefit from the AT's expertise. While other groups often support these efforts, such as parents and other health care organizations, athletic trainers need to do the significant work in this area. This may seem like a daunting task, especially when considering the busy schedules of athletic trainers, but these goals can be accomplished if all ATs work together (McKibbin and McKune 2015).

Advocacy can start with small steps that do not have to take up a large amount of time. One of the simplest things that every AT can and should do is contact his state legislators. Most states have an easy link on the state legislature page titled something like "Find my legislators." For some, there may be a separate link to find your state representative and your state senator. Typically, you just need to enter your home address and the website will show you who your legislators are and will provide you with their website's address and contact information. You should write a letter to each of your legislators to introduce yourself. This can be a simple e-mail or letter where you identify yourself as an athletic

trainer, explain where you work and what you do (or if you're a student, explain where you are enrolled), invite her to observe you on the job if possible, and thank her for the work that she does to represent you and your interests (See figure 11.4 for a sample letter). Always begin the letter by stating that you are one of her constituents, meaning that you are a voting member of her district. The legislator will likely reply with a thank you letter and may or may not accept your invitation to visit your school or workplace. Keep in mind that not all states allow legislators to accept game tickets, so she may have to observe you during practice or in a clinic setting to maintain compliance with state laws. If the legislator does accept your invitation, be sure to follow up with a thank-you letter after the visit. The legislator would likely also appreciate a picture of you with her and a public thank-you on your social media page or her social media page or both. If she is not able to accept your invitation, you could instead ask for a time to meet with her in her office, just to get acquainted (Herzog, Sedory, and McKibbin 2016).

If you are willing to support the legislator's reelection, you can also volunteer to assist with her campaign. This can be as simple as offering to put a sign in your yard, but can be as involved as attending fund-raising events, making campaign donations, making calls to potential voters, or going door to door to distribute information. The legislator will appreciate any efforts you are able to make. You can also attend town hall meetings to ask questions and to show that you are an engaged citizen. There may be many issues in your state that you care about and wish to advocate for. Communicating about all of these issues in a respectful way helps you to build a relationship with those who represent you. Legislators want to hear their constituents' opinion on the issues to ensure that they are representing the views of the voters in their district.

KEY POINT

Athletic trainers can have an impact by donating to their state association's governmental affairs efforts, directly through the association or through their **political action committee (PAC)** if they have one. Even small donations from a large number of members can add up to make a difference. To support federal legislative efforts, athletic trainers can donate to the National Athletic Trainers' Association Political Action Committee (NATAPAC).

Tyson Brown
100 Main Street
Central, UT 80001

May 15, 2018

Senator Isabel Rodriguez
100 State Capitol Drive
Capitol City, UT 80006

Dear Senator Rodriguez,

I am writing to introduce myself as one of your constituents in your district. I am an athletic trainer who provides health care services for more than 150 athletes at Central High School, where I have worked for the past eight years. I assist with preseason physical examinations, conduct baseline concussion testing, provide emergency care during sporting events and practices, develop and implement treatment and rehabilitation protocols for injured athletes, and work with other local health care professionals when needed to manage injuries and illnesses. I also serve as a preceptor (clinical supervisor) for one or two students each semester from local universities who are enrolled in athletic training graduate programs.

I would like to invite you to visit me at my high school in the next few weeks to observe how I work to protect the health and safety of youth athletes. I can show you how we assess concussions, prepare for emergencies, and rehabilitate injuries. The best times for you to come would be in the afternoons between 3:00 and 6:00 p.m. or on Thursday or Friday evenings if you'd like to observe a football game.

Thank you for all the work you do to represent our interests and work for the betterment of our state. If you would like to schedule a day and time to visit and observe the work of an athletic trainer, please contact me at 801-222-1222 or tysonbrown@email.com. I look forward to hearing from you.

Sincerely,

Tyson Brown, MS, LAT, ATC

Figure 11.4 Sample letter to legislator

Once you have established a relationship with your legislators, it is much easier to ask for their vote on proposed legislation that will affect athletic trainers. When these situations arise, be sure to follow the instructions provided by your state athletic training association. Most state associations employ a lobbyist who will provide guidance on developing the best strategies for achieving legislative goals. For example, if your state is working to ensure that every high school employs a full-time athletic trainer, it may be wise to build support with the state school board before contacting individual legislators. When you've been asked to contact your legislator to ask for support on an issue, be sure to follow the timelines provided and be both respectful and appreciative in all communications. Many legislators have full-time jobs in addition to their role in the legislature. They are also often asked to vote on a large number of bills each day during the legislative session, requiring them to work 12 to 14 hours a day for two to five months at a time.

If you would like to get more involved with legislative activities in your state, you can volunteer to serve on your state athletic training association's governmental affairs or legislative committee. These committees often organize events to raise funds to support legislative efforts and meet regularly with the association's lobbyist to develop effective strategies. They may also testify before legislative committees when needed and meet with individual legislators to discuss issues. If the state holds a Capitol Hill Day, this committee would organize that event. Even if you're not on this committee, the group might need volunteers to assist with Capitol Hill Day by talking with individuals at the capitol, passing out brochures, and so on. The group may also be looking for individuals in each district who are willing to write letters or meet with legislators to seek support for various issues and bills (McKibbin and McKune 2015).

Athletic trainers who have established relationships with legislators will often be more effective at garnering their support. An AT can write letters, meet with legislators in their offices, invite them to the AT's workplaces, and support reelection campaigns.

Athletic trainers may also have opportunities to get involved in the same ways with federal legislation. NATA has developed a webpage dedicated to advocacy that provides information about bills that it is supporting, with details and talking points for each. You can contact your national legislators in the same way that you contact your state legislators. Begin with an introductory letter or e-mail, invite them to visit you where you work, and thank them for their service. You can attend their town hall meetings and meet with them in person when they're in town. You can also sign up for NATA Capitol Hill Day, held almost every year, and visit them in their offices in Washington, D.C. (figure 11.5).

Athletic trainers can also advocate for the profession through their interactions with their patients, parents, clients, and members of the public. To prevent misconceptions, it is important that the members of the public understand the athletic trainer's vital role as a member of the health care team. This means that ATs need to dress, speak, and conduct themselves professionally at all times. Athletic trainers should look and behave like other health care providers. Athletic training clinics should look like other health care clinics. Athletic trainers serve a vital role in injury prevention and treatment and can offer this expertise through seminars and guest presentations to community groups, youth sports leagues, parent–teacher organizations (such as the PTA), and to other groups of health care professionals. The more that the public understands who athletic trainers are and what they do, the easier it is to accomplish their larger legislative goals.

Summary

It is important that athletic trainers know how to advocate for the future of the profession. This involves an understanding of the legislative process and ways in which each athletic trainer can participate in the process. Every athletic trainer has the ability to make a difference by educating the public and building relationships with legislators. It is vital that athletic trainers represent themselves in a professional manner at all times when interacting with patients, athletes, parents, clients, coaches, legislators, and so on. Athletic trainers need to show lawmakers that they appreciate the legislators' efforts on their behalf and communicate in a respectful manner. With these principles in mind, athletic trainers can make an impact on their ability to fully practice their skills and serve as effective members of the health care team.

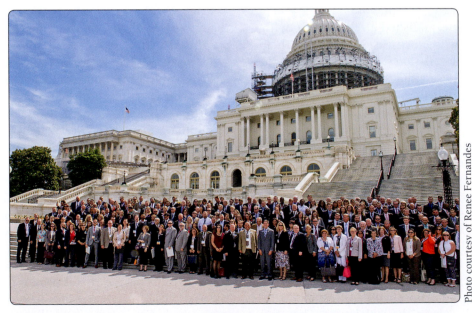

Figure 11.5 NATA members at Capitol Hill Day in Washington, D.C.

Photo courtesy of Renee Fernandes

Learning Aids

Case Study 1

Aponi had served as the head athletic trainer at Desert Canyon High School for 10 years. The school was located in southern Utah, where the summer and fall temperatures regularly exceed 100° F (38° C), so she was well versed in preventing and treating heat illness. However, in the last few years, because of increased temperatures in the summer and early fall months, the number of cases of heat illness among high school athletes in Utah had sharply increased. Several deaths resulted from these situations. In most cases, no AT was employed at the high school and in other cases, rectal thermometers and cold-water immersion were not used because of resistance by administrators.

Aponi was recently elected as president of the Utah Athletic Trainers' Association and knew that the state association could help to effect change. At the Utah Athletic Trainers' Association Annual Conference, she led a discussion to determine how to best deal with these issues statewide.

Questions for Analysis

1. For which types of initiatives would a state association be more impactful by developing a public education campaign than by supporting legislation? Are there situations in which both should be used?

2. If the association decides to pursue heat illness legislation, with whom does it need to build support for the bill?

3. What resources could the association use to convince all interested parties to take action in response to the increased incidence of heat illnesses and deaths?

4. What would you recommend and how much would it cost to implement the plan?

Case Study 2

Gabriella had recently completed her professional master's degree and passed her BOC exam. She was hired to work as an athletic trainer with an arena football team in West Virginia and was excited to get started. She submitted her registration application with the state board and was expecting to be ready to begin work in about a week. Because she couldn't do much at work until she was registered, she spent time reviewing the state association's website to see what initiatives it had been working on. She was distressed to learn that the regulation of athletic trainers had received an unfavorable review during the sunset process, which requires every professional regulation to be reviewed every seven years. The state association's website noted that its board of directors and governmental affairs committee were working to request reconsideration of the decision. They encouraged athletic trainers in the state to immediately contact their legislators to seek support for the reconsideration.

Questions for Analysis

1. How can Gabriella determine who she should contact?

2. Because Gabriella just moved to West Virginia, what is the best way for her to quickly establish a relationship with her legislators?

3. What arguments should she use to convince her legislators to support a change of decision?

Key Concepts and Review

Explain how a bill is introduced and becomes law.

Bills must first be drafted into legal language and sponsored by a legislator. The bill will begin with a brief reading either in the House or Senate, often followed by a second reading of the full bill at a later date. The bill is then referred to a committee that will study it and vote on it. If the committee votes to approve the bill, it then goes back to the same House or Senate for a vote. If that body approves it, the process is repeated in the other house and then must also be signed by the governor before becoming a law.

Explain the value and importance of youth sport safety legislation.

Youth sport safety legislation is intended to protect youth athletes from serious injuries such as concussions, heat illness, and sudden cardiac death. These laws typically establish a standard of care including the types of medical personnel and equipment that must be available to care for athletes in these situations. These laws have helped to educate schools and youth sports leagues on how to keep their athletes safe and also served to help prioritize funding for necessary resources.

Identify your state and federal representatives and senators and explain how to contact them to advocate for the athletic training profession.

Begin by searching the Internet for your state's legislature. Once on the website, look for a link for "Legislators" or "Find My Legislator." Enter your home address, including ZIP code to determine which state legislators represent you. Then, draft a letter or e-mail to each legislator to introduce yourself and the athletic training profession and request a meeting or invite them to visit you where you work.

Describe the need to advocate for the athletic training profession.

Advocating for the profession allows athletic trainers to let the public and legislators know why ATs are important members of the health care team. This can help to ensure that athletic trainers are allowed to use all their skills to provide high-quality health care to the patients they treat. ATs can help to ensure that athletes and workers have safe work environments with the necessary resources for proper care when injuries occur. They can also work to convince insurance companies to cover the services that ATs provide so that more individuals can benefit from the AT's expertise.

Administration of Clinical Policies and Procedures

Objectives

After reading this chapter, you should be able to do the following:

- Identify the components of a clinically related policy and procedure.

- Define the terms *supervision* and *direction* as they relate to athletic training.

- Establish criteria for providing appropriate medical coverage in various settings.

- Integrate policies and procedures associated with establishing a crisis intervention program, inclusive of mental health needs.

- Develop policies and procedures for athletic training services related to camp coverage.

Few duties consume more of an athletic trainer's administrative time and energy than the organization and administration of clinically related policies and procedures. Seasoned athletic trainers have experience to guide them through the many potential pitfalls involved, but new athletic trainers may require guidance in planning these important documents and activities. This chapter will help you understand and be able to apply the principles associated with establishing sound policies and procedures for clinically oriented tasks. Furthermore, implementation of these tasks will be discussed to better prepare you as an athletic trainer-administrator.

Development of a Clinical Policy and Procedure

Chapter 3 explained the development of operational plans, policies, and procedures—the higher-level guidelines that define why the department exists and its goals and operating philosophy. When it comes to developing the clinically related procedures and policies for hands-on functions and day-to-day issues, the process is similar. As you may recall, a policy is an organized plan that addresses a specific action. While chapter 3 discussed policies related more to general administrative plans of action, this chapter outlines policies that address clinical topics. Operational plans for clinical functions tend to be short and are often updated annually. Similarly, the broad statements associated with clinical policies should demonstrate the importance of recognizing the need for implementing standards associated with specific clinical issues. The written procedures address the standard of care for each clinical policy. The following sidebar provides a list of clinical topics for which athletic trainers should have policies and procedures in place. While this list is comprehensive, it may not include all the possible policies that one could determine as essential.

PEARLS OF MANAGEMENT

If NATA has published a position statement on a clinical topic, it should be standard practice for an athletic training department to adhere to such clinical policies, with the procedures also being specific to one's organization.

A handbook or manual that includes all of the clinical policies and procedures should be made available to all athletic training staff. The documents should be frequently reviewed (typically annually), with written documentation to support changes. The dates and names of people involved in the updated reviews and reviews of training should be noted. New staff, students, and others involved

in clinical decision making of any kind should be familiar with an organization's clinical policies and procedures. Again, completion of all document reviews should be put in writing and preserved as part of administrative record keeping. All clinical policies and procedures should be reviewed by the athletic trainer's team physicians in addition to the organization's legal counsel when necessary. Relatively new certified athletic trainers and athletic trainers employed in a new position may want to seek external consultation from experienced athletic trainers in an effort to establish comprehensive policies and procedures.

PEARLS OF MANAGEMENT

NATA develops official statements, which are similar to policies, but with less in-depth procedural descriptions.

Many of the clinically related policies and procedures used in athletic training programs include standard-of-care guidelines developed by experts from within the athletic training community and in collaboration with other health care experts. These standards should always serve as the foundation for organizational standards, with additional compo-

Clinical Topics for Policies and Procedures

- Crisis intervention
- Mental health (see Neal, Diamond, Goldman, Liedtka et al. 2015; Neal, Diamond, Goldman, Klossner et al. 2015)
- Management of sport concussion (see Broglio et al. 2014)
- Lightning safety (see Walsh et al. 2013)
- Hot and cold environments (see Casa et al. 2015; Cappaert et al. 2008)
- Emergency action planning (see Andersen et al. 2002)
- Helmet removal
- Spine injury (see Swartz et al. 2009)
- Bloodborne pathogens
- Appropriate medical coverage
- Preparticipation physical examinations (see Conley et al. 2014)
- Nutritional disorders (see Buell et al. 2013)

- Performance enhancing substances (see Buell et al. 2013; Kersey et al. 2012)
- Drug education and testing
- Pharmaceutical storage and dispensing
- Clinical supervision of staff
- Equipment calibration and safety training
- First aid and CPR training
- Communicable and infectious diseases
- Sickle cell trait management
- Return-to-play decision making
- Patient consent
- Release of medical records
- Medical disqualification of the student-athlete (see Conley et al. 2014)
- Pregnancy in the student-athlete
- Dental and oral injuries (see Gould et al. 2016)
- Ankle sprains (see Kaminski et al. 2013)

nents added to meet the needs of the specific program, venue, and other considerations pertinent to one's setting. It is also helpful to make these policies and procedures publicly available to stakeholders. For example, visiting teams should be familiar with an emergency action plan at a venue they are traveling to for an event. Student-athletes and all patients should be familiar with policies and procedures that pertain to their role as a stakeholder in receiving athletic training services. In many instances, the student-athlete or patient will be asked to provide a written signature acknowledging that she has read and understood the policies and procedures. For minors, it will be required for a parent or guardian to read and understand the required policies and procedures and provide a written signature of acknowledgement.

The remainder of this chapter discusses how to establish and administer clinical policies and procedures. It also offers examples of policies and procedures commonly found in athletic training settings.

Supervision

Supervision is defined differently from state to state and from program to program. For example, athletic trainers technically work under the direction of a physician as defined both by certification standards and state practice acts. The physician may fall under one of several categories: doctor of medicine (MD), doctor of osteopathic medicine (DO), and doctor of medicine in dentistry (DMD). The terms *direction* and *supervision* will also be clearly defined in the state practice act. While the policy itself will address supervision, the legal language should serve as the starting point for the procedures being drafted. How the athletic trainer will practice in his setting is not determined by his preference, but rather by the state's statute. Additional guidelines can be put in place based on standing orders established by an athletic trainer's supervising physician, although they cannot allow the athletic trainer to perform tasks not allowed by the state law.

Other forms of supervision may necessitate a policy and procedure. For example, a clinical setting may use the services of nonlicensed aides to assist with administrative functions. While such aides are not allowed to perform clinical tasks in most states, a clear written policy should be put in place to clarify the exact role of an aide in an athletic training clinic. Again, standards associated with the supervision of aides, specifically in a secondary school setting, have been published by NATA and should serve as the guiding principles for the policy. Additionally, in 2015, a similar set of guidelines was written to assist in clarifying the role of supportive personnel and athletic training aides by the College/University Athletic Trainers' Committee.

NATA has established an official statement regarding the education and supervision of secondary school students enrolled in sports medicine courses or volunteering in secondary school athletic training programs. While recognizing the value of the overall observational experience, the document offers guidance to school administrators and supervising athletic trainers as to the role of the secondary school student. The statement is rooted in the adherence to state practice acts, the BOC Standards of Professional Practice, and the NATA Code of Ethics.

Athletic training student aides must not be asked to engage in any of the following activities:

- Interpreting referrals from other health care providers
- Performing evaluations on a patient
- Making decisions about treatments, procedures, or activities
- Planning patient care
- Independently providing athletic training services during team travel

The following are examples of how supervision language is addressed through various state regulatory boards.

RHODE ISLAND

"Athletic trainers licensed in this state or any other state may discharge such responsibilities and functions as specified in section 7.3 below provided these functions are carried out upon the direction of the physician designated as the team or consulting physician to the team by an educational institution, professional and/or Board sanctioned amateur athletic association."

Reprinted from *Rules and regulations for licensing athletic trainers (R5-60-AT): State of Rhode Island and Providence Plantations* (Department of Health Board of Athletic Trainers amended 2012), Available: http://sos.ri.gov/documents/archives/regdocs/released/pdf/DOH/7000.pdf

FLORIDA

"Responsibilities of athletic trainers. An athletic trainer shall practice under the direction of a physician licensed under chapter 458, chapter 459, chapter 460, or otherwise authorized by Florida law to practice medicine. The physician shall communicate his or her direction through oral or written prescriptions or protocols as deemed appropriate by the physician for the provision of services and care by the athletic trainer. An athletic trainer shall provide service or care in the manner dictated by the physician."

Reprinted from The 2017 Florida statutes, in *Title XXXII: Athletic trainers* (Florida Department of Health, 2017), 468.713. Available: www.leg.state.fl.us/Statutes/index.cfm?App_mode=Display_Statute&Search_String=&URL=0400-0499/0468/Sections/0468.713.html

OHIO

"Athletic training means the practice of prevention, recognition, and assessment of an athletic injury and the complete management, treatment, disposition, and reconditioning of acute athletic injuries upon the referral of an individual authorized under Chapter 4731. of the Revised Code to practice medicine and surgery, osteopathic medicine and surgery, or podiatry, a dentist licensed under Chapter 4715. of the Revised Code, a physical therapist licensed under this chapter, or a chiropractor licensed under Chapter 4734. of the Revised Code. Athletic training includes the administration of topical drugs that have been prescribed by a licensed health care professional authorized to prescribe drugs, as defined in section 4729.01 of the Revised Code."

4755.64 Disciplinary actions. "Employing directing, or supervising a person in the performance of athletic training procedures who is not authorized to practice as a licensed athletic trainer under this chapter."

Reprinted from *Laws and rules regulating the practice of athletic training* (Columbus, OH: Ohio Occupational Therapy and Athletic Trainers Board, 2015). 4755.60. Available: http://otptat.ohio.gov/Portals/0/laws/Ohio%20AT%20Practice%20Act%20as%20of%20July%201%202015.pdf

COLORADO

"Direction of a Colorado-licensed or otherwise lawfully practicing physician, dentist, or health care professional" means the planning of services with a physician, dentist, or health care professional; the development and Approval by the physician, dentist, or health care professional of procedures and protocols to be followed in the Event of an injury or illness; the mutual review of the protocols on a periodic basis; and the appropriate Consultation and referral between the physician, dentist, or health care professional and the athletic trainer.

Reprinted from Professions and Occupations, ARTICLE 29.7, in Revised Statutes TITLE 12 *Athletic Trainer Practice Act*, 2016. Available: https://leg.colorado.gov/sites/default/files/documents/2016a/bills/sl/2016A_sl_264.pdf

COLORADO (RULE 5 – SUPERVISION OF STUDENT ATHLETIC TRAINERS)

For the purposes of Statute 12-29.7-109(1)(a), "immediate supervision" of a student athletic trainer by an athletic trainer registered in Colorado means the supervising, registered athletic trainer (a) is present on the premises where the services are being performed; and (b) is available for immediate consultation and to assist the person being supervised in the services being performed."

For purposes of this rule, "premises" means within the same facility or area and within close enough proximity.

To respond in a timely manner to an emergency or the need for assistance.

Reprinted from Department of Regulatory Agencies, Office of Athletic Trainer Registration, *Athletic trainer registration rules*, Rule 5. Available: https://drive.google.com/file/d/0B-K5DhxXxJZ-bZ1Vza2twUldlMkE/view

Determining how to define the terms *supervision* and *direction* is rooted in a state practice act as a foundation for clinical practice. The fact that it is defined in the law is referred to as the policy, and the explanation and guidelines that explain the definition are referred to as the procedures. Using the legal basis of the definition as a foundation, athletic trainers can further elaborate on their preferred policy based on the administrator's and organization's philosophy and preference. For example, in Colorado, immediate supervision of an athletic training student is clearly defined as having the supervising AT on premises. A Colorado clinic may in fact prefer to have its own policy dictate within visual or auditory distance, which would imply a closer line of supervision between the AT and the student.

Appropriate Medical Coverage

An important component associated with the planning and delivery of all of athletic training services is **appropriate medical coverage**. NATA has developed documents that guide an institution's abilities to deliver health care services and provide the administrative tasks associated with these functions. Simply put, these documents aim to identify how many staff members will likely be needed to perform all of the necessary functions. Tools exist for secondary schools and intercollegiate institutions to formulate comprehensive medical coverage strategy. These tools use a formula that calculates the number of **health care units (HCUs)**. For the **appropriate medical coverage for intercollegiate athletics (AMCIA)**, the formula was arbitrarily based on an academic teaching model, and states that 12 HCUs should equate to a full-time athletic trainer position (see tables 12.1 and 12.2). The number of total health care units is derived from the following factors:

- Base health care index per team (from 1 to 4 HCUs)
- Injury rates for time-loss and non-time-loss injuries
- Time required for treatment and rehabilitation
- Number of days in a season (total for official practices and competitions)
- Number of athlete exposures (number of athletes on a team multiplied by number of days in a season)
- Administrative duties
- Teaching responsibilities
- Number of athletic training facilities

- Travel requirements
- Practice and competition held at off-campus venues

When using this formula to assess the number of full-time athletic trainers a college athletics program would require, divide the total number of HCUs by 12. For example,

60 total HCUs / 12 = 5 full-time athletic trainers

Similar guidelines have been established for appropriate medical coverage in secondary school settings, although the HCU model is not used. Instead, a set of recommendations first established in 2004 serves as the standard for implementing appropriate medical coverage. First and foremost is the recommendation that every secondary school that offers an athletic program have a designated athletic health care provider, preferably an athletic trainer. This individual should be educated and qualified to do the following (National Athletic Trainers' Association 2007):

- Determine the individual's readiness to participate.
- Promote safe and appropriate practice, competition, and treatment facilities.
- Advise on the selection, fit, function, and maintenance of athletic equipment.
- Develop and implement a comprehensive emergency action plan.
- Establish protocols regarding environmental conditions.
- Develop injury and illness prevention strategies.
- Provide for on-site recognition, evaluation and immediate treatment of injury and illness, with appropriate referrals.

Administrative Duties to Consider When Developing Health Care Units

- Budget management and purchasing
- Drug education and testing
- Staff supervision and evaluation
- Clinical supervision of students
- Insurance filing and records
- Special assistance fund coordination
- Preparticipation physical examinations
- Emergency action planning

- Coordination of staff professional development
- Classroom instruction
- Facility maintenance
- Scheduling
- Team travel arrangements
- Athlete education programs

Table 12.1 Base Health Care Index by Sport

Sport	IR	TX/I	IR*TX/I	HCI
Baseball	19.3	11.5	222	1.7
Basketball-M	29.3	11.0	322	2.4
Basketball-W	32.4	16.3	528	4.0
Crew-M	7.2	12.9	93	0.7
Crew-W	22.0	13.0	286	2.2
Cross country-M	21.7	8.6	187	1.4
Cross country-W	23.7	9.4	223	1.7
Fencing-M	15.7	16.2	254	1.9
Fencing-W	24.1	12.6	304	2.3
Field hockey	34.8	10.8	376	2.8
Football	42.5	9.7	412	3.1
Golf-M	6.5	9.8	64	0.5
Golf-W	13.8	11.0	152	1.2
Gymnastics-M	29.0	16.8	487	3.7
Gymnastics-W†	48.1	27.9	1342	4.0
Ice hockey-M	33.9	7.2	244	1.8
Ice hockey-W	12.3	10.7	132	1.0
Indoor track-M	31.9	11.4	364	2.8
Indoor track-W	32.3	11.8	381	2.9
Lacrosse-M	23.9	10.0	239	1.8
Lacrosse-W	27.9	11.8	329	2.5
Outdoor track-M	18.3	8.0	145	1.1
Outdoor track-W	21.1	7.1	150	1.1
Soccer-M	35.0	10.7	375	2.8
Soccer-W	42.3	11.2	474	3.6
Softball	28.1	10.7	301	2.3
Swim and diving-M	12.8	7.6	97	0.7
Swim and diving-W	15.5	9.5	147	1.1
Tennis-M	21.7	9.3	202	1.5
Tennis-W	24.5	10.7	262	2.0
Volleyball-M†	35.0	22.7	795	4.0
Volleyball-W	36.8	12.6	464	3.5
Water polo-M	12.0	18.3	220	1.7
Water polo-W	22.2	7.9	175	1.3
Wrestling	41.8	9.1	380	2.9

M = men; W = women; IR = injury rate; TX/I = treatments/injury; HCI = health care index.

† To determine the maximum risk (value of 4), the IR*Tx/I record for each sport was divided by the highest IR*Tx/I recorded for any one sport where sufficient representative data was available (i.e., women's basketball). Sports indicated by and (†) recorded higher IR*Tx/I, but were based on limited data.

Refer to the NATA website for the most current version of the appropriate medical coverage of intercollegiate athletics.

Reprinted by permission from National Athletic Trainers' Association, Base health care index by sport, in *Recommendations and guidelines for appropriate medical coverage of intercollegiate athletics*, (Carrollton, TX: NATA, 2007), 18. Available: www.nata.org/sites/default/files/AMCIARecsandGuides.pdf

Table 12.2 Sample Worksheet: Adjustments to Base Health Care Index

A sport	B base HCI	C #days/season†	D #athletes/team	E Total athlete exposures (C*D)	F Exposure modifier (E/1,000)	G Adjusted HCI (B*F)	H % of year	I Adjusted HCI/Yr	J Travel (20 days = 1 HCU)	K Admin duties
Baseball	1.7	132	30	3960	4.0	6.7	50%	3.3	1.5	
Basketball-M	2.4	132	15	1980	2.0	4.8	50%	2.4	1.5	
Basketball-W	4.0	132	15	1980	2.0	7.9	50%	4.0	1.5	
X-country-M	1.4	144	10	1440	1.4	2.0	50%	1.0		
X-country-W	1.7	144	10	1440	1.4	2.4	50%	1.2		
Field hockey	2.8	132	25	3300	3.3	9.4	50%	4.7		
Football	3.1	120	100	12000	12.0	37.5	50%	18.7	0.5	
Gymnastics-W	4.0	144	10	1440	1.4	5.8	50%	2.9	0.5	
Lacrosse-M	1.8	132	30	3960	4.0	7.2	50%	3.6	0.5	
Outdoor track-M	1.1	132	40	4280	4.3	5.9	50%	2.9		
Outdoor track-W	1.1	132	40	4280	5.3	6.0	50%	3.0		
Rowing-M	0.7	132	50	6600	6.6	4.6	50%	2.3		
Soccer-M	3.6	132	30	3960	4.0	11.2	50%	5.6	1.0	
Soccer-W	2.8	132	30	3960	4.0	14.2	50%	3.8	1.5	
Softball	2.3	132	35	3300	3.3	7.5	50%	3.8	1.5	
Volleyball-W	3.5	132	15	1980	2.0	7.0	50%	3.5	1.0	
Wrestling	2.9	132	30	3960	4.0	11.4	50%	5.7	0.5	
Totals								75.8	11.0	
Total health care units (add all units in columns I-K)									87	
Total full-time ATs (total health care units / 12)									7.25	

†Figures represent total number of allowable practice days for both in and out of season for NCAA Division I. Individual institutional values should be adjusted based on competitive level and the extent of both traditional and non-traditional season activities.

M = men; W = women.

Reprinted by permission from National Athletic Trainers' Association, Sample worksheet, in *Recommendations and guidelines for appropriate medical coverage of intercollegiate athletics*, (Carrollton, TX: NATA, 2007), 19. Available: www.nata.org/sites/default/files/AMCIARecsand-Guides.pdf

- Facilitate rehabilitation and reconditioning.
- Provide for psychosocial consultation and referral.
- Provide scientifically sound nutritional counseling and education.
- Participate in the development and implementation of a comprehensive athletic health care administrative system (e.g., personal health information, policies and procedures, insurance, referrals).

Camp Coverage

A common type of athletic training clinical work comes in the form of providing coverage to youth participants of all ages at various types of sports camps. Under most of these circumstances, an athletic trainer simply provides first aid and emergency coverage, and is not responsible for precamp injury screening, rehabilitation of injuries, or other more in-depth tasks associated with typical everyday activities. However, thorough and detailed documentation is still important, and one may be involved with reviewing and screening medical records of camp participants in an effort to be aware of allergies or other medical conditions (e.g., diabetes, asthma) that could require an emergency response.

Few athletic trainers have established policies and procedures for the management and coverage of youth sports camps. In fact, some key questions are typically omitted:

- Does a contract exist that identifies the terms under which an ATC is employed at a camp?

- Has a directing physician or other legally appropriate supervisor been identified and contracted?

- Does the athletic trainer have professional liability insurance either as protected by his or her employer or as an independent contractor?

- Are the expectations and limitations of the duties clearly defined and agreed on?

- Is the AT allowed to practice athletic training, or first aid and emergency care, in a state other than the one the AT is licensed in?

- Do emergency action plans exist for the venues?

- Will the camp operators supply appropriate and necessary emergency equipment such as an automated external defibrillator and spine board (in addition to general first aid medical supplies, including ice, bandages, and sterile gloves)?

These are just a few of the initial considerations after agreeing to provide AT services for a sports camp. Additionally, an athletic trainer should consider the following factors that minimize legal risk:

- Are medical waivers used to allow a participant to be treated in the absence of a parent or guardian?

- Will health history forms be required for each participant and provided in enough time for the AT to review?

- Will participant identification forms be readily available to the AT with parent or guardian contact information in the case of a minor or major medical condition that arises?

- How many venues will be used? Are they all within sight and close enough that an AT can respond to an emergency?

- How many participants is the AT responsible for?

- Is the AT responsible for administering prescribed medications to camp participants?

- Is the AT responsible for overnight care?

- Do appropriate methods for communication exist between multiple venues for all ATs and staffers?

While each of these questions can be used to help an AT minimize risk while providing services for a camp, they can also help an AT establish a fair market value for his services. For example, most ATs agree to work at a sports camp for a predetermined amount of money, typically based on the number of days or hours the camp operates. Undertaking additional duties such as storing and dispensing prescribed medications, supervising staff, being responsible for more camp participants and multiple venues, and being available overnight can all justify higher wages for sports camp coverage. Designing a fee structure is a good way to reflect the relationship between responsibilities and compensation.

Fee Structure for Athletic Training Services at Sport Camp

- Single-day camp: $45 per hour for ATC
- Multiple-day camp with no overnight responsibility: $250 per day for ATC
- Multiple-day camp with overnight responsibility: $400 per day and night for ATC
- Supervision of CPR and first aid by an ATC: $60 per day for day camp, $80 per day for overnight camp
- More than 50 participants: $50 per day for additional 50
- Additional venue: $50 per day per additional venue
- Developing the written, accepted emergency action plan and standing orders: $250

The previous sidebar shows an example of a fee structure system.

While the monetary amounts identified in the sidebar are simply examples, they illustrate that one should not undervalue athletic training skills and services. They also point out the tremendous responsibility associated with the care of many minor-aged children at a sports camp, especially in the absence of knowing the past medical history of each participant. Some would argue that from a risk management perspective, being the AT responsible for care at sports camps poses as much risk, if not more, than in any other athletic training setting.

Crisis Intervention Management

As an athletic training administrator, one of your most important roles will be managing a crisis situation. As with all emergencies, the key to being prepared is grounded in the planning process. The goal of implementing a crisis intervention program is to provide the support services for student-athletes and patients and their family and friends who are in need of physical and emotional assistance as the result of a traumatic life-threatening event. When uncontrollable circumstances arise, such as a major illness, a death in the family, or other episodes of a crisis magnitude, student-athletes may feel overwhelming stress that could lead to impaired performance as a student and an athlete, and even to psychological disorders, such as posttraumatic stress disorder and depression.

Some of the most common crises for which services may be sought include nutritional disorders, death of a close friend or family member, catastrophic injury to a close friend or family member, and suicidal tendencies. Figure 12.1 is an example of an intake form used to identify a crisis.

Crisis Intervention Team Member:			Date:			
Primary reason for intake						
Check one in this column.	♀	♂	*Check one in this column.*		♀	♂
Pregnancy			Academic related			
Nutritional disorder			Sport related			
Anxiety or panic			Student life related			
Stress			Family related			
Depression or sadness						
Suicidal feelings or thoughts						
Repetitive unwanted thoughts						
Domestic violence						
Sexual assault or harassment						
Drug use or abuse						
Death or loss of family						
Death or loss of friend						
Catastrophic illness or injury to self						
Catastrophic illness or injury to family						
Catastrophic illness or injury to friend						

Age: _____ Sport: _____ (list sport)

Staff: _____ (check if applicable)

Family: _____ (check if applicable)

Friend: _____ (check if applicable)

Figure 12.1 Crisis Intervention Intake Assessment Form.

Developed by Jeff G. Konin.

Like all programs, a successful crisis intervention program requires that essential components be in place. First and foremost, a team of qualified personnel should be identified, each possessing expertise and knowledge in various aspects of planning and implementing the program. Each organization should determine the individuals that make up the team, assuring a comprehensive ability to act when called on. Members of the team may include, but are not limited to, the following:

- Athletic trainer
- Physician
- Counselor
- Dietician
- Psychologist

- Academic advisor
- Athletic director
- Communications or public relations professional
- Police or safety staff

Not all members of the team are needed in every crisis situation that may arise. However, it is important to have qualified individuals in place to appropriately respond to crises that may occur. The main role of the team as a whole is to coordinate a response to a current crisis and also to develop a plan for managing potential crisis situations. It is also important to keep in mind that many people in different capacities within an organization could be affected and may also play a role handling a crisis.

Examples of Crisis Intervention Team Member Roles

Athletic Trainer

- Be aware of the involved party and entire situation.
- Respect and maintain all privacy and confidential issues.
- Facilitate appropriate communication with stakeholders.
- Convene the crisis intervention team for debriefing.
- Ensure all written documentation is completed.

Head Coach

- Be aware of involved party and situation.
- Assist crisis management team with communication to the student-athlete's parents and fellow teammates.
- Respect and maintain all privacy and confidential issues.

Director of Athletics

- Be aware of involved party and situation.
- Communicate closely with athletic trainer managing the crisis at hand.
- Help determine the level of necessary communication.
- Keep senior leadership and administration apprised of the crisis status.

University Police

- Be aware of involved party and situation.
- If appropriate, assist crisis management team and other university officials.
- Assist with transportation needs.
- Respect and maintain all privacy and confidential issues.

University President

- Be aware of involved party and situation.
- Advise crisis management team as appropriate.
- Directly communicate with involved party to display support.
- Respect and maintain all privacy and confidential issues.
- Administer resources from administrative levels as needed.

University Public Relations

- Communicate closely with senior administration to learn facts about the involved party and situation.
- Remain informed of the status of the crisis.
- Serve as the liaison to the press and other media outlets.
- Respect and maintain all privacy and confidential issues.

In a college or university setting, these individuals may include the following:

- Parents or guardians of a student-athlete
- Head coach of a student-athlete
- Assistant coaches of a student-athlete
- Teammates of a student-athlete
- Athletics directors
- Athletic training staff
- Strength and conditioning coaching staff
- Academic advisors
- Athletic Department public relations staff
- Compliance staff
- University public relations
- University police
- University administration (e.g., presidents, deans)
- Faculty athletics representative
- Performance staff (e.g., dietician, psychologist)

The nature and timing of an incident, as well as consideration of who could be affected by the outcome, will determine which members of the crisis management team will be informed and what information will be provided to each party. Understanding each member's role and how information should be shared is essential. Examples of team member roles are defined in the previous sidebar. Team member roles should be agreed on in advance so that a timely and accurate communication can occur following a crisis situation. The key is for someone to be in charge of making these decisions, establishing a tree of communication to inform stakeholders, and simultaneously preserving the privacy and limiting information to only those who need to know and need to act on it.

Once the crisis intervention team has implemented the plan and the situation has been resolved, a debriefing meeting should take place to evaluate how the crisis was handled. Questions to consider include the following:

- Were the appropriate people informed in a timely manner?
- Was a stakeholder who should have been informed not informed?
- Were stakeholders informed who did not need to be informed?

- Does the policy need to change in any way?
- Could anything have been done differently to improve the intervention?
- What additional follow-up should occur, if any?
- Has the appropriate documentation been completed?

It may also be helpful to seek feedback from those receiving assistance. Following an appropriate amount of time after the crisis intervention, use a survey to gain feedback from the affected parties (see figure 12.2).

Additionally, a broader assessment of the crisis management plans should occur semiregularly, such as after learning new information, after a plan has been used and changes were identified, or because new research is available. In a college or university setting, for example, this assessment could include the following questions:

- Which student-athletes (based on gender, sport, age, and so on) are most likely to use a crisis intervention system?
- What are the most common crises that arise?
- Which team members have been used the most, and in what capacity?
- Should new team members be added?
- Are long-term follow-ups with the involved party effective?

Summary

One of the most important roles that an athletic trainer may hold is that of the administrator charged with developing and implementing clinical policies and procedures. This chapter has provided examples of the types of clinical policies and procedures that are commonly found in athletic training settings and discussed the importance of developing administrative documents to serve as a guide for the standard of care of services provided. Some examples include how athletic trainers are directed and supervised within the state he or she practices in, how appropriate medical coverage is determined for settings (secondary schools, colleges and universities, sports camps), and the benefits of using a formal crisis intervention team to respond to unplanned events that affect an individual and many other stakeholders.

Individual: _____ Date: _____

The following ratings reflect your perception of the guidance received through the crisis intervention program. Ratings are based on your observations and feelings about your overall interaction, the quality of the time spent, resources provided, and overall benefit of services.

Please circle the number that best reflects your experience: 5 is the highest possible rating, and 1 is the lowest.

Area of assessment	Lowest				Highest
How would you rate your initial enthusiasm about seeking assistance through this program?	1	2	3	4	5
Did the people who worked with you manage your situation in a professional way?	1	2	3	4	5
Was confidentiality maintained at all times during your crisis?	1	2	3	4	5
Were the individuals working with you respectful during all interactions?	1	2	3	4	5
Were you able to become more aware of how to manage your situation through the assistance of the program?	1	2	3	4	5
Did the professionals who assisted you appear to listen and care?	1	2	3	4	5
Were you provided additional resources and ideas beyond the assistance this program makes available to you?	1	2	3	4	5
Do you feel that the assistance you received took a caring approach?	1	2	3	4	5
Do you feel that the individuals you worked with were knowledgeable in the area that you needed assistance with?	1	2	3	4	5
Do you feel that the individuals you sought assistance from were accessible when needed?	1	2	3	4	5
Do you feel that the individuals assisting you with your crisis were sensitive to diverse circumstances?	1	2	3	4	5
How would you rate your self-esteem and self-confidence at the beginning of your interaction with the crisis intervention program?	1	2	3	4	5
How would you rate your self-esteem and self-confidence at the conclusion of your interaction with the crisis intervention program?	1	2	3	4	5
Do you feel the program has helped you with your crisis?	1	2	3	4	5
How would you rate your overall experience with the crisis intervention program?	1	2	3	4	5

Please provide written comments that may assist in the implementation of this program for the future:

_____

_____

_____

_____

_____

_____

_____

Figure 12.2 Crisis Intervention Survey.

Developed by Jeff G. Konin.

Learning Aids

Case Study 1

Andranique, who provides care for the women's soccer team at Kinkade Community College, was awakened by an unexpected phone call early Friday morning from Julia, a member of the team. As she frantically spoke, she informed Andranique that her roommate, Stephanie, was rushed to the hospital following an episode of heavy vomiting and significant difficulty in breathing. Andranique offered to meet Julia at the hospital to provide comfort. Upon arriving, he learned that tests were being performed and it would likely be many hours before a diagnosis could be made. Andranique did not know much about the ill roommate, although he came to find out that she was an incoming transfer student who was planning to try out for the basketball team.

By late afternoon, the physicians at the hospital were able to determine that a very low white blood cell count appeared to be associated with the symptoms presented. More tests were needed to determine an absolute diagnosis. Family members had been informed of the circumstances, but they live approximately 500 miles (805 km) away and would not arrive until late in the evening. Although her roommate was in stable condition, Julia remained uneasy and distraught over the incident.

Questions for Analysis

1. Assuming Andranique manages the crisis intervention plan for Kinkade Community College, what stakeholders do you think he should contact immediately? Exactly how much information should he share with each stakeholder?
2. Using a crisis intervention team, what members could best assist Julia at this time?
3. The school's women's soccer team has an away match later in the evening at a nearby school. Should Julia participate in the match? Why or why not?
4. For how long should Andranique be concerned about Julia's distress?
5. Does the crisis intervention team have a role in assisting Stephanie in this situation? If so, what role? If not, why not?

Case Study 2

Rocky Point Prep School is fortunate to employ four full-time athletic trainers to provide care and coverage for 400 student-athletes in grades 9 through 12. The athletic training staff has also assembled an athletic training aide program for students interested in sports medicine as a career path. Each of the athletic training aides is assigned responsibilities both in the athletic training clinic and with various sports teams. In addition to the learning opportunities provided to them, they serve as a tremendous asset to the overall program. Athletic administrators, student-athletes, and all others value their contributions. Some have gone on to college and studied athletic training as a major and gone on to achieve their athletic training certification. Others have studied various health care degrees and eventually entered their chosen health care profession. When surveyed after completing their first year of college, many attributed their current success in college to their experiences as an athletic training aide at Rocky Point. Notably, most referred specifically to skills they were able to perform, such as massage, preventive ankle taping, wound care, and helping to test student-athletes following an injury and determining return-to-play status.

Questions for Analysis

1. Based on the case study, do you feel proper direction and supervision was applied to the athletic training aides at Rocky Point Prep School? Why or why not?
2. In determining responsibilities that the athletic training aides perform, what documents should serve as the basis for outlining their roles?
3. Do you believe that any of the stated functions performed by the athletic training aides were inappropriate? If so, which ones? If you believe they performed inappropriate functions and these functions are removed from the responsibilities of future athletic training aides, do you believe they will be as well prepared when they enter college and choose to study a health profession major?

4. If you were hired as the new athletic trainer in charge at Rocky Point Prep School, would you change the responsibilities assigned to the athletic training aides based on the information provided in the case study?

Key Concepts and Review

Identify the components of a clinically related policy and procedure.

A clinically related policy and procedure should be developed by the stakeholders responsible for administering the policy. The policy and procedure should be frequently reviewed, with written documentation to support changes. All clinical policies and procedures should be reviewed by the athletic trainer's team physicians in additional to the organization's legal counsel when necessary. Established guidelines for standard of care should serve as the foundation, with additional components added to meet the needs of the specific program and venue and other considerations pertinent to the policy. Visitors should also have access to necessary policies and procedures. Student-athletes and all patients should also be familiar with policies and procedures that pertain to their role as a stakeholder in receiving athletic training services. In many instances, the student-athlete or patient will be asked to provide a written signature acknowledging that he or she has read and understood the policies and procedures. For minors, a parent or guardian is required to read and understand the policies and procedures and provide a written signature of acknowledgement.

Define the terms *supervision* and *direction* as they relate to athletic training.

Supervision is defined differently from state to state (in one's practice act) and from program to program. Athletic trainers work under the direction of a physician or otherwise stated health care provider according to the practice act. Additionally, athletic trainers supervise athletic training aides (ATA) who are not allowed to perform clinical tasks in most states.

Establish criteria for providing appropriate medical coverage in various settings.

An important component of the planning and delivery of all of athletic training services is referred to as appropriate medical coverage. NATA has developed documents that guide an institution's ability to deliver health care services and provide the administrative tasks associated with such functions. The goal of these documents is to identify the number of staff that is likely needed to perform all of the necessary functions. Tools exist for secondary schools and intercollegiate institutions to use to formulate a comprehensive medical coverage strategy.

Integrate policies and procedures associated with establishing a crisis intervention program, inclusive of mental health needs.

One of the most important functions that an athletic trainer will perform is managing a crisis situation. The overall goal of implementing a crisis intervention program is to provide support services to patients and student-athletes, and their family and friends, who are in need of physical and emotional assistance as the result of a traumatic life-threatening event. A successful crisis intervention program requires that essential components be in place. A team of qualified personnel should be identified, each possessing expertise and knowledge in various aspects of planning and implementing the program. Each organization should determine the individuals that make up the team, assuring a comprehensive ability to act when called on. The main role of the team as a whole is to coordinate a response to a current crisis and also to develop a plan for crisis management for potential crisis situations. Following each crisis intervention, a debriefing of the incident should occur. In addition, a broader assessment of the overall program should occur semiregularly as new research becomes available, for example.

Develop policies and procedures for athletic training services related to camp coverage.

Athletic trainers commonly provide care and coverage for different types of athletic camps. The development of policies and procedures for camp coverage should consider, at a minimum, the following: first aid responsibilities, emergency action planning, precamp participant health screening (e.g., history form), liability insurance coverage, terms of one's employment contract, equipment and supplies provided, and physician supervision guidelines.

Preparticipation Physical Examinations

Objectives

After reading this chapter, you should be able to do the following:

- Understand and support the rationale for administrating preparticipation physical examinations.

- Understand the strengths and weaknesses of the various preparticipation physical examination models.

- Organize and implement a comprehensive preparticipation physical examination program in a variety of settings.

- Identify appropriate personnel utilized in the preparticipation physical examination.

The **preparticipation physical examination (PPE)** is arguably the first step in injury prevention in amateur, scholastic, collegiate, and professional sports. Athletic trainers play an important role in helping to organize this aspect of the injury-prevention program. For the PPE to be effective, it must (1) identify disease or processes that will affect the athlete, (2) be sensitive and accurate, and (3) be practical and affordable (American Academy of Family Physicians 2010). In 2014, the National Athletic Trainers' Association published a position statement on preparticipation physical examinations and disqualifying conditions that serves as a standard of care and guiding principle for the profession (Conley et al. 2014). Athletic trainers should refer to this document regardless of the setting they are employed in. This chapter focuses on the management and administration of the process.

KEY POINT

Go online to view NATA's official position statement on preparticipation physical examinations.

Why PPEs Are Performed

Anyone with any degree of experience in sport as a participant, coach, athletic trainer, or administrator has probably asked, "Why do we have to do these physicals every year? It just seems like a formality." This is a legitimate question. PPEs take a lot of time and energy to organize. They can be time consuming and expensive to administer, despite the fact that many of the providers who participate serve in a volunteer role. They require significant effort on the part of many people, all of whom could be doing other things. Finally, athletes and coaches, who would rather spend the time practicing, often view them as no more than a necessary evil. So why are PPEs so important? PPEs are important for at least four reasons.

Injury and Illness Prevention

The most compelling reason to perform PPEs is that when properly performed and with data that are subsequently acted on, the PPE can provide information that allows an athlete to participate in sport activities with reduced risk of injury or illness. This justification for the PPE is valid, of course, only if the medical team conducting the PPE uses the data generated by the exam. If seemingly minor findings are discovered during the PPE and this is not followed up with appropriate treatment, then the PPE is more than a waste of time; it becomes a potential source of liability for the medical staff.

One of the functions of the PPE is to determine an athlete's readiness for participation in her chosen sport (National Collegiate Athletic Association 2014). On rare occasions, this may involve using the information generated by the PPE to disqualify an athlete from participation. This action should be taken only when participation in the given sport would foreseeably lead to an exacerbation of the athlete's medical condition or would cause harm to other participants. As the medical director of an institution's sports medicine program, the team physician should have the final authority to approve for or disqualify prospective athletes from participation (Herbert 1997). The wise team physician will consider the input of the athlete's personal physician, parents (especially in the case of a minor), and specialists involved in the case. The final authority, however, rests with the team physician (Herbert 1996; Herring et al. 2012). See table 13.1 for a list of **disqualifying conditions**. **Generally speaking, a** team physician has six options for determining medical qualification to participate or not (Starkey 2013):

1. *Passed.* The athlete is cleared for participation in all sports with no reservations or contraindications.
2. *Passed with conditions.* The athlete has a medical condition that requires follow-up. The athlete may participate in some activities. The

athlete may resume full activity pending satisfactory follow-up.

3. *Passed with reservations.* The athlete may not participate in contact or collision sports (whichever is appropriate).
4. *Failed with reservations.* The athlete is not cleared for his or her requested sport. Other sports may be considered. Contact or collision is not permitted.
5. *Failed with conditions.* The athlete must be reevaluated for participation after his or her medical condition is addressed and resolved.
6. *Failed.* The athlete may not participate in any sport at any level of exertion or competition.

Compliance With Association Rules

Most school- and college-based athletic programs are subject to the rules of the athletic associations of which they voluntarily choose to be members. At the high school level, the National Federation of State High School Athletic Associations (NFHS) defers on the issue of required PPEs to the various state associations. The guidelines published by these state organizations vary considerably (Caswell et al. 2015). Some require the completion of a standard form signed by a physician, whereas others have rules that are much more relaxed. Athletic trainers working in high school settings should check with their state's athletic association to become familiar with the rules specific to that state.

The National Collegiate Athletic Association (2014) also publishes guidelines for the conduct of the PPE. The NCAA instructs its member colleges to provide every student-athlete with a comprehensive PPE, complete with cardiovascular screening, upon entry to the athletic program. Updated histories and blood pressure screening should be performed annually thereafter, with additional PPEs only as warranted by these histories. This guideline reflects the modified recommendations of the American Heart Association (Mirabelli et al. 2015; Goff et al. 2014). Furthermore, with respect to privacy laws such as Health Insurance Portability and Accountability Act of 1996 (HIPAA) and Family Educational Rights and Privacy Act (FERPA), it is vital that all parties involved with the PPE process treat patient information as private and protected health information at all times. Thus, each patient should provide written authorization for the use of his data and who is allowed to have knowledge of such information. All staff associated with the

Table 13.1　Disqualifying Conditions

Condition	Contact or collision[1]	Limited contact or impact[2]	NONCONTACT		
			Strenuous[3]	Moderately strenuous[4]	Nonstrenuous[5]
Atlantoaxial instability	No	No	Yes[6]	Yes	Yes
Acute illnesses	[7]	[7]	[7]	[7]	[7]
Cardiovascular					
Carditis	No	No	No	No	No
Hypertension					
• Mild	Yes	Yes	Yes	Yes	Yes
• Moderate	[8]	[8]	[8]	[8]	[8]
• Severe	[8]	[8]	[8]	[8]	[8]
Congenital heart disease	[9]	[9]	[9]	[9]	[9]
Eyes					
Absence or loss of function of one eye	[10]	[10]	[10]	[10]	[10]
Detached retina	[11]	[11]	[11]	[11]	[11]
Inguinal hernia	Yes	Yes	Yes	Yes	Yes
Kidney: absence of one	No	Yes	Yes	Yes	Yes
Liver: enlarged	No	No	Yes	Yes	Yes
Musculoskeletal disorders	[8]	[8]	[8]	[8]	[8]
Neurologic					
History of serious head or spine trauma, repeated concussions, or craniotomy	[8]	[8]	Yes	Yes	Yes
Convulsive disorder					
• Well controlled	No	Yes	Yes	Yes	Yes
• Poorly controlled	No	No	Yes[12]	Yes	Yes[13]
Ovary: absence of one	Yes	Yes	Yes	Yes	Yes
Respiratory					
Pulmonary insufficiency	[14]	[14]	[14]	[14]	[14]
Asthma	Yes	Yes	Yes	Yes	Yes
Sickle cell trait	Yes	Yes	Yes	Yes	Yes
Skin: boils, herpes, impetigo, scabies	[15]	[15]	Yes	Yes	Yes
Spleen: enlarged	No	No	No	Yes	Yes
Testicle: absence of or undescended	Yes[16]	Yes[16]	Yes	Yes	Yes

[1]Boxing, field hockey, football, ice hockey, lacrosse, martial arts, rodeo, soccer, wrestling.

[2]Baseball, basketball, bicycling, diving, high jump, pole vault, gymnastics, equestrian, skating, softball, squash, handball, volleyball.

[3]Aerobic dance, crew, fencing, discus, javelin, shot put, running, swimming, tennis, track, weightlifting.

[4]Badminton, curling, table tennis.

[5]Archery, golf, riflery.

[6]Swimming: no butterfly, breaststroke, or diving starts.

[7]Needs individual assessment (e.g., contagiousness to others, risk of worsening illness)

[8]Needs individual assessment.

[9]Patients with mild forms can be allowed a full range of physical activities; patients with moderate or severe forms, or who are postoperative, should be evaluated by a cardiologist before athletic participation.

[10]Availability of eye guards approved by the American Society for Testing Materials (ASTM) may allow competitor to participate in most sports, but this must be judged individually.

[11]Consult ophthalmologist.

[12]No swimming or weightlifting.

[13]No archery or riflery.

[14]May be allowed to compete if oxygenation remains satisfactory during a graded exercise test.

[15]No gymnastics with mats, martial arts, wrestling, or contact sports until not contagious.

[16]Certain sports may require a protective cup.

handling of protected health information should be trained in this procedure.

Education and Counseling of Athletes

Because the PPE is frequently the only opportunity that many adolescent athletes have to interact with a physician, some have suggested that the focus of the PPE be redirected toward counseling and educating young athletes on a variety of health-related issues (Koester 1995; Corrado et al. 2008).

The ability of a health care professional to elicit high-quality information and to provide meaningful feedback regarding an adolescent's potential health risks depends on several factors. The typical **mass screening** in the gym or locker room is a poor setting for this kind of activity. The level of training and comfort of the examiner are important. Finally, young athletes are likely to open up only to those they know and trust, so it is important to use health care professionals who are familiar with this sample of athletes for this portion of the PPE.

Compliance With Standards of Practice

Although not codified in federal or state statutes, both the athletic and medical communities understand and accept the requirement to provide a PPE that at least meets minimal standards. Failure to provide such a PPE is a gross violation of the standards of practice for anyone charged with safeguarding the health of athletes.

When PPEs Should Be Conducted

The ideal time to conduct PPEs is four to six weeks before athletes intend to begin vigorous training for their sports (Conley et al. 2014). This schedule allows adequate time for remediation of most problems that the PPEs are likely to detect. An option common in many school and college settings is to conduct PPEs one season before athletes intend to participate in their sports. For example, screening of football players would occur just before the summer recess. Basketball players would be screened in early fall at the beginning of the school year. Screening for spring sport athletes would occur around the end of December. Although this system works well for high schools and small colleges that conduct sport seasons exclusively during specific times of the year, larger schools that sponsor nontraditional

seasons may have to screen all their athletes in either late spring or summer because even spring sports jump into full gear as soon as school begins in the fall. This can also pose a challenge for new athletes playing fall sports at universities if the athletes are coming from a long distance.

As discussed earlier, the frequency with which PPEs should be conducted is a matter of some debate. The least rigorous standard requires a complete and comprehensive PPE when an athlete enters an athletic program, with annual **health history updates** thereafter (see figure 13.1). Most high school programs require a PPE every year. Although athletic trainers are obligated to comply with the standards for their particular settings, the fact remains that the frequency of the PPE relates closely to its content. The more comprehensive and detailed the PPE, the less frequently it needs to be repeated. The less comprehensive and detailed the PPE, the more frequently it needs to be repeated. The nature of the sport is another factor that should influence the frequency with which PPEs should be repeated. Contact and collision sports with high injury rates may warrant more frequent repetition of the PPE than sports for which injuries are less frequent and serious. Lastly, it is recommended that individuals who increase to a higher level of participation undergo a complete PPE.

A common method for administering PPEs that is not necessarily ideal is to perform the service on the day the athletes return to their first team or individual organized practice. This day often coincides with reviewing compliance-related issues, issuing equipment, and finally holding the first practice, all within the same day. The benefit of this timing to the school and team is that all of the activities are managed within a well-organized, compact time period. However, this format can lead to challenges for the sports medicine team. Primarily, findings of concern identified through the process will require additional review, possible scheduling of further tests, and follow-up prior to granting clearance for participation. Any deficiencies identified at this time would not benefit from a period of rehabilitation before the start of the formal practice schedule as they would if the PPE were performed four to six weeks in advance. Perhaps of greatest concern is the "carte blanche" attitude that a coaching staff may take toward the PPE if it is performed just before the first practice. In this circumstance, the coaching staff is likely excited to see the athletes perform for the first time at practice after a long period away from formal competition, and any delay in this opportunity can lead to disappointment, irrational

■ PREPARTICIPATION PHYSICAL EVALUATION
HISTORY FORM

(Note: This form is to be filled out by the patient and parent prior to seeing the physician. The physician should keep this form in the chart.)

Date of Exam _____

Name _____ Date of birth _____

Sex _____ Age _____ Grade _____ School _____ Sport(s) _____

Medicines and Allergies: Please list all of the prescription and over-the-counter medicines and supplements (herbal and nutritional) that you are currently taking
_____
_____
_____

Do you have any allergies?   ☐ Yes ☐ No   If yes, please identify specific allergy below.
☐ Medicines   ☐ Pollens   ☐ Food   ☐ Stinging Insects

Explain "Yes" answers below. Circle questions you don't know the answers to.

GENERAL QUESTIONS	Yes	No
1. Has a doctor ever denied or restricted your participation in sports for any reason?		
2. Do you have any ongoing medical conditions? If so, please identify below:☐ Asthma ☐ Anemia ☐ Diabetes ☐ Infections Other: _____		
3. Have you ever spent the night in the hospital?		
4. Have you ever had surgery?		

HEART HEALTH QUESTIONS ABOUT YOU	Yes	No
5. Have you ever passed out or nearly passed out DURING or AFTER exercise?		
6. Have you ever had discomfort, pain, tightness, or pressure in your chest during exercise?		
7. Does your heart ever race or skip beats (irregular beats) during exercise?		
8. Has a doctor ever told you that you have any heart problems? If so, check all that apply: ☐ High blood pressure ☐ A heart murmur ☐ High cholesterol ☐ A heart infection ☐ Kawasaki disease Other: _____		
9. Has a doctor ever ordered a test for your heart? (For example, ECG/EKG, echocardiogram)		
10. Do you get lightheaded or feel more short of breath than expected during exercise?		
11. Have you ever had an unexplained seizure?		
12. Do you get more tired or short of breath more quickly than your friends during exercise?		

HEART HEALTH QUESTIONS ABOUT YOUR FAMILY	Yes	No
13. Has any family member or relative died of heart problems or had an unexpected or unexplained sudden death before age 50 (including drowning, unexplained car accident, or sudden infant death syndrome)?		
14. Does anyone in your family have hypertrophic cardiomyopathy, Marfan syndrome, arrhythmogenic right ventricular cardiomyopathy, long QT syndrome, short QT syndrome, Brugada syndrome, or catecholaminergic polymorphic ventricular tachycardia?		
15. Does anyone in your family have a heart problem, pacemaker, or implanted defibrillator?		
16. Has anyone in your family had unexplained fainting, unexplained seizures, or near drowning?		

BONE AND JOINT QUESTIONS	Yes	No
17. Have you ever had an injury to a bone, muscle, ligament, or tendon that caused you to miss a practice or a game?		
18. Have you ever had any broken or fractured bones or dislocated joints?		
19. Have you ever had an injury that required x-rays, MRI, CT scan, injections, therapy, a brace, a cast, or crutches?		
20. Have you ever had a stress fracture?		
21. Have you ever been told that you have or have you had an x-ray for neck instability or atlantoaxial instability? (Down syndrome or dwarfism)		
22. Do you regularly use a brace, orthotics, or other assistive device?		
23. Do you have a bone, muscle, or joint injury that bothers you?		
24. Do any of your joints become painful, swollen, feel warm, or look red?		
25. Do you have any history of juvenile arthritis or connective tissue disease?		

MEDICAL QUESTIONS	Yes	No
26. Do you cough, wheeze, or have difficulty breathing during or after exercise?		
27. Have you ever used an inhaler or taken asthma medicine?		
28. Is there anyone in your family who has asthma?		
29. Were you born without or are you missing a kidney, an eye, a testicle (males), your spleen, or any other organ?		
30. Do you have groin pain or a painful bulge or hernia in the groin area?		
31. Have you had infectious mononucleosis (mono) within the last month?		
32. Do you have any rashes, pressure sores, or other skin problems?		
33. Have you had a herpes or MRSA skin infection?		
34. Have you ever had a head injury or concussion?		
35. Have you ever had a hit or blow to the head that caused confusion, prolonged headache, or memory problems?		
36. Do you have a history of seizure disorder?		
37. Do you have headaches with exercise?		
38. Have you ever had numbness, tingling, or weakness in your arms or legs after being hit or falling?		
39. Have you ever been unable to move your arms or legs after being hit or falling?		
40. Have you ever become ill while exercising in the heat?		
41. Do you get frequent muscle cramps when exercising?		
42. Do you or someone in your family have sickle cell trait or disease?		
43. Have you had any problems with your eyes or vision?		
44. Have you had any eye injuries?		
45. Do you wear glasses or contact lenses?		
46. Do you wear protective eyewear, such as goggles or a face shield?		
47. Do you worry about your weight?		
48. Are you trying to or has anyone recommended that you gain or lose weight?		
49. Are you on a special diet or do you avoid certain types of foods?		
50. Have you ever had an eating disorder?		
51. Do you have any concerns that you would like to discuss with a doctor?		

FEMALES ONLY		
52. Have you ever had a menstrual period?		
53. How old were you when you had your first menstrual period?		
54. How many periods have you had in the last 12 months?		

Explain "yes" answers here
_____
_____
_____
_____
_____
_____
_____
_____
_____

I hereby state that, to the best of my knowledge, my answers to the above questions are complete and correct.

Signature of athlete _____ Signature of parent/guardian _____ Date _____

(continued)

Figure 13.1 Sample health history form developed collaboratively by the American Academy of Family Physicians, American Academy of Pediatrics, American College of Sports Medicine, American Medical Society for Sports Medicine, American Orthopaedic Society for Sports Medicine, and American Osteopathic Academy of Sports Medicine.

THE ATHLETE WITH SPECIAL NEEDS: SUPPLEMENTAL HISTORY FORM

Date of Exam _____

Name _____ Date of birth _____

Sex _____ Age _____ Grade _____ School _____ Sport(s) _____

1. Type of disability		
2. Date of disability		
3. Classification (if available)		
4. Cause of disability (birth, disease, accident/trauma, other)		
5. List the sports you are interested in playing		

	Yes	No
6. Do you regularly use a brace, assistive device, or prosthetic?		
7. Do you use any special brace or assistive device for sports?		
8. Do you have any rashes, pressure sores, or any other skin problems?		
9. Do you have a hearing loss? Do you use a hearing aid?		
10. Do you have a visual impairment?		
11. Do you use any special devices for bowel or bladder function?		
12. Do you have burning or discomfort when urinating?		
13. Have you had autonomic dysreflexia?		
14. Have you ever been diagnosed with a heat-related (hyperthermia) or cold-related (hypothermia) illness?		
15. Do you have muscle spasticity?		
16. Do you have frequent seizures that cannot be controlled by medication?		

Explain "yes" answers here

_____

_____

_____

_____

_____

Please indicate if you have ever had any of the following.

	Yes	No
Atlantoaxial instability		
X-ray evaluation for atlantoaxial instability		
Dislocated joints (more than one)		
Easy bleeding		
Enlarged spleen		
Hepatitis		
Osteopenia or osteoporosis		
Difficulty controlling bowel		
Difficulty controlling bladder		
Numbness or tingling in arms or hands		
Numbness or tingling in legs or feet		
Weakness in arms or hands		
Weakness in legs or feet		
Recent change in coordination		
Recent change in ability to walk		
Spina bifida		
Latex allergy		

Explain "yes" answers here

_____

_____

_____

_____

_____

I hereby state that, to the best of my knowledge, my answers to the above questions are complete and correct.

Signature of athlete _____ Signature of parent/guardian _____ Date _____

(continued)

Figure 13.1 *(continued)*

Name _____   Date of birth _____

PHYSICIAN REMINDERS

1. Consider additional questions on more sensitive issues
   - Do you feel stressed out or under a lot of pressure?
   - Do you ever feel sad, hopeless, depressed, or anxious?
   - Do you feel safe at your home or residence?
   - Have you ever tried cigarettes, chewing tobacco, snuff, or dip?
   - During the past 30 days, did you use chewing tobacco, snuff, or dip?
   - Do you drink alcohol or use any other drugs?
   - Have you ever taken anabolic steroids or used any other performance supplement?
   - Have you ever taken any supplements to help you gain or lose weight or improve your performance?
   - Do you wear a seat belt, use a helmet, and use condoms?
2. Consider reviewing questions on cardiovascular symptoms (questions 5–14).

EXAMINATION				
Height	Weight		☐ Male ☐ Female	
BP / (/) Pulse		Vision R 20/	L 20/	Corrected ☐ Y ☐ N

MEDICAL	NORMAL	ABNORMAL FINDINGS
Appearance • Marfan stigmata (kyphoscoliosis, high-arched palate, pectus excavatum, arachnodactyly, arm span > height, hyperlaxity, myopia, MVP, aortic insufficiency)		
Eyes/ears/nose/throat • Pupils equal • Hearing		
Lymph nodes		
Heart[a] • Murmurs (auscultation standing, supine, +/- Valsalva) • Location of point of maximal impulse (PMI)		
Pulses • Simultaneous femoral and radial pulses		
Lungs		
Abdomen		
Genitourinary (males only)[b]		
Skin • HSV, lesions suggestive of MRSA, tinea corporis		
Neurologic[c]		
MUSCULOSKELETAL		
Neck		
Back		
Shoulder/arm		
Elbow/forearm		
Wrist/hand/fingers		
Hip/thigh		
Knee		
Leg/ankle		
Foot/toes		
Functional • Duck-walk, single leg hop		

[a]Consider ECG, echocardiogram, and referral to cardiology for abnormal cardiac history or exam.
[b]Consider GU exam if in private setting. Having third party present is recommended.
[c]Consider cognitive evaluation or baseline neuropsychiatric testing if a history of significant concussion.

☐ Cleared for all sports without restriction

☐ Cleared for all sports without restriction with recommendations for further evaluation or treatment for _____

_____

☐ Not cleared

        ☐ Pending further evaluation

        ☐ For any sports

        ☐ For certain sports _____

        Reason _____

Recommendations _____

_____

I have examined the above-named student and completed the preparticipation physical evaluation. The athlete does not present apparent clinical contraindications to practice and participate in the sport(s) as outlined above. A copy of the physical exam is on record in my office and can be made available to the school at the request of the parents. If conditions arise after the athlete has been cleared for participation, the physician may rescind the clearance until the problem is resolved and the potential consequences are completely explained to the athlete (and parents/guardians).

Name of physician (print/type) _____   Date _____

Address _____   Phone _____

Signature of physician _____, MD or DO

Figure 13.1   *(continued)*

(continued)

■ PREPARTICIPATION PHYSICAL EVALUATION
CLEARANCE FORM

Name _____ Sex ☐ M ☐ F Age _____ Date of birth _____

☐ Cleared for all sports without restriction

☐ Cleared for all sports without restriction with recommendations for further evaluation or treatment for _____

_____

☐ Not cleared

      ☐ Pending further evaluation

      ☐ For any sports

      ☐ For certain sports _____

      Reason _____

Recommendations _____

_____

_____

_____

_____

_____

_____

I have examined the above-named student and completed the preparticipation physical evaluation. The athlete does not present apparent clinical contraindications to practice and participate in the sport(s) as outlined above. A copy of the physical exam is on record in my office and can be made available to the school at the request of the parents. If conditions arise after the athlete has been cleared for participation, the physician may rescind the clearance until the problem is resolved and the potential consequences are completely explained to the athlete (and parents/guardians).

Name of physician (print/type) _____ Date _____

Address _____ Phone _____

Signature of physician _____ , MD or DO

EMERGENCY INFORMATION

Allergies _____

_____

_____

_____

_____

Other information _____

_____

_____

_____

_____

_____

_____

_____

_____

_____

Figure 13.1 *(continued)*

bargaining, and in some cases adverse behaviors toward the medical staff for simply doing the job appropriately.

Where and How PPEs Should Be Conducted

Much debate exists regarding the optimal setting for the PPE. Before attempting to decide where and how to conduct PPEs, athletic trainers should try to answer some planning-related questions. The following list is not exhaustive, but it serves as a solid foundation for preparation:

- What kind of information do we need to get from the PPEs?
- How many people will we be able to recruit to help conduct the PPEs?
- How many of the people we recruit will be trained medical personnel with an interest and experience in sport health care?
- What options do we have in terms of physical facilities for the PPEs?
- Do the facilities to which we have access have adequate provisions for privacy?
- How much time do we have to conduct PPEs?
- What expenses will we incur?

- Will the people conducting the PPEs be volunteers, or will they expect to be paid?
- Will the individuals performing the physical examinations require background checks according to state laws?
- How many athletes will we need to service?
- What are the characteristics of the athletes to be screened? Adults? Children? Men? Women?
- Do the planned dates conflict with holidays or major local, school-related, or other events?
- Do the facilities have ample parking if large numbers of participants are expected?
- Who will manage the overall administrative responsibilities of the process?
- Who will make the final decisions regarding participation clearance?

Office-Based PPEs

Determining the methods to employ in conducting PPEs involves consideration of many important issues (see the following sidebar). All other factors being equal—which they never are—the privacy of a physician's office is probably the ideal place. This setting allows the physician to examine and counsel the athlete with a minimum of interruption and to focus on the athlete and her problems. In addition, physicians who conduct PPEs in their offices have

Strengths and Weaknesses of Office and Station PPEs

Office-Based PPE

Strengths

- Greater privacy
- Easier access to patient records
- Easier access to medical supplies and equipment
- More conducive to athlete counseling
- Less personnel required

Weaknesses

- Greater potential for breakdown in communication to school-based health care personnel
- Less potential for familiarity with specific sport demands
- Less efficient
- Incorporation of fitness testing more difficult

Station PPE

Strengths

- Greater efficiency
- Easier access to the whole sports medicine team
- Easier to include fitness testing as part of the PPE
- Use of volunteers promotes the concept of shared responsibility for safety

Weaknesses

- Little to no privacy
- Difficult to counsel athletes
- Can be noisy
- Volunteers must be recruited and trained
- Facilities and transport of supplies must be arranged
- Athletes' records are usually not available

the advantage of being able to call more easily on the wide range of medical equipment and services they may need to provide the comprehensive care the athlete requires. Accessing specialized equipment and services can be difficult in a mass screening in a gymnasium.

If an office-based PPE is the technique of choice, the next issue is to identify the appropriate physician to conduct the examination. Should all athletes be examined in the team physician's office, or should their personal physicians screen them? People disagree about this issue as well.

On one hand, the team physician is presumably more versed in sport health care issues and may be better able to make judgments regarding participation status and follow-up treatment for conditions discovered during the PPE. The team physician, as medical director of the school's athletic program, may also be legally responsible for judging an athlete's participation status. On the other hand, the athlete's family physician may be more familiar with the athlete's personal and family history. This level of familiarity can be important in establishing the confidence that the athlete will need to confide in and be receptive to the physician. In some cases, the athletic setting may play a role in this decision. For example, in a college, university, or professional setting, a contracted team physician may have the ultimate say regarding an athlete's participation, whereas in a secondary school setting, it is not uncommon for individual athletes under the age of 18 to be cleared by their own physician. In a secondary school setting absent an identified contractually bound team physician, numerous physicians could ultimately serve in the decision-making role, making it a challenge for the athletic trainer to establish ideal relationships with all of them. Finally, many would argue that the technical skills required to perform an adequate PPE are common enough that most primary care physicians have the competence required to provide this service.

In the final analysis, the nature of the patient will determine who is best suited to conduct the PPE. Personal physicians can effectively screen most young adolescents. As children grow older and routine visits to the family physician become less frequent, it may be more appropriate for the team physician to take over the administration of the PPE. Who is likely to provide athletes with the medical care they need if they become injured or ill during their seasons? For most junior and some senior high school students, this person will be the athlete's family physician. For many senior high school and most college and professional athletes, the team physician will provide medical care. Who-

ever is most likely to take care of the athletes during their seasons should probably conduct their PPEs. For the growing segment of the population without a family physician, the issue becomes more problematic. Similarly, the high school without a team physician faces difficulty in attempting to organize an effective PPE program.

Group PPEs and the Station Method

The preceding arguments in favor of office-based PPEs notwithstanding, the method that many schools employ involves screening many athletes at a common site using a variety of stations to collect information about their health. This is referred to as a **station-based PPE**. Although obtaining the privacy required for one-on-one counseling between a physician and an athlete in this setting is difficult, this method has proven to be successful in helping detect the more serious and common conditions that are likely to impair an athlete's ability to participate in sports with a relative degree of safety.

PEARLS OF MANAGEMENT

Group PPEs are excellent activities to incorporate on an interprofessional health care team.

Many nonmedical volunteers can play an important role in helping conduct an organized, efficient mass PPE. The role of the athletic trainer is to identify the number of stations, recruit an adequate number of volunteers for each station, and, where appropriate, provide the training the volunteers will need to perform their duties. Parents, coaches, and students with HIPAA training are capable of performing a variety of tasks, including checking height and weight, controlling flow through the various stations, and checking to make sure that all the required forms have been completed before the athlete leaves the examination area. For PPEs that incorporate fitness testing, coaches who have training in the techniques are an excellent choice to operate these stations. See figure 13.2 for a schematic of a typical station approach to the PPE.

What to Evaluate During the PPE

A surprising amount of disagreement exists among professionals regarding the content of the ideal PPE. Aside from following the standard of care as

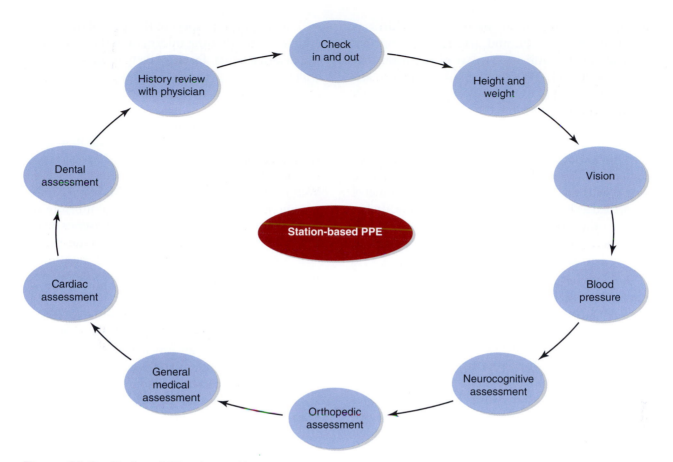

Figure 13.2 Station PPE schematic.

proposed through published position statements, athletic trainers should consider the following factors when designing the PPE.

- *Athlete age and level of competition.* Obvious differences exist between a 30-year-old professional football player and a 12-year-old seventh-grade basketball player. Although the elements of the PPE may be the same for both, the emphasis on those elements is likely to be different. The PPE for the 12-year-old, for example, should include a greater emphasis on developmental problems common to that age group. The National Football League (NFL) player will probably require a much more extensive orthopedic examination, perhaps even including magnetic resonance imaging and other imaging studies. Both athletes need an orthopedic screening, but the screening should be tailored to the athlete and will differ greatly for each.

- *Sport.* Although the PPE should include certain aspects for all athletes, the exam should be as sport specific as possible. This is especially true in the part of the PPE used to determine an athlete's physical fitness. For example, an isokinetic evaluation of a sprinter's hamstrings-to-quadriceps ratio

may yield useful information that could help the athlete undertake an exercise program designed to prevent a hamstring strain while sprinting. To do the same test on a golfer would be interesting, but not particularly useful. Similarly, the Wingate test of anaerobic power might be useful for an ice hockey player, but not that important for a 10,000-meter runner on the track team, who would benefit more from a test of his $\dot{V}O_2$max. The biomechanical movements, joint flexibility, and muscle strength expectations of a field hockey player are vastly different from those of a fencer, yet both benefit from these findings as they relate to their specific screening.

- *Follow-up.* The information collected during the PPE is valuable only if the problems discovered are acted on. Too often, the PPE becomes a routine process that collects a massive amount of information but results in no follow-up. Vision screening is useful only if athletes with problems are referred for follow-up evaluation by an optometrist or ophthalmologist. Strength and fitness screening is useful only if conditioning specialists are available to provide the athlete with feedback and advice for improvement. Questions on the medical history form designed to reveal the potential for disordered eating are useful only if the physician addresses them during the PPE and arranges appropriate referrals for the athlete. As part of the team that develops the PPE, the athletic trainer ought to ask the question "What will we do if . . . ?" for each component of the exam. If the institutional or community resources are so limited that the information collected cannot be acted on, a careful interdisciplinary review of that portion of the PPE ought to be undertaken. Examples of effective follow-up include single or group educational counseling for athletes identified as having sickle cell trait, asthma, diabetes, or other medical conditions that could affect their performance as well as their overall health status (Ferrari et al. 2015).

- *Predictability of tests.* **Few** screening activities normally undertaken during the PPE have been shown to be reliable and valid as predictors of athletic injury (Minick et al. 2010; Parchmann and McBride 2011). The orthopedic exam, especially among athletes with no previous history of injury, is a surprisingly poor predictor of future athletic injury. However, for those with preexisting orthopedic conditions, these screens should continue to be performed and should be accompanied by a thorough history that specifically relates to their musculoskeletal status. A relatively small percent (14%) of the overall findings associated with a physical examination will require follow-up prior to clearance of the athlete for participation (Joy et al. 2004). As part of the team charged with designing the PPE, the athletic trainer ought to ask "How likely is this test to uncover a problem?" for each element of the PPE.

PEARLS OF MANAGEMENT

Perhaps one of the most important administrative responsibilities is to review all of the paperwork gathered from a patient's PPE in a timely manner for appropriate follow-up about areas of concern.

The preceding cautions notwithstanding, most practitioners agree that at least five elements should be part of the PPE.

- *Health history.* The portion of the PPE that seems to have the most predictive value is the medical history (Reed 2001). The medical history, as recorded on a detailed questionnaire, constitutes the most important part of the PPE for most athletes. The answers provided on the questionnaire should guide the medical team in choosing specific tests for each athlete to address problems. Confidential-

ity is an important aspect of this part of the PPE. If athletes think that the information they record on the **health history form** is likely to be shared too widely, they may not answer the questions truthfully and completely. Athletes need to be reassured that the information will be held in confidence and will not be shared with anyone outside the medical staff unless they specifically authorize release in writing. Despite the advances in technology during the past two decades, many organizations still do not use a Web-based method to collect health history information in advance so they can screen it before the patient–practitioner interaction. All questions on the PPE history form should be relevant to the evaluation, with a plan for addressing them if the athlete's response to a specific question is not favorable for clearance to participate.

- *Physician's examination.* A physician should examine every athlete during the course of the PPE. In fact, in most states an athlete is not considered to have undergone a PPE unless a physician (or a nurse practitioner, physician assistant, or chiropractor in some states) has examined her and verified in writing that she is fit to participate. The major components of the physician's examination include a general review of systems, including examination of the head, eyes, ears, nose, throat, chest and abdomen, and genitalia (Conley et al. 2014). Every examination should include a general cardiac screening reflective of the most current standards and guidelines as established by recognized professional organizations. Although it has its limitations, the preparticipation evaluation remains the major instrument readily available for prevention of sudden cardiac death (Drezner 2000; Pfister, Puffer, and Maron 2000). Physicians (McKeag and Moeller 2007) have recommend the use of a **maturational assessment**, including **Tanner staging**, for junior and senior high school athletes, but little remains known about the usefulness of this technique in preventing injuries (Smith 1994; American Academy of Family Physicians 2005; Tanner 1994).

- *Orthopedic examination.* Although the orthopedic examination may not be a strong predictor of injury for athletes with no previous history of injury, it is an important part of the PPE for athletes who have experienced an injury. The orthopedic exam should focus on problems that the athlete identifies in the health history questionnaire using evaluation techniques specific to those body parts, as well as a general screen for all of the joints. Range of motion, flexibility, accessory joint motion, and muscle strength should be considered part of the orthopedic examination because each relates to the individual athlete's sport. Additionally, commonly performed orthopedic special tests should be included in the exam because they pertain to the more commonly involved anatomical structures for each individual and his sport. A physician need not perform the general orthopedic examination unless this is required by association rules. Athletic trainers, physical therapists, and physician assistants with the proper training can assume this responsibility.

- *Special medical tests.* This portion of the PPE will vary greatly depending on the financial resources available and the philosophy of the physician. Common special tests include simple urinalysis to detect protein or sugar. Simple tests of visual acuity using a Snellen chart can also be performed at little cost. Routine X rays and cardiovascular or other assessments are not recommended unless warranted by the health history questionnaire or the physician's examination. However, it is becoming more common to conduct cardiac screening with high school athletes. Legislation has been proposed or passed to require it in South Carolina, New Jersey, and Texas. In addition, as of 2015, 50 organizations in 26 states offer free or low-cost electrocardiogram screening to youth athletes (American Heart Association 2015).

- *Physical fitness testing.* Many athletic programs use the PPE as an opportunity to establish a baseline for the athlete's physical fitness. Although this aspect of the PPE is usually not medically necessary to clear an athlete for participation, the information obtained can be useful to athletes and staff members in providing an assessment of the athlete's conditioning status. In particular, the strength and conditioning staff can benefit from these tests, and including the staff in the development and implementation of applicable fitness testing strengthens the purpose of the exam overall. In all likelihood, the findings of the fitness performance conducted by the strength and conditioning staff will be thoroughly acted on and incorporated into the athlete's ongoing conditioning program and goals. A variety of physical fitness tests are available; listing them is beyond the scope of this text. Two important points should be made regarding this portion of the PPE.

All physical fitness tests should be designed to provide data that are important to normal physiological function for a specific sport. If fitness testing is to be included as part of the PPE, it should always be the last element completed. The athlete should always be subjected to the health history, physician's exam, and orthopedic exam before engaging in strenuous exercise so that problems that might preclude such exercise can be identified first. Positioning the fitness tests at the end of the PPE also allows examination of the athlete in a resting state, which is an important factor in the collection of baseline cardiovascular data.

Legal Considerations

The legal precautions for conducting PPEs are similar to those of other aspects of medical and allied health care practice. Athletic trainers, physicians, and other health care professionals involved in the PPE will be held to the same standards of practice for this activity as they are for other aspects of their professional practice (Oliva et al. 2017). Two areas are particularly important to emphasize: consent and waiver of liability.

Consent

As with any medical procedure, an athlete must consent to be examined during the PPE. For athletes to provide informed consent, they must be told what will happen to them during the PPE, they must understand what they were told, they should have the opportunity to ask questions, and they must sign a document indicating that they agree to submit to the procedure. The parents or guardians of minor children must provide informed consent on their behalf. Athletes who are 18 years or older can provide informed consent for themselves. See figure 13.3 for an example of an informed consent form for the PPE.

Waiver of Liability

The primary purpose of the PPE is to prevent athletes from participating when they have a medical condition that endangers their health or that of their teammates or opponents. From time to time, a team physician will decide that an athlete should not participate in a given sport. Unfortunately, this is often not the last word. Athletes and their parents frequently challenge the decision of the team physician and demand the right to participate, no matter the risk for permanent disability or death. Frequently, these athletes seek second, third, and even fourth opinions to justify their desire to participate. The actions of the medical staff, including the team physician and the athletic trainer, are important in cases like these because they can involve litigation to resolve the matter.

One approach the medical team can take is to require athletes (and their parents in the case of minors) to sign waivers when they wish to participate against the advice of the physician. Such waivers must be tailored to each specific case and should include

---

STATEMENT OF INFORMED CONSENT
TO A PREPARTICIPATION PHYSICAL EXAMINATION

It is the policy of Ohio Technological University that all students must undergo a preparticipation physical examination (PPE) by an OTU physician prior to the beginning of practice or competition in intercollegiate athletics. We insist that you undergo a PPE for the following reasons:

- We want to help you prevent injuries and illnesses.
- We want to make sure that you are ready for vigorous athletic participation.
- We want to establish a medical basis for your participation.
- We must comply with the NCAA requirement that all athletes be medically cleared for participation.
- We want to use the PPE to talk to you about your personal health issues.

The PPE has three parts:

- A health history questionnaire that you complete (please be honest and complete)
- Several special tests (e.g., vision, blood pressure, weight and height) performed by the athletic training or nursing staff
- An examination by a physician

Things you should know about your PPE:

- The information derived from the PPE is kept confidential. Only the medical staff will have access to the information unless you authorize its release to others in writing.
- You will be asked to partially undress for the physician's examination. The physician may have to touch you in private areas in order to complete the examination. If you would be more comfortable having a nurse or athletic trainer of your own gender in the room during the physician's exam, just ask and we'd be happy to do this.
- The physician may ask you a few questions that seem personal and not necessarily related to athletics. We want to use this opportunity to talk about your health because illnesses and other nonathletic problems can interfere with your season as easily as an ankle sprain or a dislocated shoulder.

I, _____, have read the statement above and understand the reasons and components of the preparticipation physical examination. I freely consent to the examination. I have had an opportunity to ask questions regarding the preparticipation physical examination. All my questions have been answered.

_____   _____   _____
Student-athlete signature   Witness signature   Date

_____   _____
Parent or guardian signature   Date

Figure 13.3 Sample informed consent form for the PPE.

a full description of the medical condition, the findings of the PPE and other associated examinations connected to the condition, and a complete list of all the possible medical complications that could arise from athletic participation, including permanent disability and death. If temporary or permanent disability is a potential outcome, the waiver should describe the financial implications of such a disability. If the athlete is married, the spouse should sign a similar document waiving her right to sue for **loss of consortium**. The waiver should be written in simple language, and all medical terms should be explained. Athletes, parents, and spouses should be offered the opportunity to ask questions regarding the contents of the waiver. The waiver should state that in signing it, the athlete admits to having read the waiver, understanding it, and agreeing to hold the institution and its medical staff harmless for any future injuries associated with the condition in question. Although some courts have upheld waivers, they are often viewed as a violation of the public interest and are frequently not upheld, no matter how detailed or explicit. For this reason, waivers are not recommended to allow athletes to participate when medical professionals have recommended against it.

The second approach the medical team should consider in these cases is simply to stick to their decision to deny medical clearance for participation and allow the athlete to bring suit. This approach forces the courts to make a decision as to the reasonableness of the physician's decision (Herbert 1997). Any orders that the court issues should be included in the athlete's medical file as a record of the facts of the case should an injury result from participation at a later date (*Penny v. Sands* 1989; *Knapp v. Northwestern* 1996; *Mobley v. Madison Square Garden* 2012).

Summary

Preparticipation physical examinations are designed to assess an athlete's health status prior to vigorous participation. These should be performed four to six weeks before the beginning of such activity, allowing for time to address concerns and complete further tests that may need to be performed. A thorough history form serves as the hallmark foundation in addition to a screening of the body's systems. The PPE can be performed in an office-based format, with assessment of one athlete at a time, or in a station-based format with multiple athletes and providers taking part in the process simultaneously. Both formats have strengths and weaknesses. Each assessment should also consider gender, sport, and level-specific needs.

Learning Aids

Case Study 1

Ghadah's phone rang in her office at Northline Sports Medicine Clinic, where she was one of several certified athletic trainers. Her supervisor, James, asked her if she would stop by his office later to discuss a new project he had in mind. When Ghadah arrived 20 minutes later, James told her that the clinic would offer a new service in the fall. "We want to expand our outreach services by offering to coordinate preparticipation physical examinations for the high schools we want to develop contracts with. We want you to pilot the program at Truman High in August. Here's the phone number of the athletic director at Truman. I've spoken with him already and he's really excited to have us doing this for him. Let me know how I can help."

Although Ghadah was excited to get started on this project, she came away from her first meeting with Truman's athletic director a bit worried. The facilities were dark, in poor repair, and dirty. The athletic training room was a converted custodial closet. The boys' locker room was next to the gym, but the girls' locker room was down the hall in another wing of the building. Truman had a doctor—the parent of one of the student-athletes—but he came only to home football games on Friday nights. The athletic director told Ghadah that he anticipated 500 students would need physical exams. The date was less than one month away.

Questions for Analysis

1. What alternatives does Ghadah have for the physical facilities she needs to be able to conduct Truman's PPEs?
2. Of all the obstacles that Ghadah faces, which are the most significant? Why?
3. Assuming that Ghadah can pull together a team of physicians for Truman's PPEs, who will decide the final participation status of each athlete? If an athlete challenges one of Ghadah's physicians on a decision to deny clearance, how should Ghadah handle it?
4. Put yourself in Ghadah's position and develop a plan to organize and administer PPEs to Truman High's 500 student-athletes. Be sure to include a floor plan of the facility you plan to use, along with staffing and supply lists. Develop all the forms you'll need to document each step of the PPE.

Case Study 2

Phil has been the only athletic trainer employed by West Kings High School since they first hired him almost 20 years ago. Since that time, much has changed in the way his job functions. For years, all of the student-athletes at West Kings High School received clearance to participate from their individual primary care physician. The school system uses standardized forms that make the process quite simple for everyone involved.

This past summer, Phil's director of athletics came to Phil with an idea to help generate revenue and asked him to look into coordinating station-based preparticipation physical examinations at the school all on the same day. She told Phil that if the school charged for them, it could serve as a small profit source for the athletics program. She also asked Phil to come up with a plan for organizing the event and securing volunteer personnel for staffing.

Questions for Analysis

1. What are the advantages and disadvantages of changing to the proposed format for the preparticipation physical examinations?

2. What specific legal issues should Phil present to his director of athletics? Will Phil take on additional liability himself if the process changes?

3. Do you think this change will generate positive or negative feedback from the stakeholders involved in the process? Who are the primary stakeholders?

Key Concepts and Review

Understand and support the rationale for administrating preparticipation physical examinations.

The preparticipation physical examination is the first step in injury prevention and a process that most athletic trainers eventually become involved with. Besides helping to prevent injury, the PPE allows institutions to comply with association rules, provides an opportunity for counseling and education, and helps improve compliance with standards of practice.

Understand the strengths and weaknesses of the various preparticipation physical examination models.

There are advantages and disadvantages to conducting PPEs in either the physician's office or in stations in a school setting. The option of using the family physician and the alternative of using the team physician both present advantages and disadvantages. Considerations for each setting include privacy, availability of equipment and supplies, and the thoroughness of the examination.

Organize and implement a comprehensive preparticipation physical examination program in a variety of settings.

PPEs should ideally be conducted six to eight weeks before the beginning of the season. The NCAA requires a comprehensive PPE only upon entry into the athletic program, whereas most state high school associations require an annual PPE. The content of the PPE should be based on the athlete's age and level of competition, the sport to be played, the level of follow-up available, and the predictability of the tests to be used. Common elements of the PPE include a comprehensive health history, physician's examination, orthopedic examination, special tests, and fitness tests. Athletes (or their parents) must give written informed consent to be examined during the PPE. Athletes who wish to challenge the judgment of the medical staff regarding their participation status should be required to sign a detailed waiver of liability. Even this, however, may not be enough to shield the medical staff from liability in the event of serious injury or illness. A more prudent approach may be to allow the courts to rule on the reasonableness of the physician's participation decision.

Identify appropriate personnel utilized in the preparticipation physical examination.

People with a healthcare background and other volunteers can be utilized to perform the preparticipation physical examination. Station-based preparticipation physical examinations will require more people to perform the various tasks as determined by those supervising the process.

Drug Education and Testing

Objectives

After reading this chapter, you should be able to do the following:

- Understand and support the rationale for administrating drug education and testing programs in athletics.

- Understand the legal ramifications of drug testing in athletic programs.

- Organize and implement a comprehensive drug education and testing program.

- Become familiar with the legalities of dispensing and prescribing medications.

This chapter provides an overview of the administrative components associated with a drug education and testing program. Drug testing itself is an issue of compliance. However, the process of drug education and the physiological and behavioral changes in clients and student-athletes who are consuming banned substances are all factors that will affect the role of the athletic trainer. Therefore, a clear understanding of how a drug education and testing program operates is essential knowledge for the practicing athletic trainer.

Why Drug Testing Should Be Performed

The reasons for drug testing are as varied as the people who have written about this controversial subject since it gained widespread attention in the 1980s. Some institutions envision drug testing as a means of promoting order and discipline on an athletic team. Others see it as a way to prevent or discourage potentially illegal activity. Yet others implement programs as a deterrent to unfair competitive advantage. One would hope that most institutions are genuinely concerned about instituting drug-testing programs as a means of helping people with chemical addictions come to grips with their problems. For all these stated reasons, and possibly more, educational components should always be a foundational part of a drug testing program (Kersey et al. 2012).

PEARLS OF MANAGEMENT

Athletic trainers in professional sports and NCAA Division I, II, and III universities are often charged with development and implementation of drug education and testing programs. These programs may occur year-round or during postchampionship events or both. Some states have enacted forms of drug testing in high schools. All athletic trainers should become familiar with the issues of organizing and administering drug education and testing programs.

Years ago, the National Collegiate Athletic Association (NCAA) identified two overarching goals for its drug-testing program, which is generally viewed as the standard for collegiate sports in the United States (National Collegiate Athletic Association 2016). The first goal is to promote fair and equitable competition. At least two objectives can be inferred from this goal. First is the proposition that all athletes should compete on a level playing field where only the sum of their training and talent determines the outcome of a contest. The second part of this goal is the idea that no athlete should feel pressure to take drugs in order to have a chance to win. The design of the drug test should ensure that these two objectives are met. Today, drug testing remains a part of compliance in medal and championship sporting events to ensure fair play. Despite the knowledge of testing, a small percentage of athletes continue to resort to banned substances and performance-enhancing drugs in an effort to obtain a competitive advantage over others (Bird et al. 2016).

The second goal that the NCAA identified is to safeguard the health and safety of athletes by discouraging drug use through drug testing. The potentially detrimental effects of drug use are well understood and universally acknowledged. The hope is that athletes who use performance-enhancing or recreational drugs will be identified so that they may be counseled and, where appropriate, receive treatment for problems their drug use may have caused. However, many, if not most, highly motivated athletes are willing to sacrifice their health for short-term glory on the athletic field. When testing programs were first implemented and athletes were asked whether they would take performance-enhancing drugs even if they knew that they would suffer serious heart or liver disease as a result, a significant percentage of athletes said they would do so (National Collegiate Athletic Association 1988). Drug testing seems like weak ammunition in a fight in which such strong motivating forces are at work. Short-term success and achievement appears to take priority over unforeseen long-term consequences. Various types of drug-testing programs have been legislatively introduced and implemented with questionable success at the secondary school level as a result of reported usage among student athletes (Bahrke 2015; Elkins, King, and Vidourek 2017; Lee 2001; *Lebron v. Secretary, Florida Department of Children and Families* 2013).

When Drug Testing Should Be Performed

Different models for the timing of drug testing account for most drug tests performed in collegiate, professional, and Olympic sports: postchampionship testing, preseason testing, and year-round testing.

- *Postchampionship testing.* Many college athletes are exposed to drug testing after their teams participate in an NCAA championship event. Choice of which athletes to test at these events can be based on random selection, position of finish, playing position, or playing time.

- *Preseason testing.* Professional athletes are frequently drug tested before their first season of competition. This test is usually part of the PPE and is considered a **preemployment test**.

- *Year-round testing.* The NCAA requires athletes in Division I and II football and baseball and Division I indoor and outdoor track and field to submit to drug testing year-round. In addition, the National Football League (NFL) and the national governing bodies for several Olympic sports require year-round testing of athletes for a variety of performance-enhancing drugs, including anabolic steroids.

- *In-house testing.* Many universities with large athletic programs also engage in year-round testing as a way to discourage off-season drug use. More and more schools, both colleges and high schools, are implementing drug screening and education programs. In the high school setting, these may be state-mandated programs designed to curtail use of both performance-enhancing and street drugs. In any case, these programs are rather expensive to implement, require extensive organizational skills and bookkeeping, and pose additional challenges when minors are being tested. Questions have arisen as to whether or not a child should be allowed to participate in state-sanctioned and state-funded high school sports that require drug testing when the parent has not consented to allow the child to be tested.

- *Union contract.* Drug testing policies and procedures on the professional level are negotiated between the league office and the players association. Thus, they become part of the collective bargaining agreement (CBA). Most policies include year-round testing for performance enhancing drugs. Testing for recreational drugs varies from league to league, but most test for recreational drug use only during the season and not year-round. Within the NFL CBA, testing for recreational drugs only occurs once a year during the off season.

PEARLS OF MANAGEMENT

Athletic trainers who are involved with drug testing as part of their job should be sure to communicate closely with their employer's legal counsel to confirm that proper procedures are in place to protect the privacy of the client or student-athlete being tested.

How Drug Testing Should Be Performed

Many important decisions regarding the mechanics of a drug-testing program will affect the eventual success or failure of the program.

Consent

All athletes should sign a consent form agreeing to submit to drug testing. Although the language of the consent form indicates that this activity is voluntary, the sanction imposed when an athlete chooses not to sign is usually athletic ineligibility. Universities that conduct their own drug-testing programs besides those required by the NCAA should develop their own consent forms (see figure 14.1) in addition to those required by the NCAA. All programs should have established policies and procedures in place and these should be clearly outlined for those who consent to the testing.

KEY POINT

The NCAA drug-testing consent forms for Division I, II, and III can be found on the NCAA website.

Selection of Subjects

Few issues related to drug testing are more riddled with potential liability than selection of the athletes to be tested. Although most drug-testing programs associated with college, professional, and Olympic sports are purported to use **random selection**, definition of this term can take many forms. Several common and accepted methods are used in an attempt to randomize subjects for drug testing. Each category has several permutations, including the following:

- *Random selection of subjects by sport.* The NCAA, some universities, and some high schools may randomly choose a sport to test during any given testing period. Under this system, athletes might be able to entirely avoid being tested during their college careers if their teams are never chosen or never participate in NCAA postseason championships.

- *Random selection of subjects by position.* Some athletes are selected for testing based on the position they play on the team. For instance, one may choose to test only the defensive players on the football team during any given testing period, saving the offensive players until another testing period.

- *Random selection of subjects by playing time or finish position.* The NCAA frequently chooses to test only within the group of athletes who contributed to the outcome of a particular contest by virtue of their playing time. A similar method involves selecting subjects who placed high in individual-sport championships, such as one of the top three places in an event.

- *Random selection of subjects by financial aid status.* In some cases, especially those involving NCAA Division I sports, subjects for drug testing are drawn from the pool of athletes on athletic scholarship. Nonscholarship athletes are often eliminated from the pool.

- *Random timing—no notice.* One method frequently used in drug testing is to conduct unannounced spot checks at random intervals. This procedure often involves taking an athlete off the field to administer a drug test with no warning. Many experts believe that this is one of the only ways to discourage cheating the system, because athletes who know when they will be tested can often mask their drug use by abstaining for as little as a few days before the test.

- *Random timing—some notice.* The alternative to unannounced random testing is to provide subjects with some notice that they will be tested. The further in advance an athlete knows about the test, however, the greater the chances that she will be able to manipulate the results. With some notice,

INDIANA UNIVERSITY DEPARTMENT OF INTERCOLLEGIATE ATHLETICS ALCOHOL AND DRUG SCREENING PROGRAM CONSENT FORM

READ CAREFULLY BEFORE SIGNING

Print name: _____

Sport: _____

1. AGREEMENT

I have carefully read the Indiana University Department of Intercollegiate Athletics Alcohol and Drug Screening Program and Policies and know the contents thereof, and I understand that by my signature, I agree to abide by the policies and I acknowledge that I have received a copy of these policies. I also understand that failure to show for a substance-screening test may be treated as a positive test result.

Student-athlete signature: _____ Date: _____

2. CONSENT TO URINALYSIS

For the 2017-18 year (which includes the summer 2018 vacation period), I hereby consent to have a sample of my urine collected and tested during my annual physical examination and at other such times as necessary or required, for the presence of certain drugs or substances in accordance with the provisions of the Indiana University Department of Intercollegiate Athletics Alcohol and Drug Screening Program and Policies.

Student-athlete signature: _____ Date: _____

Parent or guardian signature: _____ Date: _____

3. AUTHORIZATION FOR RELEASE OF INFORMATION

I further authorize you to release to the head coach of any intercollegiate sport in which I am a participant, my parent(s) or legal guardian(s), the athletic director and the team physician at Indiana University all the information and records, including test results, you may have relating to the screening or testing of my urine sample(s) in accordance with the provisions of the Indiana University Department of Intercollegiate Athletics Alcohol and Drug Screening Program and Policies. To the extent set forth in this document, I waive any privilege I may have in connection with such information.

I understand that my urine sample will be sent to the Indiana University Medical Center, Indianapolis, Indiana, for actual testing.

Student-athlete signature: _____ Date: _____

Parent or guardian signature: _____ Date: _____

4. RELEASE OF LIABILITY

The trustees of Indiana University, its officers, employees, and agents are hereby released from legal responsibility or liability for the release of such information and records as authorized by this form.

Student-athlete signature: _____ Date: _____

Parent or guardian signature: _____ Date: _____

Figure 14.1 Institutional drug-testing consent form.

Reprinted with permission from the Indiana University Athletic Department.

individuals may attempt to dilute their samples by overhydrating in an effort to mask the test results.

To demonstrate that subjects were selected for testing at random, an athletic trainer must develop a system that equalizes the probability that one athlete has as much of a chance of being tested as any other athlete. Randomization can occur in many ways. Athletes are usually assigned a number. The athletic trainer can select the number either by consulting a table of random numbers or by generating a list of random numbers from a computer statistics program. In any case, the athletic trainer must document the method used so that she can withstand challenges to the validity of the selection procedure.

Reasonable Suspicion

An alternative to random testing is to select subjects based on **reasonable suspicion**. Reasonable suspicion, also known as reasonable cause or probable cause, is based on specific signs of drug use in an individual. These signs are usually associated with observed behavior abnormalities that may or may not be related to the athlete's participation in sport. For example, an athlete may be asked to submit to a drug test after demonstrating rapid gains in muscle bulk and other signs of anabolic steroid use—a situation obviously related to the athlete's participation in sport. The same athlete may be asked to submit to drug testing after being involved in a traffic accident in which he was under the influence of drugs—an incident unrelated to the athlete's involvement in sport.

Drug testing that involves reasonable suspicion as a selection criterion should be approached with great caution. What is reasonable to one person is often unreasonable to another, especially when sanctions may be involved. Suspicious behaviors must be carefully documented. Selection by reasonable suspicion is enhanced when more than one person observes the suspicious behavior on more than one occasion. Behaviors or qualities that are measurable (documented increases in size and strength, number of motor vehicle accidents, drop in grade point average) are particularly useful in defending the reasonableness of suspicion of drug use. With a clearly written policy, individuals can be tested without notice based on reasonable suspicion. It is imperative to base such suspicion on factual information because allegations are likely to incite disagreement and anger on the part of the athlete and potentially others she communicates closely with, such a coach and parents. A policy to allow for reasonable suspicion testing within an organization should clearly identify how information is gathered, how it is acted on, and who will be made aware of the testing prior to its administration (e.g., coach, athletic director).

Notification

A person chosen to be tested should ideally be notified directly by an appropriate staff member. This is usually someone from the athletic training or compliance departments, and can occur at any time. The individual should be presented at this time with a written notification form that clearly indicates the test date, test time, and testing area. The form should also provide specific directions that may include whether or not to eat, drink, or use a bathroom prior to testing. The individual being notified for testing should have the opportunity to ask questions at that time and be sure that he or she understands the process. A signature, typically with a discreet third-party witness may also be required. Directions usually include that an unwillingness to participate or lack of appearance at the test will result in a positive test result.

Drug-Testing Methods

The most common method for drug testing in sport is urinalysis. Tests involving blood, saliva, hair, and breath analysis are also available, but are used with less frequency. A method frequently employed as a first-level screening for many drugs is the **enzyme multiplied immunoassay technique (EMIT)**. This method uses light absorption to establish the level of a drug in a subject's urine. The amount of light absorption is compared to norms for a variety of drugs commonly tested for in athletic settings. Although this method is relatively inexpensive, it may produce a high percentage of false-positive tests. For this reason, laboratories federally certified by the Substance Abuse and Mental Health Services Administration (SAMHSA) cannot report a screening result only. If a specimen screens nonnegative, it must be analyzed using a confirmatory method: either GC-MS or LC/MS/MS.

Because EMIT tests can indicate the presence of drugs in an athlete's urine at a level higher than is actually present, positive tests must be confirmed by a process known as **gas chromatography–mass spectrometry (GC-MS)**. Gas chromatography–mass spectrometry remains the standard testing of choice in the industry. This method is also the method of choice for determining the presence of anabolic steroids in the urine. The EMIT test is not sensitive to the presence of anabolic steroids. GC-MS works by separating the compounds found in the urine and developing "fingerprints" for each compound. These fingerprints can then be compared to those of known drugs. Although GC-MS is a sensitive method, athletes frequently beat the system by using "designer" drugs for which no reference fingerprints are available. **Liquid chromatography–mass spectrometry–mass spectrometry (LC/MS/MS)** is considered a more sensitive testing technology these days because testing at lower thresholds can capture designer drugs. Generally speaking, GC-MS is a more expensive form of testing than LC/MS/MS.

Specimen Handling and Chain of Custody

Although observation is distasteful to all involved, the collection, labeling, and packaging of a urine sample must be observed by a reliable witness. Otherwise, the sample is of no value. Athletes should be observed while they deliver their urine samples. This obviously requires the presence of a toilet facility in the immediate vicinity of the drug-testing area. In the event that the athlete has difficulty producing a specimen, caffeine-free and alcohol-free beverages from sealed containers should be provided. The athlete should be allowed to observe the handling of the sample until it has been transferred to an appropriate bottle provided by the testing lab. The athlete should also be allowed to observe as the bottle is sealed and labeled. After the specimen has been labeled and sealed, the athlete should sign a form indicating that the specimen she provided was indeed her own, that she did not tamper with the specimen or any of the containers used to collect or store it, that she observed the transfer of the specimen to the storage bottle and the sealing of it, and that the name on the storage bottle is hers.

Testing the Sample

Although simple immunoassay kits are available that athletic trainers can use to test urine samples in the athletic training room, this practice should be discouraged because of the potential inaccuracy of these kits. Because of the potential loss of athletic eligibility and its associated social and financial consequences, a reliable, disinterested third party should test the samples (figure 14.2). Ideally, the organization should contract with a laboratory experienced in athletic drug testing for every phase of the program, including subject selection, specimen collection, sample testing, and results reporting. The NCAA (2016) recommends that institutions contract only with labs that can provide information on **false-positive** and **false-negative** rates for the specific tests to be conducted. Using federally certified labs is also highly recommended.

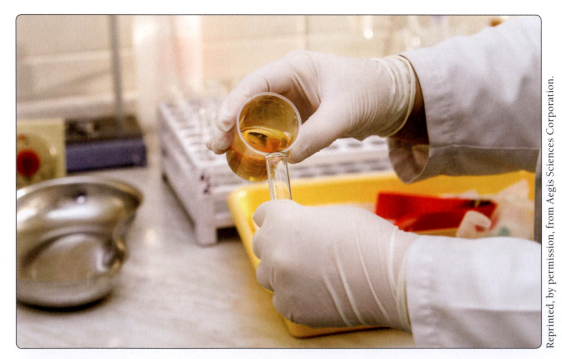

Reprinted, by permission, from Aegis Sciences Corporation.

Figure 14.2 A federally certified drug lab should be used for testing urine samples.

Results of Testing

The results of positive drug tests should be reported only to the people with a legitimate need for the information. This issue can become difficult because denial of athletic eligibility is often the result of a positive drug test. Institutions that choose to implement drug-testing programs must develop ironclad procedures regarding the dissemination of this information. People with a need to know might include the athlete, the team physician, the athletic trainer, the athletic director, and the head coach; this list will vary from institution to institution. Some may consider the strength and conditioning coaches from a safety perspective, as well as the academic advisors who may better understand a student's classroom performance as it relates to these social behaviors. Personnel who are included on the list should be warned of the potential negative consequences of releasing the information. The damage to an athlete's reputation and potential loss of income make this area especially ripe for litigation.

KEY POINT

A list of SAMHSA-certified labs can be found on its website. Labs are different from third-party administrators, which serve as an extension of a full-service lab.

Reporting the Results

Test results can be reported confidentially as being positive or negative. A negative test result is a test sample in which no evidence of a banned substance being tested for was found. A positive test means that one or more banned substances were identified at unacceptable levels. If a specimen is diluted, it may be noted as negative-dilute and a retest may be suggested. A specimen may also be canceled if there is a suspicion that it has been adulterated or manipulated.

All athletes being tested should be aware that a testing organization is not necessarily concerned with how a banned substance entered the system. It is only responsible for detecting the banned substance. Therefore, individuals should be cautious about the food, drink, supplements, and medications and anything else they put in their body. A positive report on an NCAA or International Olympic Committee (IOC) drug test could result in sanctions as significant as a minimum one-year ban from sport. For in-house institutional testing, many programs will allow up to a couple of "strikes." For example, a first-time positive test may result in a suspension of one or two games, community service, counseling, and education. A second strike may result in a longer suspension with continued rehabilitation requirements. A third strike in most programs results in a permanent suspension from the sport.

Medical Exception

Individuals taking a prescribed medication for acute or chronic medical purposes might be taking a drug that is listed on a banned substance list. In this case, a drug test would reveal a positive finding. In these cases, it is required that medical documentation, including evidence of the prescription with dates and dosages clearly identified, be on file before notification of a test. To protect themselves, individuals should inform their team physicians, athletic training staff, and compliance staff of prescribed medication usage. It is up to the testing organizers whether or not to grant an individual an exemption from a positive test.

Safe Harbor Clause

A safe harbor clause is a provision that allows an individual to self-report a substance problem without the repercussions of a positive test. Self-reporting must occur prior to formal notification of being selected for a drug test. It serves as an opportunity for an individual to seek assistance by voluntarily and privately disclosing the need for help in the event of engaging in substance abuse. The goal is to direct the individual toward professional counseling, with the intent to assess the extent to which the individual may or may not require further forms of intervention or rehabilitation. Use of a safe harbor clause is typically allowed just once during a person's involvement in an athletic program and does not exempt that individual from undergoing further drug testing. In fact, if eventually discharged from further rehabilitation, it is common to randomly test the individual to ensure he or she remains drug free. Individuals who are allowed to claim a safe harbor scenario but are not compliant with rehabilitation recommendations may also be sanctioned in some form and undergo further random testing. Safe harbor clauses are established institutionally and vary from organization to organization. This type of a policy does not exist within the NCAA or International Olympic Committee drug-testing programs.

Appeal Process

All drug-testing programs should incorporate an appeal process for individuals who receive a positive test report and want to challenge or appeal the test result. Appeals should be filed within a designated timeframe and reviewed by appropriate impartial parties as established within an institution. Appeals should be filed in writing and state clearly the reasoning behind the challenge of the test result. Appeal policies may include hearings, and individuals may be allowed, and in fact encouraged, to be present with some form of representation. A policy should also clearly outline whether or not sanctions are put in place or on hold during an appeal timeframe.

What to Test For

Which drugs should an athlete be tested for? On what basis should the list of banned drugs be developed? These policies lack consistency internationally (Petroczi et al. 2015). The two most common lists of banned drugs are those published by the NCAA and by the World Anti-Doping Agency (WADA). WADA tests for drugs in athletes who compete in the Olympic Games. The Olympic list is longer and more restrictive than the NCAA list. In general, drugs banned from use include certain kinds of stimulants (amphetamine, cocaine), anabolic agents (testosterone, clenbuterol), diuretics (acetazolamide, furosemide), street drugs (heroin, marijuana), and peptide hormones and analogs (human growth hormone, erythropoietin). In addition, some drugs are prohibited in certain sports but allowed in others. Interestingly, many institutional drug-testing programs do not test for alcohol, although this drug clearly has the greatest rate of abuse among high school and college-aged students. Both banned lists are infinite, meaning "these substance are banned but not limited to." Any substance that has a similar chemical structure or effect may also be banned.

Proceeding With Caution

Drug testing is a controversial subject. It has been widely litigated (e.g., *Todd v. Rush County Schools* 1997; *Schaill by Kross v. Tippecanoe Cty. School Corp.* 1988)—a trend that will probably continue. Legal counsel is an essential element of the drug-testing program. Athletic trainers asked to design a drug-testing program must incorporate elements that lend validity and reliability to the procedures as well as protect the rights of those to be tested. When designing a program, consider at minimum the following elements (Pickett 1986):

• *Develop written policies and procedures.* The first step in instituting a drug-testing program is

to codify the process in a written document that prescribes every step of the program. The process described in the NCAA's *Drug-Testing Program 2016-17* document (2016) is a useful template for institutions that want to implement their own programs.

• *Clearly articulate the purpose of the program.* Everyone associated with a drug-testing program must understand its purpose. If the purpose of the program is not clearly articulated, it can easily be manipulated and turned into something that its creators never intended it to be.

• *Make testing as sport specific as possible.* Defending a drug-testing program is easier if you can demonstrate that it is designed to prevent or detect problems clearly associated with a particular sport. Testing the entire cross country team for anabolic steroids and human growth hormone five times per year would be an example of testing for a problem that is unlikely to exist.

• *Use valid and reliable methods.* You must be able to prove that each positive result is associated with a particular athlete's sample through a carefully documented chain of custody. The selected laboratory must confirm all positive results with GC-MS or LC/MS/MS technology.

• *Incorporate an appeal mechanism.* If athletes have an interest in retaining their athletic scholarship, eligibility, or position on a professional team, they must have access to due process before they can be sanctioned. All athletes who test positive should be allowed to appeal the results. The more severe the sanction, the more formal the process should be. Again, the NCAA manual serves as a good resource regardless of your setting or population to be tested.

• *Protect the athlete's privacy.* Only personnel with a legitimate need to know should be informed about positive drug tests. This list should be codified in written policies and procedures. Nobody else should have access to the information without the written permission of the athlete.

• *Obtain consent.* Athletes may not be tested for drugs against their will. For the athlete's consent to be valid, the document he signs should include a detailed description of the drug-testing process and the sanctions associated with positive tests.

• *Inform recruited athletes.* Athletes being recruited to participate in an institution's athletic program should be informed that the institution has a drug-testing program to which they may be subjected. This information should be reiterated when the student enrolls. This information helps establish the evidence required to prove informed consent.

- *Inform current athletes.* All athletes with the potential to be tested should be informed, in writing, of the purposes of the program, the procedures for selection and testing, the sanctions associated with positive tests, and the appeal procedures. They should also be informed of the risk of information regarding positive tests being accessible to third parties through a court order or other legal means.

- *Train and retrain personnel.* All personnel associated with the drug-testing program should be thoroughly trained in their responsibilities. This training should occur regularly to ensure that personnel learn about changes in the program and perform their duties correctly.

- *Educate athletes.* Make readily available educational materials that athletes can access at any time. Website links, written materials, formal and informal education sessions serve a tremendous benefit. For athletes with further questions or concerns and for those who test positive, make professional counselors available to assist their needs.

One final consideration regarding drug testing for athletes in intercollegiate settings is whether or not athletic trainers should be involved in the process at all. While it could be argued that this is a health-related issue, technically speaking, whether or not one participates in accordance of the rules is a compliance issue. Furthermore, it can be argued that the athletic trainer has established a provider–client relationship and this would put the AT in a potentially compromising role. This relationship can pose tremendous ethical challenges if the athletic trainer is the only person with knowledge of a positive test of a so-called star athlete. Despite the potential conflict, many athletic trainers remain involved in supervising and administering drug testing.

Pharmacological Policy

Every program should have an approved written policy outlining procedures for handling medications, to include but not limited to storage and dispensing. The focus in this chapter is both prescription and nonprescription policies for colleges and universities and individuals of legal age. Similar medication policies for minors are much more restrictive. In general, athletic trainers should not provide prescription or nonprescription medications to a minor, unless the AT possesses full written authorization from the child's parent or guardian. The National Federation of State High School Associations' dietary supplements position statement notes that school personnel and coaches should never recommend, endorse, or encourage the use of any dietary supplement, drug, or medication for performance enhancement (2015).

Athletic trainers should also clearly understand the difference between drug administration and drug dispensing. Different laws regulate each. **Drug administration** is a process whereby one who is legally authorized and licensed as a health care practitioner administers a single dose of a medication to a client. **Drug dispensing** is the process of preparing and packaging medications for use by a client. Physicians are not legally allowed to delegate the responsibility of dispensing prescription medications to a person who is not authorized by law to dispense, including athletic trainers, unless they possess a legal dispensing license in the state that they practice in.

Prescription Medications

One way to ensure compliance with all laws governing the administration and dispensing of prescription medications is to establish policies and procedures that ban athletic trainers to store or dispense prescription medications in an athletic training facility. Athletes in need of prescription medications could still quite easily have such orders written by a team physician and filled by a local pharmacy, some of which may be located on campus. Some athletic training programs may choose to store prescription medications in an on-site athletic training facility. This is allowed and can be done legally if state and federal guidelines are strictly adhered to (Nickell 2006). External third parties (e.g., state board of pharmacy, consultants) can review a program's policies to ensure adherence to relevant laws (Huff 1998). Furthermore, regardless of what a program chooses to do, clear written guidelines should be in place, and each staff member should date and sign an agreement stating that he or she is fully aware of and understands the policies and procedures.

Prescription medications must always be kept in a locked cabinet and room with key access granted only to individuals with the current and valid licenses required to dispense the medications. It is recommended that readily accessible materials for drug referencing be nearby for questions that may arise (e.g., handouts about the drugs that are administered or *Physician's Desk Reference*). When dispensing medications, all standard state and federal labeling procedures should be followed. This includes the name of the individual for whom the medication is being prescribed, expiration date, name of medication, and dosage. Controlled substances are not to be stored or dispensed under any occasion in an athletic training facility. For traveling purposes, only individuals with appropriate credentials to maintain, prescribe, and dispense medications may carry prescription medications in a medical bag. Keep in mind, while this is an acceptable practice for many team physicians, it does pose a risk to properly securing medications, and precautions should be taken to safeguard a medical kit that contains prescribed medications.

Another key component of proper policies and procedures for handling medications is maintaining an accurate record-keeping system. In addition to a record of the individual prescriptions being dispensed, documentation must also include up-to-date inventories of all drugs in stock and signatures of receipt of each medication by the client.

In the past, it was not uncommon for athletic trainers to serve as the keeper of commonly prescribed medications that multiple athletes might be taking. Examples of medications handled this way include prescription-strength hydrocortisone cream delivered topically when using phonophoresis and epinephrine autoinjectors for individuals who may experience an anaphylactic reaction. These prescribed medications, and others like them, should be prescribed to a specific person, not the athletic trainer or athletic training room.

Nonprescription Medications

Nonprescription medications can be purchased over the counter in any pharmacy or even grocery or convenience stores. While technically, the storage and dispensation of **over-the-counter medications (OTC)** are not regulated by similarly stringent state and federal laws for prescribed medications, both the standard of care and the policies and procedures for an athletic trainer handling and dispensing OTC drugs to athletes are just as important. Stockpiling and dispensing are not recommended in an environment where athletes are minors. Best practice dictates that OTC drugs are not dispensed to minors under any circumstances.

Should you as an athletic trainer choose to store OTC drugs in your athletic training facility (and medical kit), the following guidelines are suggested:

- Maintain an accurate inventory of each OTC medication.
- Keep a log with signatures and dates of dispensing (include dosage).
- Keep a log with signatures and dates verifying an explanation of benefits, possible adverse effects, contraindications, and drug interaction warnings.
- Establish clear policies and procedures, approved by appropriate stakeholders with legal responsibilities, including any standing orders.
- Store OTC medications in a locked space.
- Ensure all OTC drugs are properly discarded if their usage date has expired. (Check local and state law for discard procedures.)
- Do not dispense beyond single-day dosage.
- Package and label in compliance with the federal law for OTC drugs.
- Review each person's medical chart before dispensing an OTC medication, reviewing for drug allergies and other reasons not to administer.

Federal OTC Drug Facts Label Requirements

The following information must appear in this order in a type size large enough to be easily read:

1. The product's active ingredients, including the amount in each dosage unit.
2. The purpose of the product.
3. The uses (indications) for the product.
4. Specific warnings, including when the product should not be used under any circumstances, and when it is appropriate to consult with a doctor or pharmacist. This section also describes side effects that could occur and substances or activities to avoid.
5. Dosage instructions—when, how, and how often to take the product.
6. The product's inactive ingredients; this is important information to help consumers avoid ingredients that may cause an allergic reaction.

Reprinted from U.S. Food & Drug Administration. Available: www.fda.gov/Drugs/ResourcesForYou/Consumers/ucm143551.htm

Summary

Athletic trainers are often involved in drug testing of student-athletes. This requires knowledge of consent procedures and the selection process. Testing may occur at random, postchampionship, or based on reasonable suspicion. Testing is performed at professional levels, for example in the National Football League, through the NCAA, and internally within school-specific programs administered under the supervision of a college or high school. Athletic trainers should be familiar with and have comprehensive policies and procedures in place regarding storing, prescribing, and dispensing of both prescribed and over-the-counter medications.

Learning Aids

Case Study 1

Mark walked into the locker room to tell Kasim that his number had come up. "Kasim," Mark began, "I know you're just a freshman on the football team, but everybody has to get drug tested if their number is drawn. Yours just came up, so I'll need a urine sample from you. Right now." "Mr. Consuelos," responded Kasim, "I've only been here five days, and besides, my religion doesn't permit me to do this. I think I should talk to my parents first." "Kasim," Mark said, "you don't have a choice. You signed the drug-testing consent form when you arrived last week, so you should have known this could happen. I don't have all day to stand here and argue. Either fill the cup, or I'll have to go to the coach." Kasim reluctantly went into the bathroom where Mark watched him provide a specimen. After he was finished, Kasim said to Mark, "Please don't let my folks know that I did this. They'd really be upset. They're pretty conservative." "If you don't test positive there's nothing to worry about," responded Mark. After that he turned and walked out of the locker room with Kasim's specimen.

Questions for Analysis

1. Based on what you read in this case, what potential flaws exist in Mark's drug-testing program? How could he correct these flaws?

2. Mark told Kasim that he had no choice but to submit to the drug test. Is he right? Why or why not?

3. Assume that Kasim's test was positive for the presence of anabolic steroids. Further assume that he was suspended for the season and that a story appeared in the newspaper reporting that Kasim was being disciplined for "violating team rules." If Kasim's parents call Mark wanting to know why their son was being suspended, how should Mark respond?

4. Would you challenge the results of this test and the resulting suspension if you were Kasim? On what grounds?

5. Design a policies and procedures manual for a drug-testing program at an NCAA Division I university. Include a comprehensive list of procedures, including subject selection, drugs to be tested for, and sample collection and chain of custody. Develop a request for proposal to send to various laboratories that might do the testing. Develop an appeal process and a list of sanctions for positive tests.

Case Study 2

Kalyn has been the athletic trainer at Washington State College, a small Division II school on the west coast, for the past five years. During this time, she has done an outstanding job establishing the trust and respect of coaches, student-athletes, colleagues, administrators, and even parents associated with the athletics programs. Simply put, she is very well liked and respected for her professionalism, work ethics, and overall leadership. Kalyn's athletic training room is a welcoming environment to those seeking treatment and care, and many student-athletes have become familiar with the facility. Therefore, Kalyn and her staff have decided to make accessible in a small countertop storage case commonly requested over-the-counter medications. Alongside the storage case is a log for individuals to sign out the name of the medication being taken, how much, and the date. All of the medications are in sample-size packets that constitute a single recommended dosage. Examples of the types of OTC medications available are aspirin, Benadryl, Tums, Visine, NyQuil, Zyrtec, Vasoline, ibuprofin, Ferrate, and bacitracin.

Questions for Analysis

1. Based on what you read in this case, would you operate an athletic training room like Kalyn has, making OTC drugs readily available for student-athletes to take as needed on their own? If so, why? If not, why not?

2. What do you see as the benefits to allowing student-athletes access to OTC drugs as needed?

3. What are the specific risks associated with allowing student-athletes access to OTC medications as needed?

4. Is the decision to leave OTC drugs openly available to student-athletes for self-usage up to Kalyn as the director of athletic training services? Should it be a staff decision? Should any other stakeholders be involved in making this decision?

Key Concepts and Review

Understand and support the rationale for administrating drug education and testing programs in athletics.

Drug testing is intended to safeguard the athlete's health while providing a level playing field for equitable competition.

Understand the legal ramifications of drug testing in athletic programs.

Athletes should be observed as they provide the specimen, and they should be allowed to witness the handling of the specimen. Reporting of positive tests should be limited to those who have a legitimate need for the information. The NCAA list of banned drugs is not as extensive as that used for Olympic athletes, but it still contains a wide range of drugs that can be abused and of performance-enhancing drugs. Athletic trainers who are charged with developing drug-testing programs should always seek legal counsel and should comply with the principles listed in the chapter.

Organize and implement a comprehensive drug education and testing program.

Drug tests are normally conducted after championship games, as part of the PPE, or as part of a year-round program. Athletes must consent to be tested, but lack of consent usually results in ineligibility. Random selection of subjects for testing is the norm, and random selection can have several permutations based on timing of the test or characteristics of the athlete. Testing based on reasonable suspicion requires identification of objective signs of drug use, preferably by more than one observer on more than one occasion. Urinalysis is the usual method employed in athletic drug-testing programs.

Become familiar with the legalities of dispensing and prescribing medications.

Drug dispensing is the process of preparing and packaging medications. Physicians are not legally allowed to delegate the responsibility of dispensing prescription medications to a person who is not authorized by law to dispense, including athletic trainers, unless they possess a legal dispensing license in the state that they practice in. Policies and procedures should be established that ban athletic trainers from storing or dispensing prescription medications in an athletic training facility. When dispensing medications, all standard state and federal labeling procedures should be followed.

Emergency Action Planning

Objectives

After reading this chapter, you should be able to do the following:

- Define and discuss the purpose of an emergency action plan.

- Identify the key components of an emergency action plan.

- Understand the role of each stakeholder in the development and operation of an emergency action plan.

- Establish a debriefing process following an emergency.

Every organization that is responsible for offering athletic-related programs and activities should have a written policy and procedure in place to address emergencies. While emergencies are not predictable, being prepared to manage all situations may serve to minimize adverse outcomes. This procedure is referred to as an **emergency action plan (EAP)** and should be in effect regardless of age and level of competition. An EAP should address all practices, competitions, conditioning sessions, and possible spectator involvement. Failure to have an approved written plan in place and disseminated is a breach of one's legal responsibility and increases the risk of exposure to injury, illness, and ultimately liability. Fulfilling the established standard of care requires that an athletic training program and its personnel be prepared for all types of emergency situations by having a workable EAP. This chapter focuses on the administrative aspects of developing an EAP, including the key stakeholders and equipment necessary for optimal preparation.

KEY POINT

Every emergency action plan should consider the following elements:

- Personnel and stakeholders directly involved
- Communication methods
- Venue specificity
- Transportation needed
- Equipment required
- Documentation
- Stakeholders affected
- Special considerations

Personnel

Many individuals may be involved with an emergency action plan. The personnel considered should fall into one of three categories: development, approval, and implementation. It is possible that some people are active in more than one category.

- *Development of plan.* Much work can go into the development of an emergency action plan. A plan designed for a secondary school or university may involve multiple venues and take a significant amount of time to coordinate. The development phase of an EAP includes all of the individuals who will actually write the plan. In most athletic organizations, this will primarily include the athletic trainers and the team physicians. Depending on the organization, the development of an EAP may also include facility staff, other first responders, police and safety personnel, and others (Kinderknecht 2016; Rubin 2004). For athletic venues that may not have regular athletic training coverage, it is also helpful to educate student-athletes on the emergency procedures and use of emergency equipment that will be on-site (see figure 15.1). While the covering athletic trainer is the one primarily responsible for

Personnel Involved in an EAP

- Athletic trainer
- Team physician
- Athletic training students
- Police and safety
- First responders (EMT and paramedics)
- Coaches
- Strength and conditioning coaches
- Athletic directors and administrators
- Principals
- Teachers
- Event staff
- Legal counsel
- Facility staff
- Hospital personnel

managing emergencies, many activities take place in the absence of an athletic trainer. In such cases, organizations may want to establish a policy of educating others on-site in general first aid and life-saving techniques (e.g., CPR, AED). This may include coaches, student-athletes, and other available staff.

- *Approval of plan.* Once a plan is developed and proposed, it should then be reviewed and receive formal approval. In most organizations, those who are ultimately in charge will have final approval. For example, in a secondary school, the athletic director and principal might have the final word on approving an EAP. In a university setting, it might be one or more of the following: director of athletics, director of sports medicine, or team physician. The individuals who make the final decision for approval will vary significantly from organization to organization. Regardless, all stakeholders that will be responsible for implementing the plan should be involved in the review process to ensure their approval and to provide an opportunity to identify concerns or challenges. It is strongly advised that every plan be reviewed and approved by an organization's legal counsel.

- *Implementation of plan.* The final phase of a successful emergency action plan is the actual implementation. A successful implementation begins long before an emergency actually occurs. First, an approved plan should be disseminated formally and directly to all stakeholders who will be responsible for enacting the steps of the plan. Electronic copies of the plan can be sent by e-mail, and hard copies can be distributed. Plans should also be available to the public through website links and posted at venues where appropriate. The stakeholders who will enact the plan should meet as a group to complete a walk-through. During the walk-through, the group should role-play various emergency scenarios. This allows for a review of the plan, collaboration with each other, and timely identification of concerns about the plan. This type of a rehearsal should occur at least once a year and every time new personnel are involved in the implementation. Walk-throughs should also occur at every venue that has an EAP. One should not assume that if a plan works at one venue it will work at another venue. Venue-specific walk-throughs can help to identify issues that may have been overlooked. Some of these will be discussed later in this chapter when special considerations of an EAP are addressed. The plan should address and the walk-through should assess on-field communication mechanisms. Whether mobile devices or landlines are used, it is important to perform a dry

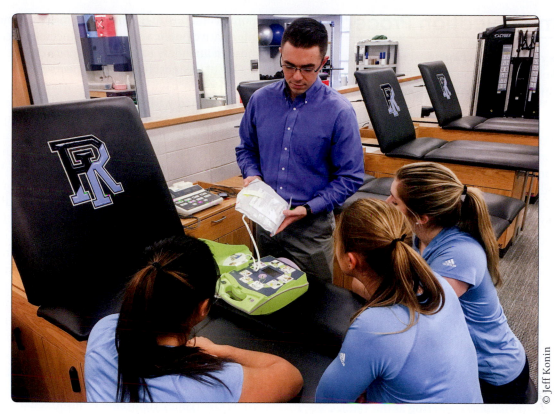
© Jeff Konin

Figure 15.1 It is important to educate student-athletes on the use of equipment in the case of an emergency.

run and ensure that a connection exists. One should be prepared for a disruption in cellular service caused by adverse weather conditions, and some venues may be located in areas where cell service is poor in general. For these reasons, one cannot rely on cell phones only in the case of an emergency and must have a backup plan. Regardless of the communication mechanism, verification of successful communication should occur prior to each and every event.

Establishing roles and responsibilities for each person involved in the implementation of an emergency action plan is important. Identifying individual roles delineates a chain of command that best matches a person's skills with the needs during an actual emergency. For example, health care providers at the scene of an emergency should be the

ones to provide immediate care. Likewise, people with no emergency health care skills can assist with communication, crowd control, and other important functions. Prior to each athletic event, event personnel should take the time to discuss and review each person's roles and responsibilities. Establishing a chain of command prevents time wasted discussing who is in charge and who will make key decisions, such as whether or not to spine-board or transport.

Likewise, visiting personnel may not be familiar with the components of the emergency action plan. It is the responsibility of personnel of the home team and venue to inform visiting team personnel of the venue-specific plan. This also includes a discussion with game officials, who play a key role in assisting in the control of an environment during emergencies. In many instances, game officials make the critical and final decisions regarding the continuance of play. For example, when an athletic trainer perceives lightning to be within a dangerous range of a playing venue, it may be the official who determines whether or not it is an emergency situation and stops play. Having these conversations before an event starts should be standard operation. The time to make such decisions is *never* during an emergency and should always be planned in advance.

Stages of an EAP

1. Development of the EAP
2. Approval of the EAP
3. Implementation of the EAP
4. Annual (at a minimum) review and update of the EAP

Communication Procedures

An emergency action plan must be communicated to all stakeholders in order to be effective. The process of communicating an EAP incorporates multiple steps, with the goal of informing as many people as possible, assuring that those who need to know the details are well informed. Once an EAP has been approved, it is safe to act as if those who will be involved with the implementation of the plan have knowledge of their role and responsibility. Each person should have a written copy of the plan, including the date most recently updated and approved. This can also be provided electronically and stored as a document on a person's mobile device. Because rescue squads will be involved in responding to emergencies at athletic venues and may have established relationships with colleges, universities, and high schools, providing a written copy of the EAP to be placed in each rescue squad vehicle is suggested. These documents can include maps of each specific venue clearly marking the venue locations and entrances. All plans should also be posted whenever possible on websites and conveyed to visitors competing at the venues.

All written EAPs should include the names and contact information of stakeholders. Not only should the names and cell phone numbers be included for stakeholders on the field, (e.g., the athletic trainers and team physicians), but also specifically how to call for emergency assistance. This may be as simple as dialing 911 for an emergency, or it may involve, for example, a university-established landline that automatically alerts all campus safety officers as well to respond. Furthermore, the plan should include a procedure for contacting administrative personnel. For example, a school principal or athletic director may not be present at every athletic event. However, should an emergency occur, she will absolutely want to know as soon as possible. Administrators may expect a direct call from the athletic trainer once the situation is under control. Different types of emergencies may call for different individuals needing to be informed. With high-profile circumstances and programs, the media may also inquire about the situation.

One small but often overlooked element of communicating an EAP is how to inform spectators of what to do in an emergency. As will be discussed later in this chapter, not all emergencies occur on a playing surface and to a participant. Some emergencies can occur to officials, coaching staff, and even spectators. Furthermore, some emergencies may be the result of inclement weather or other external variables that are not necessarily injury related. As will be explained in more detail, posting signage and making timely and informative public service announcements can alert those in attendance of an emergency event.

One of the most important aspects of communication takes place with individuals who may be related to or affiliated with an injured or ill person. It goes without saying that these folks will want to know the medical status as soon as possible. Having a plan in place to verify who you are speaking with and to appropriately share relevant information will assist in dealing with any emergency. It is important to maintain your role as a professional while balancing the delicacy of concerned family members, friends, and others. Generally, parents should be contacted prior to treatment of a minor. However, because this is not always possible, legislatures and courts have articulated the emergency medicine doctrine for minors (Martin 1994). In part, this doctrine states that medical treatment may be initiated in emergency situations "when delaying treatment to first secure parental consent would endanger the life or health of a minor." Most state laws require parental notification as soon as possible, even in states that allow emergency treatment of minors without such parental approval.

Preestablished communication with one's local hospital and rescue squads is also helpful and can improve the compliance with one's EAP. For example, managing an individual with a potential cervical spine injury requires extensive planning and interprofessional collaboration among various health care providers. Protocols regarding techniques for spine-boarding, management of the helmet and other equipment, and transferring a person from a venue to a hospital may differ. Therefore, it is essential to have well-established communication ahead of time to ensure a smooth and safe intervention (Casa et al. 2012; Courson 2007; Andersen et al. 2002).

Venue-Specific Plan

Many components of an emergency action plan for a single organization will include much of the same information. The chain of command for sharing information, how to inform caregivers of an injured individual's updated medical status, and roles and responsibilities of personnel may all be established as a standard of an approved policy and procedure. Similarly, each venue will present its own unique set of circumstances. Consider that athletic venues can be indoors, outdoors, within a pool of water, in a pole vault pit, and even through the woods during a cross country race. A venue-specific plan may differ from location to location in the following ways:

- Directions to the venue
- Venue map
- Entrance to the venue (e.g., door, gate, driveways, stairs)
- Venue surface (e.g., pool, grass, turf, court, stage)
- Locations of landlines

- Location of shelter
- List of emergency equipment available and its location (e.g., AED, spine board, oxygen)

A venue-specific emergency action plan (see figure 15.2) should also include information regarding transportation of an injured individual. It is not recommended that an athletic trainer personally

---

EMERGENCY ACTION PLAN—BUDKO STADIUM

EMERGENCY PERSONNEL
Athletic trainers and physicians on-site will assess the situation and determine whether or not to activate EMS.

EMERGENCY COMMUNICATIONS
Blue emergency phones are located at each corner of the stadium. The athletic training facility also has a landline (123) 456-7890. The athletic trainer and physician will carry a cell phone.

EMERGENCY EQUIPMENT
An AED, immobilizers, splints, and other first aid supplies are located in the athletic training facility.

FIRST RESPONDER ROLES
- Perform a primary survey (ABCs) and establish level of consciousness.
- Immediately establish the airway, breathing, and circulation of the athlete. Provide immediate care (e.g., CPR, AED, rescue breathing).
- Activate the emergency medical system (EMS).
- Call 911 and provide as much information as you can to include the following:

  Your name

  Location

  Telephone number

  General summary of what happened

  Number of victims

  Condition of victims

  Care provided thus far

  Directions to the scene (below)
- Locate and retrieve emergency equipment as needed.
- Designate an individual to meet the rescue squad at the road and direct the vehicle and personnel to the scene.
- Provide emergency personnel with the medical history of the victim if known.
- Designate one or more individuals to assist with controlling the scene.
- Notify appropriate administrators and document the occurrence.
- Communicate with family members and caretakers as appropriate.

DIRECTIONS TO BUDKO STADIUM
Enter from the main campus gates on Shero Road. Take your first left turn onto Young Lane, and proceed approximately ¼ mile to the stop sign. Turn right onto Lombardi Drive where you will enter the north end zone of the stadium and be met by a designated individual who will lead you to the scene.

Figure 15.2 Example of a venue-specific emergency action plan.

transport someone in an emergency situation. However, family members or other caregivers may request directions to the nearest emergency care facility when the injured person is transported in an ambulance. Having such information handy in written form that can be provided under circumstances of duress is helpful. Relying on oral directions, even to a facility that is close by, is not an effective way to communicate with people who are likely nervous, upset, worried, and possibly unfamiliar with the area. When a scheduled event will draw a large number of spectators, inform the local emergency care facility and hospital of the event's time. It is also suggested to provide the same facilities with a schedule of events so they can take into consideration greater activity during certain times when scheduling personnel. Lastly, providing the local rescue squad with a venue-specific emergency action plan, including aerial maps of the venues, for each vehicle is suggested.

PEARLS OF MANAGEMENT

Verify with the rescue squads that may need to enter a venue or field the width and height of their vehicles to ensure they can fit through the entry to the stadium and field.

Equipment

A critical part of planning for any emergency is to be sure that the proper equipment is available (figure 15.3). Similar to the venue-specific plan, some of the same types of emergency equipment are likely to be found at every venue, while some venues will likely require more sport- or activity-specific equipment in the case of an emergency. Determining the type of equipment needed at a venue is based on several factors including, but not limited to, environmental conditions, risk of injury with the associated sport, and venue location and setting. For example, activities held outdoors in the summer heat and in the winter cold will require different planning for extreme temperature–related emergencies. Sports like gymnastics, football, and rugby pose a greater threat of head and spinal injuries than golf and tennis do. Equipment needed to remove a facemask may be specific to football or lacrosse and should be readily accessible. Furthermore, assurance that the tools in one's possession can be used on the helmet encountered is essential. Venues on ice require different equipment for transferring an injured person safely and efficiently than venues on courts and fields. Special events and extreme sports may pose additional challenges, such as accessing elevated

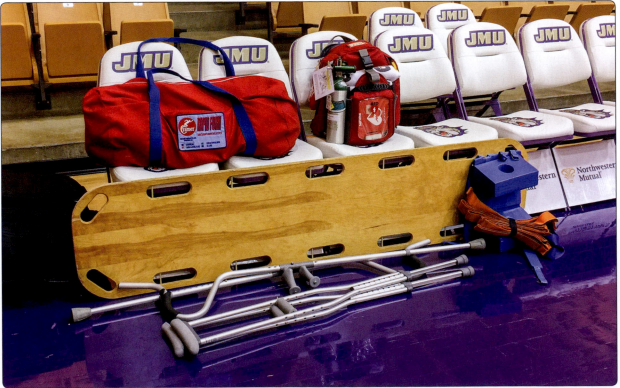

Photo courtesy of Tom Kuster

Figure 15.3 Equipment used for emergencies at athletic venues.

platforms and steep ramps. All equipment that is identified for the use of an emergency at a specific venue should be readily available and never kept in a locked place. The accessibility and working order of each piece of equipment should be verified before each event. Elements often overlooked are keys and access. For example, an ambulance might need to access the field through a locked gate, so determining who has a key to the gate in advance can save a great deal of time in an emergency.

Athletic trainers and all other personnel who will be involved in the implementation of an emergency action plan and the use of necessary equipment should maintain up-to-date certifications and credentialing. Examples of such training include administering cardiopulmonary resuscitation (CPR), operating an automated external defibrillator (AED), and implementing universal precautions for bloodborne pathogen transmission (Courson 2007). Additionally, those trained to administer oxygen, intravenous fluids, and other techniques must have up-to-date knowledge of techniques according to universal standards of care and best practices. Life-saving medications for individuals including, but not necessarily limited to, inhalers to treat asthma, epinephrine autoinjectors to manage anaphylaxis, and insulin for diabetic emergencies should also be readily available if allowed by law and appropriate guidelines for storage and dispensing are used (Rehberg 2013).

Documentation

Documentation related to emergencies can be more complex than one would initially assume. Both what is written and what is not written serve to guide policy, procedure, actions, inactions, and potential litigation. To minimize the risk of liability to an athletic trainer and to properly and thoroughly plan for the administration of the most effective emergency action plan, guidelines should be followed for documenting actions taken while developing the plan, ongoing actions during implementation, and actions taken after an emergency has occurred.

PEARLS OF MANAGEMENT

Of all the critical components of an effective emergency action plan, documentation is just as critical as any.

Thus far, we have discussed the components of an emergency action plan that should be documented before actually implementing the plan during a real-life emergency situation. This includes the process of developing the EAP and documenting the names and titles of the stakeholders who reviewed the plan, the feedback obtained from their reviews, changes made, and final approval. Dates of all exchanges of information and resulting changes should accompany all of the documentation.

Ongoing forms of documentation include walk-throughs of venue-specific emergency action plans. These should include the date, time, and individuals involved in the rehearsal. The need to document the individuals involved and the date rehearsed may seem obvious. However, the time of day may not be so obvious, but is important. For example, performing a walk-through at an outdoor stadium at noon may reveal different conditions than those encountered at an event played in the evening under the lights and in generally darker surroundings. Similarly, conditions could change during rain, snow, extreme heat, and even bright light. Most walk-throughs are performed in comfortable environments with little, if any, consideration given to how things might be different under various circumstances. Lastly, preparticipation physical exams can be considered essential documentation that will become part of an emergency situation. Catastrophic episodes, such as sudden cardiac death or heat stroke, will typically involve a review of overall medical records to determine whether preexisting signs or symptoms were identified and addressed (Hainline et al. 2016; Courson 2007; Drezner et al. 2007).

Ongoing forms of documentation typically include verification of best practices and standards. This may be a written spreadsheet that verifies communication with stakeholders if and when changes to an EAP are made. Ongoing documentation also includes verification of equipment maintenance, such as charged batteries for AEDs and adequate and appropriate storage of oxygen.

Documentation that is performed after an emergency situation is encountered is also important. Carefully putting into writing the details of the events that occurred is essential for a variety of reasons. First and foremost, being involved in an emergency situation can be extremely stressful to an athletic trainer. While focusing on the task at hand, an AT is not necessarily focused on documenting details of how things occurred or were managed. Furthermore, emergencies usually don't occur when an AT is sitting at an office desk. Rather, emergencies likely occur on a field, in a gym, or elsewhere. The athletic trainer should always be prepared regardless of where an emergency occurs. However, immediate documentation usually does not occur. Once an emergency is fully under control and the AT, along with other relevant staff, have had a chance to regain full composure, a thorough debriefing of the chain of events should be discussed and documented. Doing so allows for more accurate documentation of the episode and provides an opportunity to reflect on the emergency action plan as a whole.

While athletic trainers are frequently involved in developing EAPs, and most will experience emergencies at one time or another during a professional career, until the plan is put into place the athletic trainer does not know for sure whether it was a well-designed plan. Carefully assessing the actual execution of an emergency action plan is an important part of the process. Based on the assessment, appropriate changes can be made if necessary. Should the emergency that presented itself result in future litigation for whatever reason, thorough and detailed documentation at the time of the event is crucial. Often, notification of legal action will not occur for months, if not years, after the incident. This makes it difficult for the parties involved to remember the details of how an emergency situation presented itself and was managed.

Special Considerations

All emergency action plans should take into consideration as many possibilities as one can imagine. While some situations may occur less frequently, if at all, even the rarest of circumstances should be thought through. A few examples of special circumstances to address in an emergency action plan follow.

KEY POINT

For the complete text of NATA's position statement on emergency planning and other related papers, visit their website.

- *Weather.* The most common weather elements to trigger an EAP into effect are related to extreme heat and lightning. Emergencies related to heat illness can be life threatening, but also can be prevented with proper planning (Casa et al. 2015). Standards also exist for preparing for and managing situations that pose a risk as the result of a lightning

strike (Walsh et al. 2013). Plans will be venue specific, but it is imperative that athletic trainers follow a standardized guideline as closely as possible when they have adapted from a professional association position statement. Consideration should be given to safe evacuation from a venue and appropriate forms of shelter. Questions to consider include the following:

- Are signs posted at the venue to inform people how to evacuate?
- Has a script been written for a public service announcement to direct individuals?
- Have nearby accessible (unlocked) safe shelters been identified?

- *Team travel.* Team travel is a common responsibility of an athletic trainer. Never overlook the fact that emergencies can occur on a bus, van, or airplane or in a hotel room. What policies and procedures do you have in place in the case of an emergency while away from home? Do you travel with an accessible medical kit? Do you have standing orders from your directing physician that describe how to handle the different types of emergencies that may occur when you are traveling with a team? These are all procedural details that you should plan ahead for and have in writing. Remember, communication remains part of every emergency action plan that actively goes into effect. Thus, being sure to communicate in a timely manner with family members, administrators, and other stakeholders when on the road is important.

- *International travel.* Athletic trainers may travel to other countries with a team or individual athletes as part of a medical delegation. Furthermore, athletic trainers may travel internationally with a delegation of staff, who typically expect similar emergency and other care when necessary as a result of being away from home. Managing emergencies when away from the comfort of one's normal setting can be challenging and unique at times (Kary and Lavallee 2007). The key, like in all other situations, is to plan appropriately. Here are a few examples, but by no means an exhaustive list, of considerations to take into account:

- Communication barriers may exist with the local people when seeking assistance.
- Cell phone service may not work.
- Standard electrical wall outlets may operate with different voltage.
- Ice may not be readily available.

- Commonly used over-the-counter medications may not be found.
- Venue pathways to exit for emergencies may not be easily accessible.
- It may not be clear how the physician and emergency room visit will be paid for.
- It may not be possible to travel through airport security and country borders with all of the equipment, supplies, and medications that you would normally travel with.

● *Event spectators.* While providing athletic training services at a competition, it is not uncommon to encounter a game official experiencing a medical emergency. Similar to emergencies experienced by athletes, these can include sudden cardiac arrest, facial injuries, and diabetic comas. It is not likely that you as an athletic trainer will be aware of a game official's medical history or emergency contact information, making it more difficult in some cases during the overall assessment process. Nonetheless, a written policy should exist for managing emergency circumstances with game officials and all other individuals whose care is not technically the responsibility of the athletic trainer. As a host athletic trainer, this could also include visiting players as well as visiting coaches and staff. Historically, it has been seen as a common courtesy for a host athletic trainer to provide care for visiting parties. While it is difficult, if not unethical, to turn your back on an emergency situation for someone not directly under your care, it is imperative to have a prepared policy on such interventions. Larger-scale events, and events involving special populations, such as people with disabilities, require additional specific knowledge to plan appropriately (Motyka et al. 2005; Vasquez et al. 2015). For example, what are the ages of the participants? Do potential intellectual or physical disabilities challenge a standard emergency plan? A similar policy should exist to manage emergencies with event spectators when an on-site rescue squad is not there for that purpose. All of these considerations pertain to the liability that an athletic trainer assumes despite operating with the sole good intention to help in the event of an emergency.

● *Disaster planning.* While not typically taught as part of an athletic trainer's professional preparation, dangerous situations can occur at large-scale sporting events. These potential disasters can include terroristic acts, hostage situations, stadium collapses, and other unforeseen and unthinkable circumstances. Once again, as with all other situations, managing disasters at sporting events with mass gatherings must include detailed planning, preparation, and rehearsal to establish procedures such as proper triage and communication (Rubin 2004).

● *Clinic or hospital setting.* This chapter has focused primarily on athletic events, but emergencies can also occur in a clinic or hospital setting. The same principles outlined here can be applied to any setting. For example, if a patient in the clinic suffers a fall or cardiac event, health care providers need to know what to do, where to find the emergency equipment, how to direct emergency personnel to the correct location, and so on. Many facilities have pools that require the storage of hazardous chemicals, so emergency procedures for drownings and chemical exposure must also be in place. These same principles can also be applied to other settings where athletic trainers work, including performing arts facilities, military training sites, and factories and industrial settings.

Summary

An emergency action plan (EAP) is an essential component of all athletic training settings. The EAP is a written document that is designed to respond to unplanned emergency situations. The EAP is venue specific, and is developed, reviewed, rehearsed, and implemented with the inclusion of various stakeholders. Key components of the EAP include methods of communication, modes of transportation, required equipment, documentation, and other special considerations such as travel, weather, and spectators.

Learning Aids

Case Study 1

Justin decided that he wanted to pick up some per diem work for a local out-patient rehabilitation clinic to help pay off some of his student loans. Despite having recently graduated and having his loans deferred for a few months, he knew it would be a good idea to not only earn some extra money, but also to gain additional experience. After signing a contract to provide per diem athletic training coverage at one of the local venues, he was excited to finally put his skills to use for a good cause. During the first few events that Justin covered, he realized that there was no emergency action plan of any kind for the venue. He remembered from school how important it was to have a plan, and not only possess it, but also to ensure it was reviewed and ready at all times to implement. When Justin inquired with the employer with whom he agreed to work on a per diem basis, he wasn't too thrilled with the response he received. The clinic's director, who is not an athletic trainer, said that they are not responsible for the field, they are just there to provide first aid coverage, and that "usually nothing ever happens, so it is really easy money and good marketing for us."

Questions for Analysis

1. Should Justin be concerned that there is no EAP? Or based on what his director told him, is there no reason to worry because it is a low-risk situation?
2. If you were in Justin's position, what would you do first?
3. If Justin were to decide to develop his own EAP, what are the key steps he should consider?
4. If Justin created an EAP for this venue, how would he disseminate the information to all of the stakeholders? Who are all of the stakeholders?

Case Study 2

As an athletic training student, reflect on one of your clinical experiences that took place at a home-venue event when the visiting team did not have an on-site athletic trainer.

Questions for Analysis

1. Did you have conversations with your preceptor regarding athletic training coverage for athletes of the opposing team? Did you discuss care in the case of an emergency to staff members of the opposing team?
2. If you had a discussion, what was discussed? If you did not have a discussion, how were you planning to manage an emergency?
3. Do you know whether a written policy and procedures exist for the situation you encountered?
4. As part of this case study, review existing policy and procedures that exist at your clinical site. If one does not exist, speak with your preceptor and ask why it does not exist and how things are handled consistently in the absence of a written standard.

Key Concepts and Review

Define and discuss the purpose of an emergency action plan.

An emergency action plan (EAP) is a written policy and procedure developed to address emergencies. An EAP should address all practices, competitions, conditioning sessions, and possible spectator involvement.

Identify the key components of an emergency action plan.

Key components of an EAP include personnel and stakeholders directly involved, communication methods, venue specificity, transportation needed, equipment required, documentation, stakeholders affected, and other special considerations.

Understand the role of each stakeholder in the development and operation of an emergency action plan.

Personnel considered as stakeholders fall into one of three categories: development, approval, and implementation. It is possible that some individuals may be involved in more than one category. The development phase of an EAP includes all of the individuals who will actually write the plan. All stakeholders who will be responsible for implementing the plan should be involved in the review process to ensure their approval and to provide for an opportunity to identify concerns or challenges. It is recommended that legal counsel be included in the approval process of an EAP. Implementation stakeholders are those who would most likely be at an event when an emergency might occur. These individuals should each have a designated role in the case of an emergency, and they should have rehearsed the plan for optimal preparedness.

Establish a debriefing process following an emergency.

Once an emergency has been resolved, a thorough debriefing of the chain of events should be discussed and documented. This allows for more accurate documentation of the episode and provides an opportunity to reflect on the emergency action plan as a whole. Based on the assessment, appropriate changes can be made if necessary.

Health Care Professionals

The following is a list of professionals who may interact with an athletic trainer in a variety of settings. The list is not all-inclusive, and as the profession of athletic training grows, additional members will likely be added.

Chiropractor (DC)—treat patients with health problems of the neuromusculoskeletal system. Chiropractors use spinal adjustments and manipulation and other techniques to manage patients' health concerns, such as back and neck pain.

Dentist (DMD)—diagnose and treat problems with patients' teeth, gums, and related parts of the mouth. They provide advice and instruction for taking care of the teeth and gums and for dietary choices that affect oral health. May also assist with custom mouth guards for sport and activity.

Diagnostic medical sonographer—operate special imaging equipment to create images or to conduct tests under the direction of a physician. Diagnostic musculoskeletal ultrasound is an example.

Dietitian—expert in the use of food and nutrition to promote health and manage disease. They advise people on what to eat in order to lead a healthy lifestyle or achieve a specific health-related goal. Play key roles in assisting in the treatment of eating disorders such as anorexia and bulimia.

Emergency medical technician (EMT)—along with paramedics, respond to emergency calls, perform medical services, and transport patients to medical facilities. EMTs often are on-site at major sporting events and work closely in event planning with the athletic training staff.

Exercise physiologist—develop fitness and exercise programs that help patients recover from chronic diseases and improve cardiovascular function, body composition, and flexibility. Exercise physiologists may work with athletic trainers to establish baseline testing and performance capabilities of athletes.

Massage therapist (MT)—treat clients by using various manual therapies to the soft tissues of the body. Massage therapists may be found on staff or work with athletic trainers through consultation.

Medical laboratory technologist (MLT)—collect samples and perform tests to analyze body fluids, tissue, and other substances. While often found in a hospital or out-patient lab setting, they may also work with athletic trainers as part of an on-site primary care facility.

Mental health practitioner—psychiatrists are one example of a mental health professional who offers services for the purpose of improving an individual's mental health or to treat mental illness. As mental health concerns have become more prevalent, the addition of these practitioners in partnership with athletic training services is increasing.

Nurse practitioner (NP)—also referred to as advanced practice registered nurse (APRN), coordinate patient care and may provide primary and specialty health care. The scope of practice varies from state to state. May be found working with athletic trainers in various settings with the capacity to medically diagnose and order images and medications.

Occupational therapist (OT)—treat injured or ill patients or patients with disabilities through the therapeutic use of everyday activities. They help these patients develop, recover, and improve the skills needed for daily living and working. While not commonly seen working closely with athletic trainers, in some settings, OTs and ATs are found on the same health care team.

Ophthalmologist (OD)—specialist for care and treatment of medical and surgical needs of the eye.

Optometrist—examine the eyes and other parts of the visual system. They prescribe eyeglasses or contact lenses as needed and specialize in refractive management and medical and therapeutic care.

Orthopedic surgeon (MD)—a surgeon who has been educated and trained in the diagnosis and preoperative, operative, and postoperative treatment of diseases and injuries of the musculoskeletal system. Often serves as a team physician in an athletic setting, and the athletic trainer works under his or her direction.

Orthotist and prosthetist (O & P)—design and fabricate medical supportive devices and measure and fit patients for them. These devices include artificial limbs (arms, hands, legs, and feet), braces, and other medical or surgical devices.

Pharmacist (PharmD)—dispense prescription medications to patients and offer expertise in the safe use of prescriptions. They also may conduct health and wellness screenings, provide immunizations, and oversee the medications given to patients.

Physical therapist (PT)—enhance and restore functional ability and quality of life to those with physical impairments or disabilities. Physical therapists may be part of the rehabilitation team.

Physician assistant (PA)—practice medicine on teams with physicians, surgeons, and other health care workers. They examine, diagnose, and treat patients under the direction of a physician.

Podiatrist (DPM)—provide medical care for people with foot, ankle, and lower-leg problems. They diagnose illnesses, treat injuries, and perform surgery involving the lower extremities.

Primary care physician (PCP)—provide both the first contact for a person with an undiagnosed health concern as well as continuing care of various medical conditions. PCPs examine patients; take medical histories; prescribe medications; and order, perform, and interpret diagnostic tests. In athletic environments, PCPs often serve as the team physician.

Public health practitioner—focus on improving health among individuals, families, and communities through the prevention and treatment of diseases and promotion of healthy behaviors.

Radiologist—a physician who reads and interprets diagnostic imaging examinations, such as X rays, MRIs, and CT scans.

Registered Nurse (RN)—provide and coordinate patient care, educate patients and the public about various health conditions, and provide advice and emotional support to patients and their family members.

Social worker—community provider who facilitates the welfare of communities, individuals, families, and groups. Social workers may assist an athletic trainer in unique cases when a family may need to be involved in a situation.

Speech-language pathologist (SLP)—assess, diagnose, treat, and help prevent communication and swallowing disorders in patients. Referred to as a speech therapist.

Sport psychologist—focus on the psychological factors that affect performance and how participation in sport and exercise affect psychological and physical factors. Sport psychologists work closely with athletic trainers and athletes, especially during extended or prolonged phases of rehabilitation.

Certified strength and conditioning specialist (CSCS)—apply scientific knowledge to train athletes for the primary goal of improving athletic performance. They conduct sport-specific testing sessions, design and implement safe and effective strength training and conditioning programs, and provide guidance on nutrition and injury prevention.

SWOT Analysis
for a Sports Medicine Program

The following nine worksheets comprise a SWOT analysis for a sports medicine program. This worksheet package has been adapted from material created by D.A. Campbell and Company for Hope College.

WORKSHEET 1: BENEFITS AND CONCERNS RELATIVE TO STRATEGIC PLANNING

INSTRUCTIONS

1. List the benefits you expect from our strategic planning as well as any concerns.
2. Note possible ways to overcome each of your concerns. Circle the best ideas.

Benefits expected:

Concerns:

Ways to overcome concerns:

WORKSHEET 2: ORGANIZING THE PLANNING PROCESS

INSTRUCTIONS

Indicate how each of the following issues should be handled. Outline the steps, responsibilities, and time lines for developing the strategic plan.

1. What are we developing a strategic plan for?

   The entire sports medicine program

   Only part of the sports medicine program (which part?)

   The entire sports medicine program and each of its subprograms

   Other

2. For what period of time should we plan?

Next 2 years	Next 5 years
Next 3 years	Next 6 years
Next 4 years	Other

3. What critical issues do you hope the planning will address?

4. How much time should we spend planning?

5. Should we use a consultant or other resource person in developing our plan?

   Yes

   No

   Unsure

   If so, what kind of help do we need?

6. Who should be part of the planning team? Circle all that apply.

Athletic trainers	Consultants
Athletic administrators	Patients
Athletic training students	Team physicians
Coaches	Others

7. How many members should the planning team have?

   5-8

   9-12

   13-16

   17-20

   More than 20

8. Are there others we should involve in the development of the plan? In the review of the plan?

9. Who should manage the overall planning effort?

10. Who should lead or chair the planning meetings?

11. By what date should we have the plan completed for approval?

12. Outline the steps you envision us using as we develop our plan.
    Steps
    Person(s) responsible
    Deadline

WORKSHEET 3: HISTORY AND PRESENT SITUATION

INSTRUCTIONS

Review the history and present situation of the sports medicine program as they pertain to your area of responsibility. List any historical trends that will need attention as we plan for the future. Do not hesitate to comment on areas *outside* of your realm of responsibility if you so desire.

Historical trends

WORKSHEET 4: QUESTIONS ABOUT MISSION

1. Describe below what you understand the mission of the sports medicine program to be.

2. List questions, ideas, or concerns you have about the present mission of the sports medicine program.

3. Do you envision changes in the mission of the sports medicine program? If so, what do you want to accomplish? Who will be served by such a change?

WORKSHEET 5: CLIENT, CUSTOMER, AND STAKEHOLDER NEEDS

INSTRUCTIONS

1. List the needs of present or potential "customers" that the sports medicine program might address. Note ideas for how the sports medicine program might meet those needs.

2. List the significant groups who have a stake in what the sports medicine program does. How can the program meet their needs?

Clients and Customers

Describe existing or possible new target groups.	
Their needs:	Ways to meet those needs:

Other stakeholders	
Their needs:	Ways to meet those needs:

WORKSHEET 6: COMPETITORS AND ALLIES

INSTRUCTIONS

1. List present and potential new competitors, what the sports medicine program competes for, and our program's relative advantages and disadvantages (e.g., price, services).

2. List possible allies and how the sports medicine program might team up with each organization, person, or group.

Competitors

Existing:

New:

What we compete for

Our advantages:	Our disadvantages:
Allies of the sports medicine program:	How can we team up with our allies?

WORKSHEET 7: OPPORTUNITIES AND THREATS

INSTRUCTIONS

1. List and rank the major opportunities and threats that you believe the sports medicine program will face in the next five years that will determine its success or failure.

2. Use the information from worksheets 5 and 6 to help provide a more detailed analysis of our clients and stakeholders.

3. Be sure to consider the social, cultural, economic, political, and technological forces that may affect the sports medicine program in the next five years.

Opportunities	Threats

WORKSHEET 8: STRENGTHS AND WEAKNESSES

INSTRUCTIONS

List the major strengths and weaknesses of the sports medicine program as it looks toward the future.

Strengths and assets	Weaknesses and liabilities

WORKSHEET 9: CRITICAL ISSUES FOR THE FUTURE

INSTRUCTIONS

Review worksheets 3 through 8 and list critical issues or choices that the sports medicine program faces over the next five years.

Critical issues or choices

NATA Code of Ethics

PREAMBLE

The National Athletic Trainers' Association Code of Ethics states the principles of ethical behavior that should be followed in the practice of athletic training. It is intended to establish and maintain high standards and professionalism for the athletic training profession. The principles do not cover every situation encountered by the practicing athletic trainer, but are representative of the spirit with which athletic trainers should make decisions. The principles are written generally; the circumstances of a situation will determine the interpretation and application of a given principle and of the Code as a whole. When a conflict exists between the Code and the law, the law prevails.

1. MEMBERS SHALL PRACTICE WITH COMPASSION, RESPECTING THE RIGHTS, WELFARE, AND DIGNITY OF OTHERS

1.1. Members shall render quality patient care regardless of the patient's race, religion, age, sex, ethnic or national origin, disability, health status, socioeconomic status, sexual orientation, or gender identity.

1.2. Member's duty to the patient is the first concern, and therefore members are obligated to place the welfare and long-term well-being of their patient above other groups and their own self-interest, to provide competent care in all decisions, and advocate for the best medical interest and safety of their patient at all times as delineated by professional statements and best practices.

1.3. Members shall preserve the confidentiality of privileged information and shall not release or otherwise publish in any form, including social media, such information to a third party not involved in the patient's care without a release unless required by law.

2. MEMBERS SHALL COMPLY WITH THE LAWS AND REGULATIONS GOVERNING THE PRACTICE OF ATHLETIC TRAINING, NATIONAL ATHLETIC TRAINERS' ASSOCIATION (NATA) MEMBERSHIP STANDARDS, AND THE NATA CODE OF ETHICS

2.1. Members shall comply with applicable local, state, federal laws, and any state athletic training practice acts.

2.2. Members shall understand and uphold all NATA Standards and the Code of Ethics.

2.3. Members shall refrain from, and report illegal or unethical practices related to athletic training.

2.4. Members shall cooperate in ethics investigations by the NATA, state professional licensing/regulatory boards, or other professional agencies governing the athletic training profession. Failure to fully cooperate in an ethics investigation is an ethical violation.

2.5. Members must not file, or encourage others to file, a frivolous ethics complaint with any organization or entity governing the athletic training profession such that the complaint is unfounded or willfully ignore facts that would disprove the allegation(s) in the complaint.

2.6. Members shall refrain from substance and alcohol abuse. For any member involved in an ethics proceeding with NATA and who, as part of that proceeding is seeking rehabilitation for substance or alcohol dependency, documentation of the completion of rehabilitation must be provided to the NATA Committee on Professional Ethics as a requisite to complete a NATA membership reinstatement or suspension process.

3. MEMBERS SHALL MAINTAIN AND PROMOTE HIGH STANDARDS IN THEIR PROVISION OF SERVICES

3.1. Members shall not misrepresent, either directly or indirectly, their skills, training, professional credentials, identity, or services.

3.2. Members shall provide only those services for which they are qualified through education or experience and which are allowed by the applicable state athletic training practice acts and other applicable regulations for athletic trainers.

3.3. Members shall provide services, make referrals, and seek compensation only for those services that are necessary and are in the best interest of the patient as delineated by professional statements and best practices.

3.4. Members shall recognize the need for continuing education and participate in educational activities that enhance their skills and knowledge and shall complete such educational requirements necessary to continue to qualify as athletic trainers under the applicable state athletic training practice acts.

3.5. Members shall educate those whom they supervise in the practice of athletic training about the Code of Ethics and stress the importance of adherence.

3.6. Members who are researchers or educators must maintain and promote ethical conduct in research and educational activities.

4. MEMBERS SHALL NOT ENGAGE IN CONDUCT THAT COULD BE CONSTRUED AS A CONFLICT OF INTEREST, REFLECTS NEGATIVELY ON THE ATHLETIC TRAINING PROFESSION, OR JEOPARDIZES A PATIENT'S HEALTH AND WELL-BEING

4.1. Members should conduct themselves personally and professionally in a manner that does not compromise their professional responsibilities or the practice of athletic training.

4.2. All NATA members, whether current or past, shall not use the NATA logo in the endorsement of products or services, or exploit their affiliation with the NATA in a manner that reflects badly upon the profession.

4.3. Members shall not place financial gain above the patient's welfare and shall not participate in any arrangement that exploits the patient.

4.4. Members shall not, through direct or indirect means, use information obtained in the course of the practice of athletic training to try and influence the score or outcome of an athletic event, or attempt to induce financial gain through gambling.

4.5. Members shall not provide or publish false or misleading information, photography, or any other communications in any media format, including on any social media platform, related to athletic training that negatively reflects the profession, other members of the NATA, NATA officers, and the NATA office.

Athletic Training: State Regulation, Scope of Practice, Board and Structure, and Regulation

ALABAMA

Regulation: Licensure

Scope of practice: Practice by an athletic trainer of any of the following: a. Under physician direction or referral, or both, the prevention of athletic injuries. b. The organization and administration of athletic training programs. c. Athletic counseling and guidance and the education of athletes regarding athletics and athletic training. d. Under physician direction and referral, the rehabilitation and reconditioning of an athlete. e. Under physician supervision, the evaluation, the recognition, and the management of athletic injuries.

Board and structure: Alabama Board of Athletic Trainers (6 ATs, 1 PT, 3 physicians)

Regulatory requirements: Annual application and fee

ALASKA

Regulation: Licensure

Scope of practice: The practice of an athletic trainer includes: (1) the treatment of an athlete for an athletic injury or illness prevention, (2) the clinical evaluation and assessment of an athlete for an athletic injury or illness sustained or exacerbated while participating in an athletic or sport-related exercise or activity, (3) the immediate care and treatment of an athlete for an athletic injury or illness sustained or exacerbated while participating in an athletic or sport-related exercise or activity, and (4) the rehabilitation and reconditioning of an athlete from an athletic injury or illness sustained or exacerbated while participating in an athletic or sport-related exercise or activity

Board and structure: Alaska Department of Commerce, Community, and Economic Development

Regulatory requirements: Biennial application and fee

ARIZONA

Regulation: Licensure

Scope of practice: Athletic training includes the following performed under the direction of a licensed physician and for which the athletic trainer has received appropriate education and training as prescribed by the board: (a) The prevention, recognition, examination, evaluation, rehabilitation, and management of athletic injuries. (b) The prevention, evaluation, immediate care, and monitoring of athletic illnesses. (c) The referral of a person receiving athletic training services to appropriate health care professionals, as necessary. (d) The use of heat, cold, water, light, sound, electricity, passive or active exercise, massage, mechanical devices, or any other therapeutic modality to prevent, treat, rehabilitate, or recondition athletic injuries. (e) The planning, administration, evaluation, and modification of methods for prevention and risk management of athletic injuries and athletic illnesses. (f) Education and counseling related to all aspects of the practice of athletic training. (g) The use of topical pharmacological agents in conjunction with the administration of therapeutic modalities and pursuant to a prescription issued pursuant to the laws of this state and for which an athletic trainer has received appropriate education and training.

Board and structure: Arizona Board of Athletic Training (3 ATs and 2 public members)

Regulatory requirements: Annual application and fee

ARKANSAS

Regulation: Licensure

Scope of practice: *Athletic training* means the prevention, recognition, evaluation, treatment, and rehabilitation of an athletic injury or illness and the organization and administration of exercise, conditioning, and athletic training programs.

Board and structure: Arkansas Board of Athletic Training (4 ATs and 1 public member)

Regulatory requirements: Annual application and fee

CALIFORNIA

Regulation: No Regulation

Scope of practice: None

Board and structure: No Regulation nor board

Regulatory requirements: Not available

COLORADO

Regulation: Registration

Scope of practice: (a) Athletic training includes services appropriate for the prevention, recognition, assessment, management, treatment, rehabilitation, and reconditioning of injuries and illnesses sustained by an athlete (I) engaged in sports, games, recreation, or exercise requiring physical strength, flexibility, range of motion, speed, stamina, or agility; or (II) that affect an athlete's participation or performance in such sports, games, recreation, or exercise. (b) Athletic training includes (I) the planning, administration, evaluation, and modification of methods for prevention and risk management of injuries and illnesses; (II) the identification and appropriate care and referral of medical conditions and disabilities associated with athletes; (III) the recognition, assessment, treatment, management, prevention, rehabilitation, reconditioning, and appropriate referral of injuries and illnesses; (IV) the use of therapeutic modalities for which the athletic trainer has received appropriate training and education; (V) the use of conditioning and rehabilitative exercise; (VI) the use of topical pharmacological agents, in conjunction with the administration of therapeutic modalities and pursuant to prescriptions issued in accordance with the laws of this state, for which the athletic trainer has received appropriate training and education; (VII) the education and counseling of athletes concerning the prevention and care of injuries and illnesses; (VIII) the education and counseling of the general public with respect to athletic training services; (IX) the referral of an athlete receiving athletic training services to appropriate health care personnel as needed; and (X) the planning, organization, administration, and evaluation of the practice of athletic training.

Board and structure: Colorado Board of Medical Examiners (Office of Athletic Trainer Registration: 1 director)

Regulatory requirements: Biennial application and fee

CONNECTICUT

Regulation: Licensure

Scope of practice: *Athletic training* means the application or provision, with the consent and under the direction of a health care provider, of (A) principles, methods and procedures of evaluation, prevention, treatment and rehabilitation of athletic injuries sustained by athletes, (B) appropriate preventative and supportive devices, temporary splinting and bracing, physical modalities of heat, cold, light massage, water, electric stimulation, sound, exercise and exercise equipment, (C) the organization and administration of athletic training programs, and (D) education and counseling to athletes, coaches, medical personnel, and athletic communities in the area of the prevention and care of athletic injuries.

Board and structure: Connecticut Department of Public Health

Regulatory requirements: Biennial application and fee

DELAWARE

Regulation: Licensure

Scope of practice: *Athletic training* means the prevention, evaluation, and treatment of athletic injuries by the utilization of therapeutic exercises and modalities such as heat, cold, light, air, water, sound, electricity, massage, and nonthrust mobilizations.

Board and structure: Delaware Examining Board of Physical Therapy (4 PTs, 1 PTA, 2 ATs, 3 pubic members)

Regulatory requirements: Biennial application and fee

DISTRICT OF COLUMBIA

Regulation: Licensure

Scope of practice: *Practice of athletic training* means any of the following: (i) The treatment of an athletic injury that is (I) for an athlete whose condition is within the professional and educational ability of the licensed athletic trainer; and (II) performed under the general supervision of a physician who has issued any written order, protocol, or recommendation for an athletic injury; (ii) the immediate treatment of athletic injuries, including common emergency medical situations; (iii) the provision of education, guidance, and counseling to athletes, coaches, parents of athletes, and athletic communities regarding athletic training and the prevention, care, and treatment of athletic injuries; and (iv) the organization and administration of athletic training programs.

Board and structure: Board of Physical Therapy (4 PTs and 1 public member)

Regulatory requirements: Awaiting regulatory phase

FLORIDA

Regulation: Licensure

Scope of practice: *Athletic training* means the recognition, prevention, and treatment of athletic injuries.

Board and structure: Florida State Health Department (Florida Board of Athletic Trainers; 5 ATs, 2 physicians, 2 public members)

Regulatory requirements: Biennial application and fee

GEORGIA

Regulation: Licensure

Scope of practice: *Athletic trainer* means a person with specific qualifications, who, upon the advice and consent of a physician, carries out the practice of prevention, recognition, evaluation, management, disposition, treatment, or rehabilitation of athletic injuries, and, in carrying out these functions, the athletic trainer is authorized to use physical modalities, such as heat, light, sound, cold, electricity, or mechanical devices related to prevention, recognition, evaluation, management, disposition, rehabilitation, and treatment.

Board and structure: Georgia Board of Athletic Trainers (2 ATs, 1 physician, and 1 public member)

Regulatory requirements: Biennial application and fee

HAWAII

Regulation: Registration

Scope of practice: *Practice of athletic training* refers to the application by an athletic trainer, whether or not registered under this chapter and without regard to certification by any certifying body, of principles and methods to (1) prevent athletic injuries; (2) recognize, evaluate, and assess athletic injuries and conditions; (3) provide immediate care of athletic injuries, including common emergency medical care; (4) treat, rehabilitate, and recondition athletic injuries; (5) administer athletic training services and organization; and (6) educate athletes.

Board and structure: Hawaii Department of Commerce and Consumer Affairs

Professional and Vocational Licensing (1 director)

Regulatory requirements: Triennial application and fee

IDAHO

Regulation: Licensure

Scope of practice: *Athletic training* means the application by a licensed athletic trainer of principles and methods of (a) prevention of athletic injuries; (b) recognition, evaluation, and assessment of athletic injuries and conditions; (c) immediate care of athletic injuries including common emergency medical situations; (d) rehabilitation and reconditioning of athletic injuries; (e) athletic training services administration and organization; and (f) education of athletes.

Board and structure: Idaho State Board of Medicine (Board of Athletic Trainers; 3 ATs and 1 public member)

Regulatory requirements: Annual application and fee

ILLINOIS

Regulation: Licensure

Scope of practice: *Licensed athletic trainer* means a person licensed to practice athletic training and with the specific qualifications who, upon the direction of his or her team physician or consulting physician, carries out the practice of prevention/emergency care or physical reconditioning of injuries incurred by athletes participating in an athletic program conducted by an educational institution, professional athletic organization, or sanctioned amateur athletic organization employing the athletic trainer; or a person who, under the direction of a physician, carries out comparable functions for a health organization-based extramural program of athletic training services for athletes.

Board and structure: Illinois Department of Professional Regulation (Illinois Board of Athletic Training; 4 ATs, 2 physicians, 1 public member)

Regulatory requirements: Biennial application and fee

INDIANA

Regulation: Licensure

Scope of practice: *Athletic training* means the practice of prevention, recognition, assessment, management, treatment, disposition, and reconditioning of athletic injuries under the direction of a licensed physician, osteopath, podiatrist, or chiropractor. However, in a clinic accessible to the general public, the term means practicing athletic training only upon the referral and order of a licensed physician, osteopath, podiatrist, or chiropractor. The term includes the following:

(1) Practice that may be conducted by an athletic trainer through the use of heat, light, sound, cold, electricity, exercise, rehabilitation, or mechanical devices related to the care and the conditioning of athletes. (2) The organization and administration of educational programs and athletic facilities. (3) The education and the counseling of the public on matters related to athletic training.

Board and structure: Indiana Athletic Trainers Board (4 ATs, 2 physicians, and 1 public member)

Regulatory requirements: Biennial application and fee

IOWA

Regulation: Licensure

Scope of practice: *Practice of athletic training* means the prevention, physical evaluation, emergency care, and physical reconditioning relating to injuries and illnesses incurred through sports-induced trauma, which occurs during the preparation for or participation in a sports competition or during a physical training program, either of which is sponsored by an educational institution, amateur or professional athletic group, or other recognized organization, by a person who uses the title of licensed athletic trainer.

Board and structure: Iowa Board of Athletic Training (3 ATs, 3 physicians, 1 public member)

Regulatory requirements: Biennial application and fee

KANSAS

Regulation: Licensure

Scope of practice: *Athletic training* means the practice of injury prevention, physical evaluation, emergency care, and referral or physical reconditioning relating to athletic activity.

Board and structure: Kansas State Board of the Healing Arts (Athletic Training Council: 3 ATs, 2 physicians, and 1 chiropractor)

Regulatory requirements: Annual application and fee

KENTUCKY

Regulation: Licensure

Scope of practice: *Athletic trainer* means a person with specific qualifications, who, upon the advice and consent of a team physician, carries out the practice of prevention or physical rehabilitation, or both, of injuries incurred by participating athletes at an educational institution, professional athletic organization, or other bona fide athletic organization. In carrying out these functions the athletic trainer is authorized to use whatever physical modalities as are deemed necessary by a team physician.

Board and structure: Kentucky Board of Medical Licensure (Athletic Training State Advisory Council: 5 ATs, 2 physicians, 1 board member, and 1 public member)

Regulatory requirements: Triennial application and fee

LOUISIANA

Regulation: Licensure

Scope of practice: *Athletic trainer* means an individual licensed by the board as an athletic trainer with the specific qualifications who, under the general supervision of a physician carries out the practice of prevention, emergency management, and physical rehabilitation of injuries and sports-related conditions incurred by athletes. In carrying out these functions, the athletic trainer shall use whatever physical modalities are prescribed by a team physician or consulting physician, or both.

Board and structure: Louisiana State Board of Medical Examiners

Regulatory requirements: Biennial application and fee

MAINE

Regulation: Licensure

Scope of practice: *Athletic training* means a. prevention of athletic injuries; b. recognition and evaluation of athletic injuries; c. management, treatment, and disposition of athletic injuries; d. rehabilitation of athletic injuries; e. organization and administration of an athletic training program; and f. education and counseling of athletes, recreational athletes, coaches, family members, medical personnel and communities in the area of care and prevention of athletic injuries.

Board and structure: Maine Department of Professional and Financial Regulation

Regulatory requirements: Annual application and fee

MARYLAND

Regulation: Licensure

Scope of practice: *Athletic training* means (1) application of the following principles and methods for managing athletic injuries for active individuals and athletes in good overall health under the supervision of a licensed physician: (I) prevention; (II) clinical evaluation and assessment; (III) immediate care; and (IV) treatment, rehabilitation and reconditioning, (2) (I) organization and administration of an athletic training program; and (II) instruction to coaches athletes, parents, medical personnel and community members regarding the care and prevention of athletic injuries.

Board and structure: Maryland Board of Physicians

Regulatory requirements: Biennial application and fee

MASSACHUSETTS

Regulation: Licensure

Scope of practice: *Athletic training* includes the application of principles, methods, and procedures of evaluation and treatment of athletic injuries; preconditioning, conditioning, and reconditioning of the athlete through the use of appropriate preventive and supportive devices; temporary splinting and bracing; physical modalities of heat, cold, massage, water, electric stimulation, sound, exercise, and exercise equipment under the discretion of a physician. Athletic training includes instruction to coaches, athletes, parents, medical personnel, and communities in the area of care and prevention of athletic injuries.

Board and structure: Massachusetts Division of Professional Licensure

Regulatory requirements: Biennial application and fee

MICHIGAN

Regulation: Licensure

Scope of practice: *Practice of athletic training* means the treatment of an individual for risk management and injury prevention, the clinical evaluation and assessment of an individual for an injury or illness, or both, the immediate care and treatment of an individual for an injury or illness, or both, and the rehabilitation and reconditioning of an individual's injury or illness and performed under the direction and supervision of a licensed physician.

Board and structure: Michigan Department of Community Health

Regulatory requirements: Initial license issued for one year with application and fee, and then triennial application and fee

MINNESOTA

Regulation: Registration

Scope of practice: An athletic trainer shall (1) prevent, recognize, and evaluate athletic injuries; (2) give emergency care and first aid; (3) manage and treat athletic injuries; and (4) rehabilitate and physically recondition athletic injuries. The athletic trainer may use modalities such as cold, heat, light, sound, electricity, exercise, and mechanical devices for treatment and rehabilitation of athletic injuries to athletes in the primary employment site.

Board and structure: Minnesota Athletic Trainers' Advisory Council – State Board of Medical Practice

Regulatory requirements: Annual application and fee

MISSISSIPPI

Regulation: Licensure

Scope of practice: *Athletic trainer* means a person licensed by the State Department of Health as an athletic trainer after meeting the requirements of this chapter and rules and regulations promulgated pursuant to this chapter, who, upon the advice, consent, and oral or written prescriptions or referrals of a licensed physician, nurse practitioner, or physician assistant, carries out the practice of athletic training, and in carrying out these functions, the athletic trainer is authorized to use physical modalities, such as heat, light, sound, cold, electricity, or mechanical devices related to prevention, recognition, evaluation, management, disposition, rehabilitation, and treatment. An athletic trainer shall practice only in those areas in which the athletic trainer is competent by reason of training or experience that can be substantiated by records or other evidence found acceptable by the board in the exercise of the board's considered discretion.

Board and structure: Mississippi State Department of Health (Athletic Trainers Advisory Council: 5 ATs)

Regulatory requirements: Annual application and fee

MISSOURI

Regulation: Licensure

Scope of practice: *Athletic trainer* means a person who meets qualifications and who, upon the direction of the team physician or consulting physician, or both, practices prevention, emergency care, first aid, treatment, or physical rehabilitation of injuries incurred by athletes in the manner, means, and methods deemed necessary to effect care or rehabilitation, or both.

Board and structure: Missouri Athletic Trainer Advisory Committee (3 ATs, 1 physician, and 1 public member)

Regulatory requirements: Annual application and fee

MONTANA

Regulation: Licensure

Scope of practice: *Athletic training* means the practice of prevention, recognition, assessment, management, treatment, disposition, and reconditioning of athletic injuries. The term includes the following: (a) the use of heat, light, sound, cold, electricity, exercise, reconditioning, or mechanical devices related to the care and conditioning of athletes; and (b) the education and counseling of the public on matters related to athletic training.

Board and structure: Montana Board of Athletic Trainers (3 ATs, 1 physician, and 1 public member)

Regulatory requirements: Annual renewal

NEBRASKA

Regulation: Licensure

Scope of practice: *Athletic trainer* means a person who is responsible for the prevention, emergency care, first aid, treatment, and rehabilitation of athletic injuries under guidelines established with a licensed physician.

Board and structure: Nebraska Department of Health and Human Services Regulation and Licensure (Board of Athletic Training: 3 ATs and 1 public member)

Regulatory requirements: Biennial application and fee

NEVADA

Regulation: Licensure

Scope of practice: *Practice of athletic training* means (a) the prevention, recognition, assessment, management, treatment, disposition, or reconditioning of the athletic injury of an athlete: (1) whose condition is within the professional preparation and education of the licensed athletic trainer; and (2) that is performed under the direction of a physician; (b) the organization and administration of programs of athletic training; (c) the administration of an athletic training room; (d) the provision of information relating to athletic training to members of the public; or (e) any combination of the activities described in paragraphs (a) to (d), inclusive.

Board and structure: Nevada State Board of Athletic Training (3 ATs, 1 PT, and 1 public member)

Regulatory requirements: Annual application and fee

NEW HAMPSHIRE

Regulation: Licensure

Scope of practice: *Athletic training* means the practice, with respect to injuries or conditions incurred by participants in organized or recreational sports, of (a) prevention; (b) assessment and evaluation; (c) acute care, management, treatment, and disposition; (d) rehabilitation and

reconditioning; and (e) education, counseling and program administration, provided such care is within the professional preparation and education of athletic trainers and under the direction of a physician licensed in any state or in Canada.

Board and structure: New Hampshire Office of Allied Health Professionals (Board of Athletic Trainers: 3 ATs, 1 physician, and 1 public member)

Regulatory requirements: Biennial application and fee

NEW JERSEY

Regulation: Licensure

Scope of practice: *Athletic training* means and includes the practice of physical conditioning and reconditioning of athletes and the prevention of injuries incurred by athletes. Athletic training shall also include the application of physical treatment modalities to athletes under a plan of care designed and overseen by a physician licensed in this state, as recommended by the advisory committee and defined in regulation by the board.

Board and structure: New Jersey State Board of Medical Examiners (Athletic Training Advisory Committee: 4 ATs and 1 physician)

Regulatory requirements: Biennial application and fee

NEW MEXICO

Regulation: Licensure

Scope of practice: *Athletic trainer* means a person who, with the advice and consent of a licensed physician, practices the treatment, prevention, care, and rehabilitation of injuries incurred by athletes.

Board and structure: New Mexico Regulation and Licensing Department (Athletic Training Practice Board: 3 ATs and 2 public members)

Regulatory requirements: Annual application and fee

NEW YORK

Regulation: Certification

Scope of practice: The practice of the profession of athletic training is defined as the application of principles, methods, and procedures for managing athletic injuries, which shall include the preconditioning, conditioning, and reconditioning of an individual who has suffered an athletic injury through the use of appropriate preventive and supportive devices, under the supervision of a physician and recognizing illness and referring to the appropriate medical professional with implementation of treatment pursuant to physician's orders. Athletic training includes instruction to coaches, athletes, parents, medical personnel and communities in the area of care and prevention of athletic injuries.

Board and structure: New York Division of Professional Licensing Services (State Committee for Athletic Trainers: 5 ATs)

Regulatory requirements: Triennial application and fee

NORTH CAROLINA

Regulation: Licensure

Scope of practice: *Athletic trainer* is a person who, under a written protocol with a licensed physician, carries out the practice of care, prevention, and rehabilitation of injuries incurred by athletes, and who, in carrying out these functions, may use physical modalities, including heat, light, sound, cold, electricity, or mechanical devices related to rehabilitation and treatment.

Board and structure: North Carolina Board of Athletic Trainer Examiners (4 ATs, 2 physicians, and 1 public member)

Regulatory requirements: Annual application and fee

NORTH DAKOTA

Regulation: Licensure

Scope of practice: *Athletic training* means the practice of prevention, recognition, evaluation, management, treatment, and disposition of athletic injuries. The term also means rehabilitation of athletic injuries, if under the order of a licensed physician. The term includes organization and administration of educational programs, athletic facilities, and the education and counseling of the public.

Board and structure: North Dakota Board of Athletic Trainers (1 physician, 3 ATs, 1 public member)

Regulatory requirements: Annual application and fee

OHIO

Regulation: Licensure

Scope of practice: *Athletic training* means the practice of prevention, recognition, and assessment of an athletic injury and the complete management, treatment, disposition, and reconditioning of acute athletic injuries upon the referral of an individual authorized to practice medicine and surgery, osteopathic medicine and surgery, podiatry, a dentist licensed, a physical therapist, or a chiropractor. Athletic training includes the administration of topical drugs that have been prescribed by a licensed health care professional authorized to prescribe drugs. Athletic training also includes the organization and administration of educational programs and athletic facilities, and the education of and consulting with the public as it pertains to athletic training.

Board and structure: Ohio Occupational Therapy, Physical Therapy, and Athletic Trainers Board (Joint Board: 4 OTs, 1 OTA, 9 PTs [5 with voting privileges], 1 public member, 4 ATs, and 1 physician

Regulatory requirements: Biennial application and fee

OKLAHOMA

Regulation: Licensure

Scope of practice: *Athletic trainer* means a person with the qualifications specified of this title, whose major responsibility is the rendering of professional services for the prevention, emergency care, first aid, and treatment of injuries incurred by an athlete by whatever methods are available, upon written protocol from the team physician or consulting physician to effect care, or rehabilitation.

Board and structure: Oklahoma Board of Medical Licensure and Supervision (Athletic Trainers Advisory Committee: 2 ATs, 2 physicians, and 1 member from Oklahoma Coaches Association)

Regulatory requirements: Annual application and fee

OREGON

Regulation: Registration

Scope of practice: *Practice athletic training* means the application by a registered athletic trainer of principles and methods of (a) prevention of athletic injuries; (b) recognition, evaluation, and immediate care of athletic injuries; (c) rehabilitation and reconditioning of athletic injuries; (d) health care administration; and (e) education and counseling.

Board and structure: Oregon Department of Human Resources (Board of Athletic Trainers: 3 ATs, 1 physician, and 1 public member)

Regulatory requirements: Annual application and fee

PENNSYLVANIA

Regulation: Licensure

Scope of practice: *Athletic training services* means the management and provision of care of injuries to a physically active person, with the direction of a licensed physician. (i) The term includes the rendering of emergency care, development of injury prevention programs, and providing appropriate preventive and supportive devices for the physically active person. (ii) The term also includes the assessment, management, treatment, rehabilitation, and reconditioning of the physically active person whose conditions are within the professional preparation and education of a licensed athletic trainer. (iii) The term also includes the use of modalities such as mechanical stimulation, heat, cold, light, air, water, electricity, sound, and massage and the use of therapeutic exercise, reconditioning exercise, and fitness programs. (iv) The term does not include surgery, invasive procedures, or prescription of any medication or controlled substance.

Board and structure: Pennsylvania State Board of Osteopathic Medicine and Pennsylvania State Board of Medicine (each board: 6 physicians, 2 public members, 1 rotating allied health professional, 1 secretary of health representative, and 1 commissioner)

Regulatory requirements: Biennial application and fee

RHODE ISLAND

Regulation: Licensure

Scope of practice: *Athletic trainer* means a person with the specific qualifications who, upon the direction of his or her team physician or consulting physician, or both, carries out the practice of athletic training to athletic injuries incurred by athletes in preparation of or participation in an athletic program being conducted by an educational institution under the jurisdiction of an interscholastic or intercollegiate governing body, a professional athletic organization, or a board-sanctioned amateur athletic organization; provided, that no athlete shall receive athletic training services if classified as geriatric by the consulting physician. No athlete shall receive athletic training services if nonathletic or age-related conditions exist or develop that render the individual debilitated or nonathletic. To carry out these functions, the athletic trainer is authorized to utilize modalities such as heat, light, sound, cold, electricity, exercise, or mechanical devices related to care and reconditioning. The athletic trainer, as defined in this chapter, shall not represent himself or herself or allow an employer to represent him or her to be any other classification of health care professional governed by a separate and distinct practice act. This includes billing for services outside of the athletic trainer's scope of practice, including, but not limited to, services labeled as physical therapy.

Board and structure: Rhode Island Department of Health (Rhode Island Board of Athletic Trainers: 3 ATs, 1 physician, and 1 public member)

Regulatory requirements: Biennial application and fee

SOUTH CAROLINA

Regulation: Certification

Scope of practice: *Athletic trainer* means a person with specific qualifications who, upon the advice and consent of a licensed physician, carries out the practice of care, prevention, and physical rehabilitation of athletic injuries, and who, in carrying out these functions, may use physical modalities, including, but not limited to, heat, light, sound, cold, electricity, or mechanical devices related to rehabilitation and treatment.

Board and structure: South Carolina Department of Health and Environmental Control (Athletic Training Advisory Committee: 2 Department of Health, 1 physician, 4 ATs, 2 public members)

Regulatory requirements: Biennial application and fee

SOUTH DAKOTA

Regulation: Licensure

Scope of practice: *Athletic trainer* means a person whose responsibility is the prevention, evaluation, emergency care, treatment, and reconditioning of athletic injuries under the direction of the team or treating physician. The athletic trainer may use cryotherapy, which includes cold packs, ice packs, cold-water immersion, and spray coolants; thermotherapy, which includes topical analgesics, moist hot packs, heating pads, infrared lamp, and paraffin bath; hydrotherapy, which includes whirlpool; and therapeutic exercise common to athletic training, which includes stretching and those exercises needed to maintain condition, in accordance with a physician's written protocol. Any rehabilitative procedures recommended by a physician for the rehabilitation of athletic injuries that have been referred and all other physical modalities may be administered only following the prescription of the team or referring physician.

Board and structure: South Dakota Board of Medical and Osteopathic Examiners (Athletic Training Committee: 3 ATs)

Regulatory requirements: Annual application and fee

TENNESSEE

Regulation: Licensure

Scope of practice: *Athletic trainer* means a person with specific qualifications, who, upon the advice, consent, and oral or written prescriptions or referrals of a physician licensed under this title, carries out the practice of prevention, recognition, evaluation, management, disposition, treatment, or rehabilitation of athletic injuries, and, in carrying out these function, the athletic trainer is authorized to use physical modalities, such as heat, light, sound, cold, electricity, or mechanical devices related to prevention, recognition, evaluation, management, disposition, rehabilitation, and treatment; an athletic trainer shall practice only in those areas in which such athletic trainer is competent by reason of training or experience that can be substantiated by records or other evidence found acceptable by the board in the exercise of the board's considered discretion.

Board and structure: Tennessee Health Related Boards (Board of Athletic Trainers: 3 ATs, 1 physician, and 1 public member)

Regulatory requirements: Biennial application and fee

TEXAS

Regulation: Licensure

Scope of practice: *Athletic training* means the form of health care that includes the practice of preventing, recognizing, assessing, managing, treating, disposing of, and reconditioning athletic injuries under the direction of a physician licensed in this state or another qualified, licensed health professional who is authorized to refer for health care services within the scope of the person's license.

Board and structure: Texas Advisory Board of Athletic Trainers (Advisory Board of Athletic Trainers: 3 ATs, 2 public members)

Regulatory requirements: Biennial application and fee

UTAH

Regulation: Licensure

Scope of practice: The *practice of athletic training* means the application by a licensed and certified athletic trainer of principles and methods of (a) prevention of athletic injuries; (b) recognition, evaluation, and assessment of athletic injuries and conditions; (c) immediate care of athletic injuries, including common emergency medical situations; (d) rehabilitation and reconditioning of athletic injuries; (e) athletic training services administration and organization; and (f) education of athletes.

Board and structure: Utah Division of Occupational and Professional Licensing

(Athletic Training Licensing Board: 4 ATs, 1 physician, and 1 public member)

Regulatory requirements: Biennial application and fee

VERMONT

Regulation: Licensure

Scope of practice: *Athletic training* means the application of principles and methods of conditioning; the prevention, immediate care, recognition, evaluation, assessment, and treatment of athletic and orthopedic injuries within the scope of education and training; the organization and administration of an athletic training program; and the education and counseling of athletes, coaches, family members, medical personnel, and communities in the area of care and prevention of athletic and orthopedic injuries. Athletic training may only be applied in the traditional setting and the clinical setting: (A) without further referral, to athletes participating in organized sports or athletic teams at an interscholastic, intramural, instructional, intercollegiate, amateur, or professional level; (B) with a referral from a physician, osteopathic physician, dentist, or chiropractor, to athletes or the physically active who have an athletic or orthopedic injury and have been determined, by a physician's examination, to be free of an underlying pathology that would affect treatment.

Board and structure: Vermont Secretary of State's Office (Athletic Training Advisors to the Office of Professional Regulation: 2 ATs)

Regulatory requirements: Biennial application and fee

VIRGINIA

Regulation: Licensure

Scope of practice: *Practice of athletic training* means the prevention, recognition, evaluation, and treatment of injuries or conditions related to athletic or recreational activity that requires physical skill and utilizes strength, power, endurance, speed, flexibility, range of motion, or agility or a substantially similar injury or condition resulting from occupational activity immediately upon the onset of such injury or condition; and subsequent treatment and rehabilitation of such injuries or conditions under the direction of the patient's physician or under the direction of any doctor of medicine, osteopathy, chiropractic, podiatry, or dentistry, while using heat, light, sound, cold, electricity, exercise or mechanical or other devices.

Board and structure: Virginia Department of Health Professions (Athletic Trainers Advisory Board: 3 ATs, 1 physician, and 1 public member)

Regulatory requirements: Biennial application and fee

WASHINGTON

Regulation: Licensure

Scope of practice: *Athletic training* means the application of the following principles and methods as provided by a licensed athletic trainer: (i) risk management and prevention of athletic injuries through preactivity screening and evaluation, educational programs, physical conditioning and reconditioning programs, application of commercial products, use of protective equipment, promotion of healthy behaviors, and reduction of environmental risks; (ii) recognition, evaluation, and assessment of athletic injuries by obtaining a history of the athletic injury, inspection and palpation of the injured part and associated structures, and performance of specific testing techniques related to stability and function to determine the extent of an injury; (iii) immediate care of athletic injuries, including emergency medical situations through the application of first aid and emergency procedures and techniques for non-life-threatening or life-threatening athletic injuries; (iv) treatment, rehabilitation, and reconditioning of athletic injuries through the application of physical agents and modalities, therapeutic activities and exercise, standard reassessment techniques and procedures, commercial products, and educational programs, in accordance with guidelines established with a licensed health care provider; and (v) referral of an athlete to an appropriately licensed health care provider if the athletic injury requires further definitive care or the injury or condition is outside an athletic trainer's scope of practice.

Board and structure: Washington State Department of Health (Athletic Training Advisory Committee: 4 ATs and 1 public member)

Regulatory requirements: Annual application and fee

WEST VIRGINIA

Regulation: Registration

Scope of practice: None

Board and structure: West Virginia Board of Physical Therapy (5 PTs, 1 PTA, and 1 public member)

Regulatory requirements: Biennial application and fee

WISCONSIN

Regulation: Licensure

Scope of practice: *Athletic training* means doing any of the following: (a) Preventing, recognizing, and evaluating injuries or illnesses sustained while participating in physical activity. (b) Managing and administering the initial treatment of injuries or illnesses sustained while participating in physical activity. (c) Giving emergency care or first aid for an injury or illness sustained while participating in physical activity. (d) Rehabilitating and physically reconditioning injuries or illnesses sustained while participating in physical activity. (e) Rehabilitating and physically reconditioning injuries or illnesses that impede or prevent an individual from returning to participation in physical activity, if the individual recently participated in and intends to return to participation in physical activity. (f) Establishing or administering risk management, conditioning, and injury prevention programs.

Board and structure: Wisconsin Department of Regulation and Licensing (Athletic Training Affiliated Credentialing Board: 4 ATs, 1 physician, and 1 public member)

Regulatory requirements: Biennial application and fee

WYOMING

Regulation: Licensure

Scope of practice: *Practice of athletic training* means the application of the principles and methods of prevention; recognition, evaluation, and assessment of athletic injuries and illnesses; immediate care of athletic injuries, including common injuries, medical emergencies, psychosocial intervention and referral; conditioning and rehabilitative exercise; nutritional aspects of injuries and illnesses; the use of therapeutic modalities; proper health care administration; professional development; and the understanding and education of applications, precautions, interactions, indications, and contraindications of pharmacology for athletes.

Board and structure: Wyoming Athletic Training Board (2 ATs and 1 physician)

Regulatory requirements: Triennial application and fee

Glossary

90th-percentile fee—The fee below which 90% of all other medical vendors in a particular geographic area charge for a specific service.

abandonment—The desertion of a patient by the health care provider without the consent of the patient.

accreditation—Formal recognition provided to an organization or one of its programs indicating that it meets certain prescribed quality standards.

accuracy standards—Performance evaluation standards intended to improve the validity and reliability of the employee appraisal process.

actual cause—The degree to which a health care practitioner's actions are associated with the adverse outcomes of a patient's care.

adversaries—People who are unsupportive of both a program and a particular plan related to the program.

agreement–trust matrix—A model that identifies and types the most important people in developing support for a plan.

allies—People who exhibit a high level of support for a plan.

allocator of resources—A type of decisional role in which the leader exercises authority to determine how organizational assets will be deployed.

amendment—A proposed change to a bill or law, which can be a minor edit, major edit, addition, or deletion of language in the bill or law.

analytical listening—A type of listening approach in which one is open minded despite listening for specific words or terms.

appropriate medical coverage—The appropriate number of staff that is likely needed to perform all of the necessary athletic training–related functions.

appropriate medical coverage for intercollegiate athletics (AMCIA)—Document developed by NATA to assess how much staffing is required based on health care units (HCU) in a college or university athletic setting.

approved provider—A provider of continuing education for athletic trainers that has met all of the requirements of the BOC to offer CEUs to ATCs.

assumption of risk—A legal defense that attempts to claim that an injured plaintiff understood the risk of an activity and freely chose to undertake the activity regardless of the hazards associated with it.

athletic accident insurance—A type of insurance policy intended to reimburse medical vendors for the expenses associated with acute athletic accidents.

authority—The aspect of power, granted to either groups or individuals, that legitimizes the right of the group or individual to make decisions on behalf of others.

bedfellows—People who exhibit support for a particular plan, but who have a history of untrustworthy behavior and vacillation.

benchmarking—To associate a recognized comparison of one's own program to the best in the industry.

bicameral legislature—A state legislature consisting of two regulatory bodies, both of which must pass bills before they move to the governor's office to be signed into law, typically called a House of Representatives and a Senate (or House and Assembly)

bidding—A process whereby vendors provide cost quotations for goods and services they want to sell.

bidding documents—The package of materials prepared by the architect and sent to contractors, including the invitation to bid, the bid form, and special bidding instructions.

Board of Certification (BOC)—The organization that creates and delivers the national certification exam for athletic trainers; manages continuing education for athletic trainers.

BOC Athletic Trainer Regulatory Conference—An event focused on state regulatory issues affecting athletic trainers.

breach of confidentiality—Violation of a commitment to privacy and protection of information or communications.

breach of contract—An unexcused failure to perform the services specified in a contract, either formal or informal.

breach of duty—When an athletic trainer does not exercise the standard of care that other reasonably prudent athletic trainers would have exercised under the circumstances.

budget—An organized plan for coordinating resources, revenues, and expenditures.

business plan—Plan used by commercial loan officers to assess the viability of a business. Includes a written description of the activities the business will engage in, a market analysis, historical and projected financial statements, and other associated information.

capital campaign—A program, usually of fixed length, designed to raise funds for program creation, development, and improvement.

capitation—A system whereby medical vendors receive a fixed amount per patient.

CARF International—A nonprofit agency that sets quality standards for rehabilitation services and facilities.

carrier—Charge-based provider contracted by the federal government, charged with reviewing Medicare claims made by physicians or other health care providers.

catastrophic insurance—A type of accident insurance designed to provide lifelong medical, rehabilitation, and disability benefits for a victim of devastating injury.

certification—A form of title protection, established by state law or sponsored by professional associations, designed to ensure that practitioners have essential knowledge and skills sufficient to protect the public.

charting by exception—A type of medical record that notes only those patient responses that vary from predefined norms.

clinical education—The application of athletic training knowledge, skills, and clinical abilities on an actual patient base that is evaluated and the feedback provided by a preceptor.

clinical practice guidelines (CPGs)—Systematic algorithm-like procedures that are universally followed in an effort to provide standardized clinical care and interventions.

conduct—The behavior of an athletic trainer in ethical and legal terms.

CMS 1500—The form that private-practice clinics should use when filing a claim with an insurance company. Originally developed by the Health Care Financing Administration (now known as the Centers for Medicare and Medicaid Services) for Medicare claims.

code of ethics—A systematized set of standards or principles that defines ethical behavior appropriate for a profession. Moral values determine the standards and principles.

collegial culture—A type of organizational culture characterized by consensus, teamwork, and participatory decision making.

commercial loan—An amount of money borrowed from a lending institution for the purpose of establishing, improving, or maintaining a business.

commission—An action that violates a legal duty.

Commission on Accreditation of Athletic Training Education (CAATE)—Sets accreditation standards and awards accreditation to professional, postprofessional, and residency programs.

Committee on Practice Advancement (COPA)—NATA committee that supports ATs in emerging settings and works on reimbursement issues.

comparative negligence—A legal doctrine intended to determine the degree to which a plaintiff contributed to the harm caused by a defendant.

conflict of interest—Situation in which the interests of one individual or group are discordant or in competition with those of another individual or group.

construction documents—The highly detailed technical drawings that a contractor uses to determine building costs and guide construction.

construction management—A method that involves the general contractor as part of the design team from the beginning of the building process.

Convention Program Committee (CPC)—NATA committee that plans and runs the NATA Annual Meeting and Clinical Symposia each year.

copayment—The percentage of a medical bill not paid by the insurance company and that the patient is responsible for.

counterpower—The potential to influence the behavior of a superior.

criteria—Quantifiable measures used to determine whether a particular objective has been accomplished.

cultural awareness—A set of behaviors that an individual or group of individuals (organizations, businesses) possesses and implements through consistent actions that demonstrate appropriate behavior of diverse cultures.

cultural competence—One's ability to successfully incorporate a set of behaviors that demonstrate appropriate behavior when interacting with diverse cultures.

culture—The shared values, beliefs, traditions, customs, and values of a particular group.

Current Procedural Terminology (CPT)—A coding system applied to medical procedures to standardize the language associated with third-party reimbursement.

curriculum vitae (CV)—A longer version of an individual's resume, typically used for academic positions. In addition to items included on a resume, a CV also includes more details, such as a list of publications, classes taught, committees that the individual has served on, and awards received.

damage—The legal harm found associated with negligence, commonly in the form of any one or more of the following: physical injury, monetary loss, and emotional distress.

data port—A dedicated phone line or network terminal used to connect computers in different locations.

decisional role—The portion of a manager's work that requires her to use authority to make decisions.

dependent care initiatives—Measures meant to provide employees the ability to manage their family responsibilities.

deposition—A process of discovery, where facts regarding the case are formally gathered through questioning of an individual under oath.

design–build—A construction method that uses only one firm both to design and to construct a new building.

developmental supervision—A supervisory model that emphasizes collaboration between supervisors and supervisees to help them solve problems and develop professionally.

diagnostic—Referring to a specific medical finding for the purposes of identification.

dictation—The act of orally recording, on a cassette tape or directly into a computer, the details of a health care assessment or treatment for later transcription and filing.

disability insurance—Insurance designed to protect an athlete against future loss of earnings because of a disabling injury or sickness.

disqualifying conditions—Injuries, illnesses, or other medical conditions that pose an undue risk to athletes, their teammates, or their competitors.

disseminator—An informational role that requires the leader to communicate with members of the group.

disturbance handler—A type of decisional role in which the leader manages conflict.

drug administration—Provision of a single dose of medication to a patient by order of a physician.

drug dispensing—Preparing and packaging medication for subsequent use by a patient.

duty—A contract between the athletic trainer and employer to provide athletic training services to the clientele served by the employer.

elective—Referring to a surgical procedure that is not required but that one chooses to undergo.

emergency action plan (EAP)—A blueprint for handling emergencies that helps establish accountability for their management.

endowment—The portion of an institution's assets in cash and investments not normally used for operational purposes.

employee assistance program (EAP)—An on-site workplace program that is designed to assist and support employees who may need short-term counseling.

entrepreneurial role—A type of decisional role in which the leader initiates and designs controlled change within an organization.

enzyme multiplied immunoassay technique (EMIT)—A first-line screening procedure designed to detect abuse of drugs or the presence of performance-enhancing drugs by testing an athlete's urine.

ergonomics—The scientific study of human work or the "scientific discipline concerned with the understanding of interactions among humans and other elements of a system, and the profession that applies theory, principles, data and methods to design in order to optimize human well-being and overall system performance."

ethics—The rules, standards, and principles that dictate right conduct among members of a society or profession. Ethics are based on moral values.

Ethnic Diversity Advisory Committee (EDAC)—NATA committee formed to study the issues affecting minorities and to enhance minority involvement in the profession of athletic training.

evidence-based medicine—The type of medicine that considers scientific findings, experience of the clinician, and considerations of the patient in an effort to provide the best care.

exclusions—Situations or circumstances specifically not covered by an insurance policy.

exclusive provider organization (EPO)—A type of preferred provider organization in which medical services are reimbursed only if the patient uses contracted providers.

exculpatory clause—A signed release from a patient or parents that waives all future legal claims against an athletic trainer or the employing institution.

excuse—A reason that is considered justifiable.

exemption—A legislative mechanism used to release members of one profession from the liability of violating another profession's practice act.

experimental treatments—Therapies not proved effective.

explanation of benefits form (EOB)—A summary prepared by an insurance company, and sent to a policyholder, that documents how the insurance policy covered the charges associated with a particular claim.

exploitation—Using another person for selfish purposes, particularly when it comes at the expense of that person or without the person's knowledge or full informed consent.

express warranty—An explicit statement specifying the conditions, circumstances, and terms under which a vendor will replace or repair a product if it is found to be faulty.

external chart audit—A technique for patient records review, performed by an accreditation agency or a payer, intended to ensure that patient care is appropriate and meets certain minimum standards.

external evaluators—Experts not affiliated with an organization who are retained to assess the various programs within the organization.

Fair Labor Standards Act (FLSA)—Congressional act responsible for establishing minimum wage and overtime pay guidelines for employees.

false-negative—The results of a drug test that indicate either the absence of a banned compound or its presence below an acceptable level, when in fact the compound is present above acceptable levels.

false-positive—The results of a drug test that indicate the presence of a banned compound above an acceptable level, when in fact the compound is either absent or present below acceptable levels.

feasibility standards—Performance evaluation standards intended to help foster practicality in the employee appraisal process.

Federal Legislative Council—NATA committee focused on national legislative efforts.

federal Anti-Kickback Statute—Similar to Stark Law, prevents athletic trainers from self-referring to entities with whom they or their family have a financial relationship.

fee-for-service plan—Also known as an indemnity plan. A type of traditional medical insurance whereby patients are free to seek medical services from any provider. The plan covers a portion of the cost of covered procedures, and the patient is responsible for the balance.

Family Educational Rights and Privacy Act (FERPA)—Sometimes referred to as the Buckley Amendment. A 1974 federal law requiring student authorization to release educational records to a third party and ensuring access for students to their records.

figurehead role—An interpersonal role that requires the authority holder to represent the group, usually in a visible public capacity.

first reading—The first time a bill is introduced or "read" in the legislature; may include just a reading of the bill number and title or may also include an overview of the bill's intent.

fixed budgeting—A method in which expenditures and revenues are projected on a monthly basis, thereby providing an estimate of cash flow.

flexible work arrangements—Employment arrangements that allow employees to establish their own work schedules.

FOB point—Freight-on-board point. The point at which the title for shipped goods passes from vendor to purchaser.

focus charting—A medical record that registers a patient's complaint data, the health care practitioner's actions, and the patient's response.

forbidden knowledge—Information about a situation that an athletic trainer is forbidden to act on.

forecast—A prediction of future conditions based on various statistics and indicators that describes an athletic training program's past and present situations.

foreseeability—The ability to project the likely outcome of an act.

formalistic culture—A type of organizational culture characterized by a clear chain of command and well-defined lines of formal authority.

formative evaluation—An assessment designed primarily for improvement of a program.

fraud—Criminal misrepresentation for the purpose of financial gain.

Free Communications Committee—NATA Foundation committee that reviews case reports and research submissions for presentation at the NATA Clinical Symposia each year.

gas chromatography–mass spectrometry (GC-MS)—A highly accurate method for detecting the presence of performance-enhancing and other drugs, including anabolic steroids, in an athlete's urine.

general contractor—The company responsible for coordinating the construction of a building.

goals—General statements of program intent.

Good Samaritan laws—Statutes intended to shield certain health care practitioners from certain types of legal liability when they voluntarily come to the aid of injured or ill persons under specific circumstances.

Government Affairs Committee (GAC)—NATA committee that supports state legislative efforts and awards grants to states to help fund these efforts.

ground fault interrupter (GFI)—A highly sensitive device designed to discontinue the flow of electricity in an electrical circuit during a power surge.

guardian—A person who has legal responsibility for the care and decisions of someone who is incompetent to act for himself or who is a minor.

health history form—A detailed questionnaire designed to document an athlete's previous injuries, illnesses, and other medical conditions. This form often serves as the basis for additional medical follow-up and evaluation.

health history update—A brief questionnaire designed to determine whether an athlete has suffered injuries or developed medical conditions since the last comprehensive PPE.

health insurance—A type of policy designed to reimburse the cost of preventive as well as corrective medical care.

health maintenance organization (HMO)—A type of health insurance plan that requires policyholders to use only those medical vendors approved by the company. All medical services are coordinated by a primary care physician, who acts as a gatekeeper to specialty services.

health care initiatives (wellness programs)—Initiatives or programs or both aimed at improving the quality of life for employees.

health care units (HCUs)—The unit make-up of a formula arbitrarily based on an academic teaching model, used to identify appropriate staffing of athletic trainers, stating that 12 HCUs should equate to one full-time athletic trainer position.

high-risk behaviors—Behaviors that expose a person to an unnecessarily high degree of physical or psychological jeopardy.

Health Insurance Portability and Accountability Act (HIPPA)—Act that helps employees transfer their health insurance when they switch employers, ensures that their health information will remain private, and gives people more access to their own health care information.

Hippocratic Oath—The foundation for ethical practice for physicians.

honeymoon effect—The period of time, usually immediately after arriving in a new position, in which people are more likely to be granted extra authority to make decisions.

implied warranty—An unstated understanding that a vendor will "make good" if a product is faulty.

individual practice association (IPA)—A managed care model whereby an HMO provides health care services through a network of individual medical practitioners. Care is provided in a physician's office as opposed to a large, multifunctional medical center.

informational role—The function that requires the manager to collect, use, and disseminate information.

inspection–production—A supervisory model that emphasizes the use of formal authority and managerial prerogatives to improve employee efficiency and efficacy.

insurance claim tracking form—A worksheet that aids in tracking the progress of an insurance claim through the entire process.

Intercollegiate Council for Sports Medicine (ICSM)—NATA committee that focuses on issues faced by athletic trainers working in the college and university setting.

interference—Anything, including environmental elements or characteristics of the communication medium, that distorts the message sent from the sender to the receiver.

intermediary—Cost-based provider contracted by the federal government and charged with reviewing Medicare claims made by hospitals.

internal chart audit—A technique for patient records review performed by the sports medicine staff as part of a quality assurance program.

internal influencers—Organization decision makers.

International Classification of Diseases (ICD-10-CM)—A coding system applied to illnesses, injuries, and other medical conditions to standardize the language associated with third-party reimbursement.

International Committee (IC)—NATA committee that supports athletic trainers working outside of the United States.

interpersonal role—A managerial role, emanating from the possession of formal authority, that requires the manager to interact and form relationships with others in the organization.

inventory management—The process of controlling equipment and supply stocks so that services can be provided without interruption while the use of institutional resources is maximized.

job description—A written description of the specific responsibilities a position holder will be accountable for in an organization.

job specification—A written description of the requirements or qualifications a person should have in order to fill a particular role in an organization.

Joint Commission—The oldest and largest health care standards organization in the country. The Joint Commission accredits ambulatory health care facilities.

laws—The rules and regulations governing the affairs of a community or society.

layered coverage—A method of using different insurance companies to underwrite different levels of coverage in a common policy.

leadership—A subset of power that involves influencing the behavior and attitudes of others to achieve intended outcomes.

leave of absence—Time allowed away from work for an employee.

legal structure—A process that regulates the business operations; identifies who the business owner is; and ensures a method for tax collection, employee wages and protection, and fair practice acts.

liaison role—An interpersonal role that requires the leader to interact with others in the group, including superiors, subordinates, and coequals.

licensure—A form of state credentialing, established by statute and intended to protect the public, that regulates the practice of a trade or profession by specifying who may practice and what duties they may perform.

line-item budgeting—A method that allocates a fixed amount of money for each subfunction of a program.

liquid chromatography–mass spectrometry–mass spectrometry (LC/MS/MS)—A method of drug testing used to indicate the presence of drugs in an athlete's urine.

lobbyist—An individual hired and typically paid by a business or organization to advocate for particular issues with the legislature at the state or federal level or both.

loss of consortium—A legal claim of damages for injuries to a spouse or for alienation of a spouse's affection.

lump-sum bidding—A process whereby general contractors provide cost quotations for the right to construct or renovate a building.

lump-sum budgeting—A method that allocates a fixed amount of money for an entire program without specifying how the money will be spent.

malfeasance—When an individual performs an improper act, such as something that is not within that individual's scope of practice.

malpractice—Liability-generating conduct associated with the adverse outcome of patient treatment.

managed care—A growing concept in the insurance industry emphasizing cost control through coordination of medical services, for example with an HMO or PPO.

management—The element of leadership that involves planning, decision making, and coordination of the activities of a group.

manipulate—Shrewdly or deviously influence or control another person or a situation. When the influence or control is motivated by self-interest, it can be exploitative.

market analysis—Analysis that includes a written description of the competitive advantages of a business, analysis of the competition, pricing structure, and marketing plan.

mass screening—A method of preparticipation physical examination whereby many athletes are screened simultaneously, usually in a school gymnasium or locker room.

matrix structure—A type of organizational model that defines relationships in terms of both functions and services.

maturational assessment—A medical screening procedure based on Tanner's stages of maturational development. It is often used to classify children and adolescents for the purpose of matching them with appropriate athletic opponents.

medical ethics—The process by which one determines right from wrong when medical care is involved.

medical insurance—A type of insurance that a patient purchases in the form of a policy from a health insurance company for the purpose of covering medically related expenses.

medical practice act—A state law regulating the practice of medicine, usually by specifying who may practice and under what circumstances.

medical record—Cumulative documentation of a person's medical history and health care interventions.

minor—A person under legal age to take on adult responsibilities and make adult decisions.

minimal qualifications—The essential skills and experiences required to perform a specific job.

misfeasance—When an individual improperly performs a legal act such as spine-boarding incorrectly.

mission statement—A written expression of an organization's philosophy, purposes, and characteristics.

mixing valve—A type of plumbing fixture designed to blend hot and cold water, eliminating the need for separate hot- and cold-water controls.

mobile workplace—An arrangement that allows an employee the chance to work remotely.

monitor—A type of informational role that requires the leader to observe and keep abreast of changes that will affect the group and its activity.

narrative charting—A method of recording the details of a patient's assessments and treatments using a detailed, prose-based format.

National Athletic Trainers' Association (NATA)—A professional membership organization for certified athletic trainers and others who support the athletic training profession.

NATA Research and Education Foundation (NATA Foundation)—An entity that awards research grants and scholarships, and manages Free Communications and the NATA Quiz Bowl.

National Provider Identifier (NPI) number—A unique 10-digit identification number used in standard health care transactions, issued by the Centers for Medicare and Medicaid Services (CMS) to health care professionals and covered entities in the United States that transmit standard HIPAA electronic transactions.

natural lighting—Outside light used to illuminate indoor spaces, usually through windows or skylights.

need—Something essential or important.

needs assessment—A systematic set of procedures undertaken to set organizational or programmatic priorities based on identified needs.

negligence—A type of tort in which an athletic trainer fails to act as a reasonably prudent athletic trainer would act under the circumstances.

negotiation—The process of bargaining.

negotiator—A type of decisional role in which the leader uses authority to bargain with members of the internal or external audience.

nonfeasance—When an individual does not perform an act that he or she should, such as not performing CPR when indicated.

nonmedical correspondence—Letters and memoranda not associated with a specific patient's health status.

numeric analysis—The process of determining a staff member's workload by calculating and comparing the amount of time a person spends on certain tasks with the outputs that result from those tasks.

objectives—Specific statements of how a program intends to accomplish a particular goal.

omission—A failure to act when there was a legal duty to do so.

operational plan—A type of plan that defines organizational activities in the short term, usually no longer than two years.

opponents—People who support a particular program but dispute the implementation of a plan related to that program.

organizational chart—A graphic representation of an organization's structure, usually arranged by function, by service, or in a matrix format.

organizational culture—The values, beliefs, assumptions, and norms that form the infrastructure of the organizational ethos.

organizational structure—A model that defines the relationships among the members of an organization.

OSHA's Bloodborne Pathogen standard—Federal government rules that require employers to protect employees against the accidental transmission of bloodborne pathogens, especially HIV and hepatitis B.

outcomes assessment—An evaluation method used in health care that seeks objective evidence that the care provided by the athletic trainer enhanced a patient's functional ability.

over-the-counter medication (OTC)—A medication that can be purchased without a physician's prescription.

patient encounter—Any interaction that an athletic trainer has with a patient that is related to that patient's medical history.

performance budgeting—A method that allocates funds for discrete activities.

performance evaluation—The process of placing a value on the quality of an employee's work.

perpetrator—The person who is responsible for or has committed an act or both.

personalistic culture—A type of organizational culture characterized by autonomy in decision making and problem solving.

personal power—The potential to influence others by virtue of personal characteristics and personality attributes.

person specification—A specific delineation, based on the job specification, of the qualities, skills, and characteristics a person must have to fill a particular role.

Peter Principle—A concept that states that in a hierarchy, every employee tends to rise to his level of incompetence.

planning—A type of decision-making process in which a course of action is determined in order to bring about a future state of affairs.

planning committee—A group of institutional employees who work with an architect to develop the design of a building.

plumbing fixtures—The external hardware used to control the flow and temperature of water.

point-of-service plan (POS)—Managed care plans that are similar to PPOs, except that primary care physicians are assigned to patients to coordinate their care.

policy—A type of plan that expresses an organization's intended behavior relative to a specific program subfunction.

political action committee (PAC)—An organization that accepts donations used to support legislative efforts, often used for campaign contributions to key legislators to garner support for important issues at state or national levels.

pooled buying consortium—A group of similar institutions that merge resources to purchase goods in large quantities in order to receive volume discounts.

position description—A formal document that describes the qualifications, work content, accountability, and scope of a job.

position power—The power vested in people by virtue of the roles they play in an organization.

postprofessional education—A degree program, typically master's or doctoral, designed for students who have already completed a professional education program and are already certified as athletic trainers; teaches knowledge and skills beyond entry level.

power—The potential to influence others.

practice—The action that takes place in response to administrative problems.

preceptor—A certified or licensed professional who teaches or evaluates students, or both, in a clinical setting using an actual patient base.

preemployment test—Any procedure (including a drug test) conducted on a potential employee that is used to determine the applicant's suitability for employment.

preferred qualifications—The additional skills and experiences possessed by a candidate beyond meeting all minimum qualifications.

preferred provider organization (PPO)—A type of health insurance plan that provides financial incentives to encourage policyholders to use medical vendors approved by the company.

premium—The invoiced cost of an insurance policy.

preparticipation physical examination (PPE)—A medical screening procedure designed to determine an athlete's readiness for participation in a specific sport at a specific level of competition.

primary care provider—The physician, selected by an HMO member, who acts as the first source of medical service for the patient. Most HMOs require members to seek a referral from the primary care provider before seeking care from another medical vendor.

primary coverage—A type of health, medical, or accident insurance that begins to pay for covered expenses immediately after a deductible has been paid.

primary party—A person directly involved as a participant in an activity.

problem-oriented medical record (POMR)—A system of medical record keeping that organizes information around a patient's specific complaints.

procedure—A type of operational plan that provides specific directions for members of an organization to follow.

proceedings—A book containing the abstracts or outlines of each speaker's presentation.

process—A collection of incremental and mutually dependent steps designed to direct the most important tasks of an organization.

process analysis—A technique for streamlining the number and complexity of steps needed to provide a service to a customer.

professional education—A degree that is designed for students not yet certified as athletic trainers, which leads to eligibility for certification.

program administration records—Documentation of the activities of a program.

program evaluation—A systematic and comprehensive assessment of the worth of a particular program.

propriety standards—Performance evaluation standards intended to help ensure that a process is legal and fair.

proximate (legal) cause—The degree to which the harm caused by a health care practitioner was foreseeable.

purchase order—A document that formalizes the terms of a purchase and transmits the intentions of the buyer to purchase goods or services from a vendor.

purchasing—The process that athletic trainers use to implement the budget plan.

random selection—A method for choosing subjects for drug testing based on permutations of timing, subject characteristics, or both. Implies an equal probability of choosing any subject within a given population for testing.

reason—The basis or explanation for an action.

reasonable suspicion—A basis for selecting subjects for drug testing, taking into account observable signs of drug use. Also known as reasonable cause or probable cause.

receiving—The process of accepting delivery of goods purchased from a vendor.

recruitment—The process of planning for human resources needs and identifying potential candidates to meet those needs.

registration—A type of state credentialing that requires qualified members of a profession to register with the state in order to practice.

relative value—The value of the overall cost of providing a service.

reliability (in staff selection)—Consistency of staff selection procedures.

request for quotation (RFQ)—A document that provides vendors with the specifications for bidding on the sale of goods and services.

request for proposal (RFP)—Notice from internal and external funding sources announcing the details of a grant program.

requisition—A type of formal or informal communication, usually written, used for requesting authorization to purchase goods or services.

rider—Additions to a standard insurance policy that provide coverage for conditions not normally covered.

right conduct—Behavior that is fitting or proper or conforms to legal or moral expectations.

rights—Moral or legal privileges inherent in being a member of a community or society.

risk management—A process designed to prevent losses of all kinds for everyone associated with an organization, including its directors, administrators, employees, and clients.

safe harbor clause—A provision that allows an individual to self-report a substance problem without repercussions of a positive test. Self-reporting must occur before formal notification of being selected for a drug test.

schematic drawings—A graphic representation, derived from the program statement, that illustrates the relationships among the principal functions of a building.

secondary coverage—A type of health, medical, or accident insurance that begins to pay for covered expenses only after all other sources of insurance coverage have been exhausted. Also known as excess insurance.

Secondary School Athletic Trainers' Committee (SSATC)—NATA committee that works on issues specific to ATs working in secondary schools.

self-determination—Freedom to judge for oneself, to determine one's own course of action, and to manage one's own affairs.

SOAP note—Medical appraisal organized by subjective and objective evaluation, assessment of the patient's problem, and development of a plan for treatment.

sovereign (governmental) immunity—A legal doctrine that holds that neither governments nor their agents can be held liable for negligent actions.

span of control—The number of subordinates supervised by a particular individual in an organizational setting.

spending-ceiling model—A type of expenditure budgeting that requires justification only for expenses that exceed those of the previous budget cycle. Also known as the *incremental model*.

spending-reduction model—A type of budgeting used during periods of financial retrenchment that requires reallocation of institutional funds, resulting in reduced spending levels for some programs.

spokesperson role—An informational role that requires communication with organizational influencers and members of the organization's public.

staff selection—The procedures used as the basis for any employment decision, including recruitment, hiring, promotion, demotion, retention, and performance evaluation.

standard of care—The legal duty to provide health care services consistent with what other health care practitioners of the same training, education, and credentialing would provide under the circumstances.

standards of practice—Widely accepted principles intended to guide the professional activities of a health care practitioner.

standing orders—A written document in which a physician provides operational directions for an athletic trainer to adhere to.

standpipe drain—A type of drain that is raised above floor level.

Stark Law—Physician self-referral law; prevents health care practitioners from referring patients to entities with whom they or their family members have a financial relationship.

State Association Advisory Committee (SAAC)—NATA committee that supports state leaders to help them better manage their state associations.

station-based PPE—A group screening process whereby information for individual athletes is collected at a variety of stations staffed by a combination of medical and nonmedical personnel, usually in the context of a school environment.

statutes of limitations—Laws that fix a certain length of time beyond which legal actions cannot be initiated.

strategic planning—A type of planning that involves critical self-examination to bring about organizational improvement.

Student Leadership Committee (SLC)—NATA committee made up of noncertified athletic training students to represent student interests and plan the student portion of the NATA Clinical Symposia each year.

subcontractor—A company hired by a general contractor to complete a particular portion of a building project. The subcontractor's work is usually devoted to a particular skilled trade, such as plumbing, electrical, or landscaping.

subpoena—The legal authority used to compel a person to provide testimony.

summative evaluation—An assessment designed primarily to describe the effectiveness or accomplishments of a program.

supervision—A process whereby authority holders observe the work activities of an employee to improve the outcomes of the employee's work or to improve the employee's professional development.

SWOT analysis—An acronym for strengths, weaknesses, opportunities, and threats. Sometimes referred to as WOTS UP.

Tanner staging—A method for assessing physical maturation by categorizing the development of secondary sexual characteristics.

tax-exempt bonds—Bonds authorized and sold by governmental agencies to provide funding for construction projects.

testimony—Legally binding statements offered as evidence to the facts in a legal proceeding.

third party—(1) A medical vendor with no binding interest in a particular insurance contract. (2) A party affected by, but not directly involved in, a situation. Professionals who simply have knowledge of an unethical act can be affected by it because they have a professional responsibility to act on such knowledge.

third-party reimbursement—The process by which medical vendors receive reimbursement from insurance companies for services provided to policyholders.

Title IX legislation—Part of the United States Education Amendments of 1972 that made it illegal to discriminate based on gender in educational institutions.

tort—A legal wrong, other than breach of contract, for which a remedy will be provided, usually in the form of monetary damages.

Total Quality Management (TQM)—Also known as continuous quality improvement. A management system that emphasizes continuous improvement in the process by which work is accomplished to create improvements in a product. A continuous focus on the needs and desires of clients is a major focus of TQM.

traffic patterns—The anticipated flow of people from one area of a building to another.

transactional leadership—The simple exchange of one thing for another in a relationship between two people.

transformational leadership—The aspect of leadership that uses both change and conflict to elevate the standards of the social system.

UB-04 (also known as the CMS 1450)—Insurance claim form that hospitals should use.

usual, customary, and reasonable (UCR)—The charge consistent with what other medical vendors would assess.

utility standards—Performance evaluation standards intended to help ensure that employee appraisal is useful to workers, employers, and others who need to use the information.

validity (in staff selection)—The employment of criteria that predict how well a candidate will perform in a role.

variable budgeting—A method requiring adjustment of monthly expenditures so that they do not exceed revenues.

vision statement—A concise statement that describes the ideal state to which an organization aspires.

whistle-blowing—The reporting of others who are perceived to have violated a set of rules by an individual believed to be doing the right thing.

work–life balance—A theory that focuses on the blending of and prioritizing between an individual's work and lifestyle.

World Federation of Athletic Training and Therapy (WFATT)—An organization that brings together ATs and similar health care professionals from around the world to share ideas and support one another.

WOTS UP (SWOT) analysis—A data collection and appraisal technique designed to determine an organization's weaknesses, opportunities, threats, and strengths in order to facilitate planning. UP stands for underlying planning, indicating that it is used for strategic planning purposes.

Young Professionals' Committee (YPC)—NATA committee that supports newly certified ATs.

zero-based budgeting—A model that requires justification for every budget line item without reference to previous spending patterns.

References

Chapter 1

Board of Certification. 2007. *The BOC exam: The first 40 years.* Lincoln, NE: Jacob North Printing.

Board of Certification. n.d. www.bocatc.org (accessed October 1, 2016).

Carpenter, L.J., and Acosta, R.V. 2005. The law. In L.J. Carpenter, and R.V. Acosta (Eds.), *Title IX* (3-33). Champaign, IL: Human Kinetics.

Commission on Accreditation of Athletic Training Education. n.d.-a. https://caate.net/caate-decision-regarding-masters-degree-name-new-standards/ (accessed October 8, 2017)

Commission on Accreditation of Athletic Training Education. n.d.-b. The professional degree. www.caate.net/the-professional-degree (accessed May 2, 2017).

Ebel, R.G. 1999. *Far beyond the shoe box: Fifty years of the National Athletic Trainers' Association.* New York: Forbes Custom Publishing.

National Athletic Trainers' Association. 2016. *NATA Financial Report.* Dallas, TX: Author.

National Athletic Trainers' Association. n.d.-a. www.nata.org/about (accessed June 15, 2017).

National Athletic Trainers' Association. n.d.-b. Volunteer committees. www.nata.org/membership/get-involved/volunteer-committees (accessed May 2, 2017).

National Athletic Trainers' Association. n.d.-c. www.nata.org/membership/honors-and-awards/EDAC-Bill-Chisolm (accessed October 1, 2017).

Sitzler, B. 2016. Leadership emphasized during NATAPAC breakfast. *NATA News.* 28(8): 40-41.

Webber, M.J. 2013. *Dropping the bucket and sponge: A history of early athletic training 1881-1947.* Prescott, AZ: Athletic Training History Publishing.

Chapter 2

Bass, B.M. 2008. *Bass handbook of leadership.* 4th Ed. New York: Free Press.

Chicago Tribune. January 15, 2016. NCAA autonomy group approves new concussion protections. www.chicagotribune.com/sports/college/ct-colleges-ncaa-convention-concussions-spt-20160115-story.html (accessed October 16, 2016).

Drafke, M.W. 2002. *Working in health care: What you need to know to succeed.* 2nd Ed. Philadelphia: F.A. Davis.

Fayol, H. 1949. *General and industrial management.* London: Pitman & Sons.

Fisher, A. 2015. How to build a reputation as an expert. *Fortune Magazine.* http://fortune.com/2015/07/09/reputation-building-expertise-networking (accessed August 4, 2016).

Gillies, D.A. 1994. *Nursing management: A systems approach.* 3rd Ed. Philadelphia: Saunders.

Gulick, L., and Urwick, L., Eds. 1977. *Papers on the science of administration.* Fairfield, NJ: Kelley.

Helmrich, B. 2016. 33 ways to define leadership. *Business News Daily.* www.businessnewsdaily.com.

Konin, J.G. 1997. *Clinical athletic training.* Thorofare, NJ: Slack.

Mintzberg, H. 1973. *The nature of managerial work.* New York: Harper & Row.

Peter, L.J., and Hull, R. 2011. *The peter principle.* New York: HarperBusiness Publishers.

Smith, E. 1975. Improving listening effectiveness. *Texas Medicine* 71: 98-100.

Surbhi, S. 2015. Difference between transactional and transformational leadership. http://keydifferences.com/difference-between-transactional-and-transformational-leadership.html (accessed August 6, 2016).

Yukl, G.A. 2012. *Leadership in organizations.* 8th Ed. Boston: Pearson.

Chapter 3

Albohm, M.J., and Wilkerson, G.B. 1999. An outcomes assessment of care provided by certified athletic trainers. *Journal of Rehabilitation Outcomes Measurement* 3(3): 51-56.

Belanger, A.Y. 2002. *Evidence-based guide to therapeutic physical agents.* Baltimore: Lippincott Williams & Wilkins.

Block, P. 2016. *The empowered manager: Positive political skills at work.* 2nd Ed. Hoboken, NJ: Wiley.

Burns, H.K., and Foley, S.M. 2005. Building a foundation for an evidence-based approach to practice: Teaching basic concepts to undergraduate freshman students. *Journal of Professional Nursing* 21(6): 351-357.

Campbell, D. 1999. Researchers update data from athletic training outcomes study. *NATA News* (April): 26-27.

Cliska, D. 2005. Educating for evidence-based practice. *Journal of Professional Nursing* 21(6): 345-350.

Denegar, C.R., and Hertel, J. 2002. Clinical education reform and evidence-based clinical practice guidelines. *Journal of Athletic Training* 37(2): 127-128.

Esposto, L. 1993. Applying functional outcome assessment to Medicare documentation. In *Documenting functional outcomes in physical therapy,* edited by D.L. Stewart and S.H. Abeln, 135-174. St. Louis: Mosby.

Field, M.J., and Lohr, K.N., Eds. 1990. *Clinical practice guidelines: Directions for a new program.* Washington, DC: National Academy Press.

Fineout-Overholt, E., Melnyk, B.M., and Schultz, A. 2005. Transforming health care from the inside out: Advancing evidence-based practice in the 21st century. *Journal of Professional Nursing* 21(6): 335-344.

Friedman, S.D., and Greenhaus, J.H. 2000. *Allies or enemies? What happens when business professionals confront life choices.* New York: Oxford University Press.

Gibson, C.K., Newton, D.J., and Cochran, D.S. 1990. An empirical investigation of the nature of hospital mission statements. *Health Care Management Review* 15(3): 35-45.

Haynes, B., and Haynes, A. 1998. Barriers and bridges to evidence based clinical practice. *British Medical Journal (Clinical Research Edition)* 317(7153): 273-276.

Hertel, J. 2005. Research training for clinicians: The crucial link between evidence-based practice and third-party reimbursement. *Journal of Athletic Training* 40(2): 69-70.

Hootman, J.M. 2004. New section in JAT: Evidence-based practice. *Journal of Athletic Training* 39(1): 9.

Keirns, M.A., Knudsen, L., and Webster, K.J. 1997. Outcomes assessment in athletic training. In *Clinical athletic training,* edited by J.G. Konin, 245-253. Thorofare, NJ: Slack.

Law, M. 2002a. Building evidence in practice. In *Evidence-based rehabilitation: A guide to practice,* edited by M. Law, 185-194. Thorofare, NJ: Slack.

Law, M. 2002b. Introduction to evidence-based practice. In *Evidence-based rehabilitation: A guide to practice,* edited by M. Law, 3-12. Thorofare, NJ, Slack.

Lencioni P. 2004. *Death by meeting.* San Francisco: Jossey Bass.

Maher, C.G., Sherrington, C., Elkins, M., Herbert, R.D., and Mosely, A.M. 2004. Challenges for evidence-based physical therapy: Accessing and interpreting high-quality evidence on therapy. *Physical Therapy* 84(7): 644-654.

Moses, H., Dorsey E.R., Matheson, D.H., and Their, S.O. 2005. Financial anatomy of biomedical research. *Journal of the American Medical Association* 294(11): 1333-1342.

Neal, T., and Konin, J.G. 2017. Protect yourself with policy. *Sports Medicine Legal Digest* 1(2): 2-3.

Sackett, D.L., Rosenberg, W.M., Gray, J.A., Haynes, R.B., and Richardson, W.S. 1996. Evidence based medicine: What it is and what it isn't. *British Medical Journal (Clinical Research Edition)* 312(7023): 71-72.

Steiner, G.A. 1979. *Strategic planning.* New York: The Free Press.

Steves, R., and Hootman, J.M. 2004. Evidence-based medicine: What is it and how does it apply to athletic training? *Journal of Athletic Training* 39(1): 83-87.

Streator, S., and Buckley, W.E. 2000. Clinical outcomes in sports medicine. *Athletic Therapy Today* 5(5): 57-61.

Tropman, J.E. 2003. *Making meetings work: Achieving high quality group decisions.* 2nd Ed. Thousand Oaks, CA: Sage.

Watkins, P. 2003. A conference planner's 8 worst nightmares. www.gotkeynote.com/8_worst_nightmares.php (accessed May 30, 2003).

Chapter 4

Athletic Trainers' Society of New Jersey. 2014. Summative Performance Report. www.atsnj.org/documents/protected/pdf/DOE/ATSNJ_Licensed_Athletic_Trainer_Summative_Performance_Report.pdf (accessed April 22, 2017).

Bazigos, M. and Harter, J. 2016. Revisiting the matrix organization. McKinsey Quarterly. www.mckinsey.com/business-functions/organization/our-insights/revisiting-the-matrix-organization (accessed April 23, 2017).

Bennis, W., and Nanus, B. 2007. *Leaders: Strategies for taking charge.* New York: Collins Business Essentials.

Commission on Accreditation of Athletic Training Education. 2012. *Standards for the accreditation of professional athletic training programs.* https://caate.net/pp-standards.

Dixon, M.A., and Bruening, J.E. 2007. Work-family conflict in coaching I: A top-down perspective. *Journal of Sport Management* 21(3): 377-406.

Drafke, M.W. 2002. *Working in health care: What you need to know to succeed.* 2nd Ed. Philadelphia: F.A. Davis.

Dunne, G.D. 2002. *The nursing job search.* Philadelphia: University of Pennsylvania Press.

Equal Employment Opportunity Commission. n.d. *Uniform guidelines on employee selection procedures.* Washington, DC: Bureau of National Affairs, www.eeoc.gov/laws/regulations (accessed August 10, 2016).

Falcone, P. 2008. *96 great interview questions to ask before you hire.* New York: AMACOM.

Fry, R. 2016. *101 Smart questions to ask on your interview.* 4th Ed. Wayne, NJ: Career Press Publishers.

Goode, W.J. 1960. A theory of role strain. *American Sociological Review* 25(4): 483-496.

Greenhaus, J.H., and Beutell, N.J. 1985. Sources of conflict between work and family roles. *Academy of Management Review* 10(1), 76-88.

Greenhaus, J.H., and Powell, G.N. 2006. When work and family are allies: A theory of work-family enrichment. *The Academy of Management Review* 31(1): 72-92.

Hammer, L., Kossek, E., Yragui, N., Bodner, T., and Hansen, G. 2009. Development and validation of a multi-dimensional scale of family supportive supervisor behaviors (FSSB). *Journal of Management* 35: 837-856.

Harris, M.E. 2009. Implementing portfolio assessment. *Young Children,* 64(3), 82-85.

Joint Committee on Standards for Educational Evaluation. 2017. The personnel evaluation standards. www.jcsee.org/personnel-evaluation-standards (accessed September 15, 2017).

Kalliath, T., and Brough, P. 2008. Work-life balance: A review of the meaning of the construct. *Journal of Management and Organization* 14: 323-327.

Konin, J.G. 1997. *Clinical athletic training.* Thorofare, NJ: Slack.

Kossek, E., and Hammer, L. 2008. Work/life training for supervisors gets big results. *Harvard Business Review* November: 36.

Kossek, E., and Lautsch, B. 2008. *CEO of me: Creating a life that works in the flexible job age.* Englewood Cliffs, NJ: Pearson/Wharton School.

Kossek, E.E, Baltes, B.B., and Matthews, R.A. 2011. How work–family research can finally have an impact in organizations. *Industrial and organizational psychology* 4(3): 352-369.

Kossek, E.E., Hammer, L.B., Kelly, E.L., and Moen, P. 2014. Designing work, family, and health organizational change initiatives. *Organizational Dynamics* 43(1): 53-63.

Kossek, E.E., Lewis, S., and Hammer, L.B. 2010. Work–life initiatives and organizational change: Overcoming mixed messages to move from the margin to the mainstream. *Human Relations; Studies Towards the Integration of the Social Sciences* 63(1): 3-19. doi:10.1177/0018726709352385.

Lencioni, P. 2002. *The five dysfunctions of a team.* San Francisco: Jossey-Bass.

Mayo, D., and Goodrich, J. 2002. *Staffing for results.* Chicago: American Library Association.

Mazerolle, S.M., Bruening, J.E., and Casa, D.J. 2008. Work-family conflict part I: Antecedents of work-family conflict in National Collegiate Athletic Association Division I-A certified athletic trainers. *Journal of Athletic Training* 43(5): 505-512.

Mazerolle, S.M., Pitney, W.A., Casa, D.J., and Pagnotta, K.D. 2011. Assessing strategies to manage work and life balance of athletic trainers working in the National Collegiate Athletic Association Division I setting. *Journal of Athletic Training* 46(2): 1941205. doi: 10.4085/1062-6050-46.2.194

Morash, R., Brintnell, J., and Rodger, G.L. 2005. A span of control tool for clinical managers. *Nursing Leadership* 18(3):83-93.

Myers, O.J. 1985. Myths concerning employees' performance appraisal. *Supervision* 47(12): 14-16.

National Athletic Trainers' Association. 2016. June 2016 NATA membership by class and district. https://members.nata.org/members1/documents/membstats/2016-06.htm (accessed March 28, 2017).

Nelson, S., Altman, E., and Mayo, D. 2000. *Managing for results.* Chicago: American Library Association.

Owens, R.G. and Valesky, T.C. 2014. *Organizational behavior in education.* 11th Ed. Englewood Cliffs, NJ: Pearson.

Parks, J. 1977. Athletic trainer evaluation. *Athletic Training* 12(2): 92-93.

Penman, K.A., and Adams, S.H. 1980. *Assessing athletic and physical education programs.* Boston: Allyn & Bacon.

Perez, P.S., Hibbler, D.K., Cleary, M.A., and Eberman, L.E. 2006. Gender equity in athletic training. *Athletic Therapy Today* 11(2): 66-69.

Porter, L., Bigley G., and Steers, R.M. 2002. *Motivation and work behavior.* 7th Ed. New York: McGraw-Hill.

Raab S., Wolfe, B.D., Gould, T.E., and Piland, S.G. 2011. Characteristics of a quality certified athletic trainer. *Journal of Athletic Training* 46(6): 672-679.

Rapoport, R., Bailyn, L., Fletcher, J.K., and Pruitt, B.H. 2002. *Beyond work-family balance: Advancing gender equity and workplace performance.* San Francisco: Jossey-Bass.

Ray, R.R. 1991. Performance evaluation in athletic training: Perceptions of athletic trainers and their supervisors. *Dissertation Abstracts International* 51: 5053. (Doctoral dissertation, Western Michigan University, 1990).

Reinhardt, C. 1985. The state of performance appraisal: A literature review. *Human Resource Planning* 8(2): 105-110.

Tanner, D.T., and Tanner, L.N. 1987. *Supervision in education: Problems and practices.* New York: Macmillan.

United States Department of Labor. 2011. The Fair Labor Standards Act of 1938, As Amended. www.dol.gov/whd/regs/statutes/fairlaborstandact.pdf (accessed August 7, 2016).

Yate, M. 2002. *Resumes that knock 'em dead.* Avon, MA: Adams Media Corporation.

Chapter 5

Barnes, R.P. 1997. Fiscal management. *Clinical athletic training,* edited by J. Konin, 77-86. Thorofare, NJ: Slack.

Bass, B. n.d. Incremental budgeting formula. *Small Business.* http://smallbusiness.chron.com/incremental-budgeting-formula-23138.html (accessed August 10, 2016).

Cashmore, J. 2006. There's more than one way to effectively maintain equipment. *Materials Management in Health Care* 15(2): 60.

Kujawa, J.A., and Short, J.R. 2005. Six steps to managing service contracts effectively. *Biomedical Instrumentation & Technology* 39(3): 200-201.

National Collegiate Athletic Association. n.d. Finances of Intercollegiate Athletics. www.ncaa.org/about/resources/research/finances-intercollegiate-athletics (accessed December 5, 2016).

Ray, R.R. 1990. An injury-free budget. *College Athletic Management* 2(l): 42-45.

Ray, R.R. 1991. Training room efficiency. *Athletic Business* 15(l): 46-49.

Stiefel, R.H. 2002. Developing an effective inspection and preventive maintenance program. *Biomedical Instrumentation & Technology* 36(6): 405-408.

Witkin, B.R., and Altschuld, J.W. 1995. *Planning and conducting needs assessments: A practical guide.* Thousand Oaks, CA: Sage.

Chapter 6

Accreditation Association for Ambulatory Health Care. n.d. www.aaahc.org/en/news/press/archives/2016/Study-of-US-Ambulatory-Health-Care-Facilities-/ (accessed October 6, 2016).

American Institute of Architects. n.d. How Design Works For You. http://howdesignworks.aia.org/tools.asp (accessed August 21, 2016).

Clover, J. 1997. Clinical marketing. *Clinical athletic training,* edited by J. Konin, 107-120. Thorofare, NJ: Slack.

International Ergonomics Association. n.d. www.iea.cc/whats (accessed August 21, 2016).

Kesler, S.P., and Fagan, D. 2005. Firm foundation, successful facility expansion is built on robust MEP master planning. *Health Facilities Management* 18(6): 31-33.

Knight, K.L., and Draper, D.O. 2012. *Therapeutic modalities: The art and science.* 2nd Ed., 315. Philadelphia: Lippincott Williams & Wilkins.

Knowles, J.M. 1997. Planning a new athletic therapy facility. In *Clinical athletic training,* edited by J.G. Konin, 55-66. Thorofare, NJ: Slack.

Secor, M.R. 1984. Designing athletic training facilities or "Where do you want the outlets?" *Athletic Training* 19(l): 19-21.

Snider, S.W. 1982. Planning a new building? Consider design/build. *Athletic Purchasing and Facilities* 50-51.

Stiefel, R.H. 2002. Developing an effective inspection and preventive maintenance program. *Biomedical Instrumentation & Technology* 36(6): 405-408.

Chapter 7

Abdenour, T.E. 1982. Computerized training room records. *Athletic Training* 17(3): 91.

Allan, J., and Englebright, J. 2000. Patient-centered documentation: An effective and efficient use of clinical information systems. *Journal of Nursing Administration* 30(2): 90-95.

Atkins v. Swimwest Family Fitness Center, 03-2487-FT (Wis. 2005).

Hrysomallis, C., and Morrison, W.E. 1997. Sports injury surveillance and protective equipment. *Sports Medicine* 24(3): 181-183.

Joint Commission. 2010. *Health care staffing certification: Written documentation.* www.jointcommission.org/assets/1/18/2010%20Written%20Documentation%20Requirements1.PDF (accessed May 15, 2017).

Kerr, N. 2013. Creating a protective picture: A grounded theory of RN decision making when using a charting-by-exception documentation system. *Medical Surgical Nursing* 22(2): 110-8.

Kettenbach, G. 2003. *Writing SOAP notes.* 3rd Ed. Philadelphia: F.A. Davis.

Konin, J.G., and Frederick, M. 2018. *Documentation for athletic training.* 3rd Ed. Thorofare, NJ: Slack Inc.

Konin, J.G., and Neal, T. 2017 Standing orders: What do they mean and do I need them? *Sports Medicine Legal Digest* 1(1):11-12.

Lam, K.C., Valier, A.R., Anderson, B.E., and McLeod, T.C. 2016. Athletic training services during daily patient encoun- ters: A report from the athletic training practice-based research network. *Journal of Athletic Training* 51(6): 435-41.

Lampe, S. 1997. *Focus charting: Documentation for patient centered care.* 7th Ed. Minneapolis, MN: Creative Health Care Management.

Makoul, G., Curry, R.H., and Tang, P.C. 2001. The use of electronic medical records: Communication patterns in outpatient encounters. *Journal of the American Medical Informatics Association* 8(6): 610-615.

Mehta, R., Radhakrishnan, N.S., Warring, C.D., Jain, A., Fuentes, J., Dolganiuc, A., Lourdes, L.S., Busigin, J., and Leverence, R.R. 2016. The use of evidence-based, problem-oriented templates as a clinical decision support in an inpatient electronic health record system. *Applied Clinical Informatics* Aug 17;7(3): 790-802.

Murphy, J., and Burke, L.J. 1990. Charting by exception. *Nursing 90* 20(5): 65-69.

Occupational Safety and Health Administration. 2016. Occupational exposure to bloodborne pathogens. www.osha.gov/pls/oshaweb/owadisp.show_document?p_table=STANDARDS&p_id=10051 (accessed August 29, 2016).

Panettieri, M. 2000. If it's not documented, you didn't do it: Documentation in school nursing practice. *School Nurse News* 17(1): 10.

Powell v. American Health Fitness Center of Fort Wayne, Inc., 02A05-9705-CV-192 (Ind. Ct. App. 1998).

Stolle, D.P., and Slain, A.J. 1997. Standard form contracts and contract schemas: A preliminary investigation of the effects of exculpatory clauses on consumers' propensity to sue. *Behavioral Sciences and the Law* Winter;15(1): 83-94.

Wolters Kluwer Health. 2008. *Complete Guide to Medical Documentation.* 2nd Ed., 70-72. Philadelphia: Lippincott Williams & Wilkins.

Chapter 8

Albohm, M.J., Campbell, D., and Konin, J.G. 2001. *Reimbursement for athletic trainers.* Thorofare, NJ: Slack.

Albohm, M.J., and Wilkerson, G.B. 1999. An outcomes assessment of care provided by certified athletic trainers. *Journal of Rehabilitation Outcomes Measurement* 3(3): 51-56.

DeCarlo, M.S. 1997. Reimbursement for health care services. In *Clinical athletic training,* edited by J. Konin, 89-104. Thorofare, NJ: Slack.

Dixon, C.L. 2015. When student-athletes get injured, who pays? www.noodle.com/articles/when-student-athletes-get-injured-who-pays134 (accessed September 5, 2016).

Garner, S. 2016. Measuring the return on investment for a clinical athletic trainer. *NATA News* Aug./Sept.: 60-61.

Grantham, J. 2017. Reimbursement pilot project records encouraging results. *NATA News* 28:5, 30-31.

Keeley, K., Walker, S.E., Hankemeier, D.A., Martin, M. and Cappaert, T.A. 2016. Athletic Trainers' beliefs about and implementation of evidence-based practice. *Journal of Athletic Training* 51(1): 35-46.

Konin, J.G., and Frederick, M. 2018. *Documentation for athletic training*. 3rd Ed. Thorofare, NJ: Slack.

Manspeaker, S., and Van Lunen, B. 2011. Overcoming barriers to implementation of evidence-based practice concepts in athletic training education: Perceptions of select educators. *Journal of Athletic Training* 46(5):514-22.

Matney, M., and Husen, K. n.d. Contract services: What you need to know. www.nata.org/sites/default/files/contract-services-fact-sheet.pdf (accessed May 17, 2017).

National Collegiate Athletic Association. n.d. Student-athlete insurance programs. www.ncaa.org/about/resources/insurance/student-athlete-insurance-programs (accessed September 5, 2016).

Nicolello, T.S., Pecha, F.Q., Omdal, R.L., Nillson, K.J., and Homaechevarria, A.A. 2017. Patient throughput in a sports medicine clinic with the implementation of an athletic trainer: A retrospective analysis. *Sports Health* 9(1): 70-74.

Ray, R.R. 1996. Create your own HMO. *Athletic Therapy Today* 1(4): 11-12.

U.S. Department of Health and Human Services. 2015. About the affordable care act. www.hhs.gov/healthcare/about-the-law/read-the-law (accessed September 5, 2016).

Chapter 9

Alford, C.F. 2001. *Whistleblowers: Broken lives and organizational power*. Ithaca, NY: Cornell University Press.

Bigby, J. 2003a. Advocating for health care systems that meet the needs of diverse populations. In *Cross-cultural medicine*, edited by J. Bigby, 269-275. Philadelphia: American College of Physicians.

Bigby, J. 2003b. Beyond cultures: Strategies for caring for patients from diverse racial, ethnic, and cultural groups. In *Cross-cultural medicine*, edited by J. Bigby, 1-28. Philadelphia: American College of Physicians.

Bok, S. 2004. Whistleblowing and professional responsibility. In *Taking sides: Clashing views on controversial issues in business ethics and society*. 8th Ed., edited by L.H. Newton and M.M. Ford, 174-181. Guilford, CT: McGraw-Hill and Dushkin.

Callister, L.C. 2005. What has the literature taught us about culturally competent care of women and children. *MCN: The American Journal of Maternal Child Nursing* 30(6): 380-388.

Campbell, A.V., Gillett, G., and Jones, D.G. 2005. *Medical ethics*. 4th Ed. Oxford, New York: Oxford University Press.

Campinha-Bacote, J. 2003. *The process of cultural competence in the delivery of healthcare services: A culturally competent model of care. 4th Ed.* Cincinnati, OH: Transcultural C.A.R.E. Associates.

Caswell, S.V., and Gould, T.E. 2008. Individual moral philosophies and ethical decision making of undergraduate athletic training students and educators. *Journal of Athletic Training* 43(2): 205-214.

Chambers, D.W. 2004. The professions. *The Journal of the American College of Dentists* 71(4): 57-64.

Cohen, J.J. 2006. Professionalism in medical education, an American perspective: From evidence to accountability. *Medical Education* 40(7): 607-617.

Craig, D.J. 2006. Learning professionalism in athletic training education. *Athletic Training Education Journal* 1(1): 8-11.

Cruess, S.R., and Cruess, R.L. 2012. Teaching professionalism – why, what, and how. *OBGYN* 4(4), 259-265.

Davidoff, F. 2000. Changing the subject: Ethical principles for everyone in health care. *Annals of Internal Medicine* 133(5): 386-389.

DeRosa, G.P. 2006. Professionalism and virtues. *Clinical Orthopaedics and Related Research* 449: 28-33.

Doherty, R.F., and Purtilo, R.B. 2016. *Ethical dimensions in the health professions*. 6th Ed. St. Louis, MO: Elsevier.

Geisler, P.R. 2003. Multiculturalism and athletic training education: Implications for educational and professional progress. *Journal of Athletic Training* 38(2): 141-151.

Gibson, J.M. 2002. Deciding values. In *The tracks we leave: Ethics in healthcare management*, edited by F. Perry, 17-30. Chicago: Health Administration Press.

Griffin, L. 2005. The ethical health lawyer: Watch out for whistleblowers. *Journal of Law, Medicine and Ethics* 33(1): 160-163.

Institute of Medicine. 2002. What health care system administrators need to know about racial and ethnic disparities in healthcare. www.iom.edu/CMS/3740/4475/14973.aspx (accessed May 16, 2010).

Isear, J.A. 1997. Clinical professionalism. In *Clinical athletic training*, edited by J.G. Konin, 150-157. Thorofare, NJ: Slack.

Jette, D.U., and Portney, L.G. 2003. Construct validation of a model for professional behavior in physical therapist students. *Physical Therapy* 83(5): 432-443.

Johnson, R.L., Saha, S., Arbelaez, J.J., Beach, M.C., and Cooper, L.A. 2004. Racial and ethnic differences in patient perceptions of bias and cultural competence in health care. *Journal of General Internal Medicine* 19(2): 101-110.

Juckett, G. 2005. Cross-cultural medicine. *American Family Physician* 72(11): 2267-2274.

Kroshus, E., Baugh, C.M., Daneshvar, D.H., Stamm, J.M., Laursen, R.M., and Austin, S.B. 2015. Pressure on sports medicine clinicians to prematurely return collegiate athletes to play after concussion. *Journal of Athletic Training* 50(9): 944-51.

Magee, M. 2010. What ever happened to the Tavistock Principles and what is the consumer's role in defining professionalism? *Health Commentary*. http://healthcommentary.org/?page_id=1798 (accessed March 25, 2010).

Makarowski, L.M., and Rickell, J.B. 1993. Ethical and legal issues for sport professionals counseling injured athletes. In *Psychological bases of sport injuries,* edited by D. Pargman, 45-65. Morgantown, WV: Fitness Information Technology, Inc.

Marra, J., Covassin, T., Shingles, R.R., Canady, R.B., and Mackowiak, T. 2010. Assessment of certified athletic trainers' levels of cultural competence in the delivery of health care. *Journal of Athletic Training* 45(4); 380-385.

Nath, C., Schmidt, R., and Gunel, E. 2006. Perceptions of professionalism vary most with educational rank and age. *Journal of Dental Education* 70(8): 825-834.

National Athletic Trainers' Association. 2016. *NATA code of ethics*. www.nata.org/membership/about-membership/member-resources/code-of-ethics (accessed November 16, 2016).

Nynas, S.M. 2015. The assessment of athletic training students' knowledge and behavior to provide culturally competent care. *Athletic Training Education Journal* Vol 10, No 1, 82-90.

Perrin, D.H. 2015. Seeking greater relevance for athletic training education within American higher education and the health care professions. *Athletic Training Education Journal*, Vol 15, No 4, 323-328.

Ratanawongsa, N., Bolen, S., Howell, E.E., Sisson, S.D., and Larriviere, D. 2006. Residents' perceptions of professionalism in training and practice: Barriers, promoters, and duty hour requirements. *Journal of General Internal Medicine* 21(7): 758-763.

Riendeau, C., Parent-Houle, V., Lebel-Gabriel, M.E., Gauvin, P., Liu le, Y., Pearson, L., Hunt, M.R. 2015. An investigation of how university sports team athletic therapists and physical therapists experience ethical issues. *Journal of Orthopaedic and Sports Physical Therapy* 45(3): 198-206.

Padela, A.I., and del Pozo, P.R. 2010. Muslim patients and cross-gender interactions in medicine: An Islamic bioethical perspective. *Journal of Medical Ethics*. doi: 10.1136/jme.2010.037614.

Rubin, R.H. 2002. Ethical issues in managed care. In *The tracks we leave: Ethics in healthcare management*, edited by F. Perry, 51-69. Chicago: Health Administration Press.

Salimbene, S. 2015. *What language does your patient hurt in? A practical guide to culturally competent patient care.* 3rd Ed. Amherst, MA: Diversity Resources.

Schlabach, G.A., and Peer, K.S. 2008. *Professional ethics in athletic training.* St. Louis, MO: Mosby/Elsevier Science.

Spector, R.E. 2016. *Cultural diversity in health and illness.* 9th Ed. Upper Saddle River, NJ: Pearson.

Strategic Alliance. n.d. Strategic Alliance Statement – Duty to Report. http://atstrategicalliance.org/strategic-alliance-statement-duty-report (accessed November 16, 2016).

Stuart, B.K., Cherry, C., and Stuart, L. 2011. *Pocket guide to culturally sensitive health care.* Philadelphia: F.A. Davis.

Swick, H.M. 2000. Toward a normal definition of medical professionalism. *Academic Medicine* 75(6): 612-616.

Taylor, S.L., and Lurie, N. 2004. The role of culturally competent communication in reducing ethnic and racial healthcare disparities. *The American Journal of Managed Care* 10 Spec No. SP1-SP4.

Testoni, D., Hornik, C.P., Smith, P.B., Benjamin Jr., D.K., and McKinney Jr., R.E. 2013. Sports medicine and ethics. *American Journal of Bioethics* 13(10): 4-12.

U.S. Department of Health and Human Services. n.d. National culturally and linguistically appropriate services standards. www.thinkculturalhealth.hhs.gov/clas/standards (accessed June 16, 2017).

Volberding, J.L. 2013. Perceived cultural competence levels in undergraduate athletic training students. *Athletic Training Education Journal* Vol 8, No 3, 66-70.

Weuve, C., Pitney, W.A., Martin, M., and Mazerolle, S.M. 2014. Perceptions of workplace bullying among athletic trainers in the collegiate setting. *Journal of Athletic Training* 49(5): 706-718.

Chapter 10

Andersen, J.C., Courson, R.W., Kleiner, D.M., and McLoda, T.A. 2002. National Athletic Trainers' Association position statement: Emergency planning in athletics. *Journal of Athletic Training* 37: 99-104.

Benda, C. 1991. Sideline Samaritans. *The Physician and Sportsmedicine* 19(11): 132-142.

Brodsky, S.L. 2012. *Testifying in court: Guidelines and maxims for the expert witness.* 2nd Ed., Washington, DC: American Psychological Association.

Colberg, S.R., Sigal, R.J., Fernhall, B., Regensteiner, J.G., Blissmer, B.J., Rubin, R.R., Chasan-Taber, L., Albright, A.L., and Braun, B. 2010. Exercise and Type 2 Diabetes: American College of Sports Medicine and the American Diabetes Association: Joint Position Statement. *Medicine and Science in Sports and Exercise* 42(12): 2282-2303.

Feinman, J.M. 2006. *Law 101: Everything you need to know about the American legal system.* 3rd Ed. New York: Oxford University Press.

Florida Statute 90.702. 2016. Testimony by experts. www.leg.state.fl.us/Statutes/index.cfm?App_mode=Display_Statute&URL=0000-0099/0090/Sections/0090.702.html (accessed September 10, 2016).

Garza v. Edinburg Consolidated Independent School District, 576 S.W.2d. 916 (Tx. 1979).

Gieck, J., Lowe, J., and Kenna, K. 1984. Trainer malpractice: A sleeping giant. *Athletic Training* 19(l): 41-46.

Graham, J.D., and Rhomberg, L. 1996. How risks are identified and managed. *Annals of the American Academy of Political and Social Science,* edited by H. Kunreuter and P. Slovic, 545 (May 1996): 15-24.

Graham, L.S. 1985. Ten ways to dodge the malpractice bullet. *Athletic Training* 20(2): 117-119.

Killion, S.W., and Depmski, K.M. 2000. *Legal and ethical issues.* Thorofare, NJ: Slack.

Lowe v. Texas Tech University, 540 S.W.2d. 297 (Tx. 1976).

Mulder, S. 2003. Computer-aided planned maintenance system for medical equipment. *Journal of Medical Systems* 27(4): 393-398.

National Athletic Trainers' Association. 2016. National Athletic Trainers' Association Official Statement in Support of New NCAA Autonomous 5 (aka Power 5) Conferences' Independent Medical Care Rules. www.nata.org/sites/default/files/power-5-official-statement.pdf (accessed June 7, 2017).

Pearsall, A.W., 4th, Kovaleski, J.E., and Madanagopal, S.G. 2005. Medicolegal issues affecting sports medicine practitioners. *Clinical Orthopaedics and Related Research* Apr;(433): 50-7.

Pozgar, G.D. 2016. *Legal and ethical issues for health professionals.* 4th Ed. Burlington, MA: Jones and Bartlett Learning.

Rankin, J.M., and Ingersoll, C. 2001. *Athletic training management: Concepts and applications.* 2nd Ed. New York: McGraw-Hill.

Root, B.C. 2009. How the promises of riches in collegiate athletics lead to the compromised long-term health of student-athletes: Why and how the NCAA should protect its student-athletes' health. *Health Matrix Cleveland* 19(1): 279-315.

Salyanarayana Rao, K.H. 2008. Informed consent: An ethical obligation or legal compulsion. *Journal of Cutaneous and Aesthetic Surgery* 1(1): 33-35.

Sanders, A.K., Boggess, B.R., Koenig, S.J., and Toth, A.P. 2005. Medicolegal issues in sports medicine. *Clinical Orthopaedics and Related Research* Apr;(433): 38-49.

Sorey v. Kellett, 849 F.2d. 429 (5th Cir. 1988).

Suk, M. 2012. Sovereign immunity: Principles and application in medical malpractice. *Clinical Orthopaedics and Related Research.* 470(5): 1365-1369.

van der Smissen, B. 2001. Tort liability and risk management. In *The management of sport: Its foundation and application.* 3rd Ed. Edited by B.L. Parkhouse, 177-198. New York: McGraw-Hill.

Chapter 11

Centers for Disease Control and Prevention. n.d. Heads Up. www.cdc.gov/HeadsUp (accessed November 28, 2016).

HB 204 – Protection of Athletes with Head Injuries. 2011. http://le.utah.gov/~2011/bills/static/HB0204.html (accessed April 5, 2017).

Herzog, V., Sedory, A., and McKibbin, J. 2016. Legislative Process and Strategies. Presentation at the National Athletic Trainers' Association 67th Clinical Symposia on June 25, 2016 in Baltimore, MD.

McKibbin, J., and McKune, R. 2015.The lights are on. Somebody's home...but are they listening? Effectively communicating your message with lawmakers, legislators, and stakeholders. Presentation at the Mid-America Athletic Trainers' Association Symposium on March 21, 2015 in Omaha, NE.

National Athletic Trainers' Association. n.d.-a, Advocacy. www.nata.org/advocacy (accessed May 15, 2017).

National Athletic Trainers' Association. n.d.-b, Legislative toolkit. www.nata.org/sites/default/files/legislative-grassroots-toolkit.pdf (accessed May 8, 2017).

National Athletic Trainers' Association. 2016. Capitol Hill Day. *NATA News.* Aug./Sept.: 22.

S.436 – SAFE PLAY Act. 2016. www.congress.gov/bill/114th-congress/senate-bill/436/text (accessed April 5, 2017).

Vote Smart. n.d. Government 101: How a bill becomes law. https://votesmart.org/education/how-a-bill-becomes-law#.WRCq8ogrI54 (accessed May 8, 2017).

Youth Sports Safety Alliance. n.d. http://youthsportssafety-alliance.org (accessed November 22, 2016).

Chapter 12

Andersen, J.C., Courson, R.W., Kleiner, D.M., and McLoda, T.A. 2002. National Athletic Trainers' Association position statement: Emergency planning in athletics. *Journal of Athletic Training* 37: 99-104.

Broglio, S.P., Cantu, R.C., Gioia, G.A., Guskiewicz, K.M., Kutchner, J., Palm, M., and Valovich McLeod, T.C. 2014. National Athletic Trainers' Association position statement: Management of sport concussion. *Journal of Athletic Training* 49(2): 245-165.

Buell, J.L., Franks, R., Ransone, J., Powers, M.E., LaQuale, K.M., and Carlson-Phillips, A. 2013. National Athletic Trainers' Association position statement: Evaluation of dietary supplements for performance. *Journal of Athletic Training* 48(1): 124-136.

Cappaert, T.A., Stone, J.A., Castellani, J.W., Krause, B.A., Smith, D., and Stephens, B.A. 2008. National Athletic Trainers' Association position statement: Environmental cold injuries. *Journal of Athletic Training* 43(6): 640-658.

Casa, D.J., DeMartini, J.K., Bergeron, M.F., Csillan, D., Eichner, E.R., Lopez, R.M., Ferrara, M.S., Miller, K.C., O'Connor, F., Sawka, M.N., and Yeargin, S.W. 2015. National Athletic Trainers' Association position statement: Exertional heat illnesses. *Journal of Athletic Training* 50(9): 986-1000.

Conley, K.M., Bolin, D.J., Carek, P.J., Konin, J.G., Neal, T.L., and Violette, D. 2014. National Athletic Trainers' Association position statement: Pre-participation physical examinations and disqualifying conditions. *Journal of Athletic Training* 49(1): 102-120.

Gould, T.E., Piland, S.G., Caswell, S.V., Ranalli, D., Mills, S., Ferrara, M., and Courson, R. 2016. National Athletic Trainers' Association position statement: Preventing and managing sport-related dental and oral injuries. *Journal of Athletic training* 51(10): 821-839.

Kaminski, T.W., Hertel, J., Amendola, N., Docherty, C.L., Dolan, M.G., Hopkins, J.T., Nussbaum, E., Poppy, W., and Richie, D. 2013. National Athletic Trainers' Association position statement: Conservative management and prevention of ankle sprains in athletes. *Journal of Athletic Training* 48(4): 528-545.

Kersey, R.D., Elliot, D.L., Goldberg, L., Kanayama, G., Leone, J.E., Pavlovich, M., and Pope, H.G. 2012. National Athletic

Trainers' Association position statement: Anabolic-androgenic steroids. *Journal of Athletic Training* 47(5): 567-588.

National Athletic Trainers' Association. 2007. Recommendations and guidelines for appropriate medical coverage of intercollegiate athletics. www.nata.org/sites/default/files/amciarecsandguides.pdf (accessed August 9, 2016).

Neal, T.L., Diamond, A.B., Goldman, S., Liedtka, K.D., Mathis, K., Morse, E.D., Putukian, M., Quandt, E., Ritter, S.J., Sullivan, J.P., and Welzant, V. 2015. Interassociation recommendations for developing a plan to recognize and refer student-athletes with psychological concerns at the secondary school level: A consensus statement. *Journal of Athletic Training* 50(3): 231-249.

Neal, T.L., Diamond, A.B., Goldman, S., Klossner, D., Morse, E.D., Pajak, D.E., Putukian, M., Quandt, E., Sullivan, J.P., Wallack, C., and Welzant, V. 2015. Interassociation recommendations for developing a plan to recognize and refer student-athletes with psychological concerns at the collegiate level: An executive summary of a consensus statement. *Journal of Athletic Training* 48(5): 716-720.

Swartz, E.E., Boden, B.P., Courson, R.W., Decoster, L.C., Horodyski, M.B., Norkus, S.A., Rehberg, R.S., and Waninger, K.N. 2009. National Athletic Trainers' Association position statement: Acute management of the cervical spine-injured athlete. *Journal of Athletic Training* 44(3): 306-331.

Walsh, K.M., Cooper, M.A., Holle, R., Rakov, V.A., Roederll, W.P., and Ryan, M. 2013. National Athletic Trainers' Association position statement: Lightning safety for athletics and recreation. *Journal of Athletic Training* 48(2): 258-270.

Chapter 13

American Academy of Family Physicians, American College of Sports Medicine, American Academy of Pediatrics. 2010. *Preparticipation physical evaluation.* 4th Ed. Elk Grove Village, IL: American Academy of Pediatrics.

American Academy of Family Physicians. 2005. *Preparticipation physical evaluation.* 2nd Ed. Minneapolis: McGraw-Hill and Physician and Sportsmedicine.

American Heart Association News. 2015. *Screening young athletes for heart disease.* http://news.heart.org/screening-young-athletes-for-heart-disease (accessed December 18, 2016).

Caswell, S.V., Cortes, N., Chabolla, M., Ambegaonkar, J.P., Caswell, A.M., and Brenner J.S. 2015. State-specific differences in school sports preparticipation physical evaluation policies. *Pediatrics* 135(1): 26-33.

Conley, K.M., Bolin, D.J., Carek, P.J., Konin, J.G., Neal, T.L., and Violette, D. 2014. National Athletic Trainers' Association position statement: Preparticipation physical examinations and disqualifying conditions. *Journal of Athletic Training* 49(1): 102-120.

Corrado, D., Basso, C., Schiavon, M., Pelliccia, A., and Thiene, G. 2008. Pre-participation screening of young competitive athletes for prevention of sudden cardiac death. *Journal of the American College of Cardiology* 52(24): 1981-1989.

Drezner, J.A. 2000. Sudden cardiac death in young athletes: Causes, athlete's heart, and screening guidelines. *Postgraduate Medicine* 108(5): 37-44, 47-50.

Ferrari, R., Parker, L.S., Grubs, R.E., and Krishnamurti, L. 2015. Sickle cell trait screening of collegiate athletes: Ethical reasons for program reform. *Journal of Genetic Counseling* 24(6): 873-877.

Goff, D.C., Lloyd-Jones, D.M., Bennett, G., Coady, S., D'Agostino, R.B., Gibbons, R., Greenland, P., Lackland, D.T., Levy, D., O'Donnell, C.J., Robinson, J.G., Sanford Schwartz, J., Shero, S.T., Smith, S.C., Sorlie, P., Stone, N.J., and Wilson, P.W.F. 2014. ACC/AHA guideline on the assessment of cardiovascular risk: A report of the American College of Cardiology/American Heart Association Task Force on practice guidelines. *Circulation* 129: S49-S73.

Herbert, D.L. 1996. Athlete's exclusion from participation does not violate Federal Rehabilitation Act. *Sports Medicine Standards and Malpractice Reporter* 8: 40-43.

Herbert, D.L. 1997. Sports medicine physician has "final say" in exclusion of athlete from participation. *Sports Medicine Standards and Malpractice Reporter* 9(17): 20-23.

Herring, S.A., Kibler, W.B., and Putukian, M. 2012. The team physician and the return-to-play decision: A consensus statement—2012 update. *Medicine and Science in Sports and Exercise* 44(12): 2446–2448.

Joy, E.A., Paisley, T.S., Price Jr., R., Rassner, L., and Thiese, S.M. 2004. Optimizing the collegiate preparticipation physical evaluation. *Clinical Journal of Sports Medicine* 14(3): 183-187.

Knapp v. Northwestern University, 96-3450 (7th Cir. 1996).

Koester, M.C. 1995. Refocusing the adolescent preparticipation physical evaluation toward preventive health care. *Journal of Athletic Training* 30: 352-360.

McKeag, D.B., and Moeller J.L. 2007. *ACSM's primary care sports medicine.* 2nd Ed. Philadelphia: Lippincott Williams & Wilkins.

Minick, K., Kiesel, K., Lee, B., Taylor, A., Plisky, P., and Butler, R. 2010. Interrater Reliability of the Functional Movement Screen. *Journal of Strength & Conditioning Research* 24(2): 479-486.

Mirabelli, M.H., Devine, M.J., Singh, J., and Mendoza, M. 2015. The preparticipation sports evaluation. *American Family Physician* 92(5): 371-376.

Mobley v. Madison Square Garden LP, 11-Civ-8290 (DAB) (S.D.N.Y. 2012).

National Collegiate Athletic Association. 2014. *2014-2015 NCAA sports medicine handbook.* Overland Park, KS: Author.

Oliva, A., Grassi, V.M., Campuzano, O., Brion, M., Arena, V., Partemi, S., Coll, M., Pascali, V.L., Brugada, J., Carracedo, A., and Brugada, R. 2017. Medico-legal perspectives on sudden cardiac death in young athletes. *International Journal of Legal Medicine* 131(2): 393-409.

Parchmann, C., and McBride, J.M. 2011. Relationship between functional movement screen and athletic performance. *Journal of Strength & Conditioning Research* 25(12): 3378-3384.

Penny v. Sands, H89-280 (D. Conn. 1989).

Pfister, G.C., Puffer, J.C., and Maron, B.J. 2000. Preparticipation cardiovascular screening for US collegiate student-athletes. *Journal of the American Medical Association* 283(12): 1597-1599.

Reed, F.E. 2001. Improving the preparticipation exam process. *The Journal of the South Carolina Medical Association* 97(8): 342-346.

Smith, D.M. 1994. Pre-participation physical evaluations: Development of uniform guidelines. *Sports Medicine* 18: 293-300.

Starkey, C. 2013. *Athletic training and sports medicine: An integrated approach.* 5th Ed. Park Ridge, IL: American Academy of Orthopaedic Surgeons.

Tanner, S.M. 1994. Preparticipation exam targeted for the female athlete. *Clinics in Sports Medicine* 13(2): 337-353.

Chapter 14

Bahrke, M.S. 2015. Drug testing US student athletes for performance-enhancing substance misuse: A flawed process. *Substance Use Misuse* 50(8-9): 1144-7.

Bird, S.R., Goebel, C., Burke, L.M., and Greaves, R.F. 2016. Doping in sport and exercise: Anabolic, ergogenic, health and clinical issues. *Annals of Clinical Biomechanics* 53(Part 2): 196-201.

Elkins, R.L., King, K., and Vidourek, R. 2017. School and parent factors associated with steroid use among adolescents. *Journal of School Health* 87(3): 159-166.

Huff, P.S. 1998. Drug distribution in the training room. *Clinics in Sports Medicine* 17: 211-228.

Kersey, R.D., Eliot, D.L., Goldberg, L., Kanayama, G., Leone, J.E., Pavlovich, M., and Pope, H.G. 2012. National Athletic Trainers' Association position statement: Anabolic-androgenic steroids. *Journal of Athletic Training* 47(5): 567-588.

Lee, B. 2001. Drug testing and the confused athlete: A look at the differing athletic drug testing programs in high school, college, and the Olympics. *Florida Coastal Law Journal* 3: 91.

Lebron v. Secretary, Florida Department of Children and Families, 11–15258 (11th Cir. 2013).

National Collegiate Athletic Association, Committee on Competitive Safeguards and Medical Aspects of Sports. 1988. *Drugs and the intercollegiate athlete.* Indianapolis: Author.

National Collegiate Athletic Association. 2016. *Drug-testing program 2016-17.* www.ncaa.org/sites/default/files/2016SSI_DrugTestingProgramBooklet_20160728.pdf (accessed October 25, 2016).

National Federation of State High School Associations. 2015. Dietary supplements position statement. www.nfhs.org/media/1015652/dietary-supplements-position-statement-2015.pdf (accessed October 29, 2016).

Nickell, R. 2006. Eight important principles for managing prescriptions in the athletic training room. *NATA News* 30-32.

Pickett, A.D. 1986. Drug testing: What are the rules? *Athletic Training* 21: 331-336.

Petroczi, A., Backhouse, S.H., Barkoukis, V., Brand, R., Elbe, A.M., Lazuras, L., and Lucidi, F. 2015. A call for policy guidance on psychometric testing in doping control in sport. *International Journal of Drug Policy* 26(11): 1130-9.

Schaill by Kross v. Tippecanoe Cty. School Corp., 679 F. Supp. 833 (N.D. Ind. 1988).

Todd v. Rush County Schools, 983 F. Supp. 799 (S.D. Ind. 1997).

Chapter 15

Andersen, J.C., Courson, R.W., Kleiner, D.M., and McLoda, T.A. 2002. National Athletic Trainers' Association position statement: Emergency planning in athletics. *Journal of Athletic Training* 37: 99-104.

Casa, D.J., DeMartini, J.K., Bergeron, M.F., Csillan, D., Eichner, E.R., Lopez, R.M., Ferrara, M.S., Miller, K.C., O'Connor, F., Sawka, M.N., and Yeargin, S.W. 2015. National Athletic Trainers' Association position statement: Exertional heat illnesses. *Journal of Athletic Training* 50(9): 986-1000.

Casa, D.J., Guskiewicz, K.M., Anderson, S.A., Courson, R.C., Heck, J.F., Jimenez, C.C., McDermott, B.P., Miller, M.G., Stearns, R.L., Swartz, E.E., and Walsh, K.M. 2012. National Athletic Trainers' Association position statement: Preventing sudden death in sports. *Journal of Athletic Training* 47(1): 96-118.

Courson, R. 2007. Preventing sudden death on the athletic field: The emergency action plan. *Current Sports Medicine Reports* 6(2): 93-100.

Drezner, J.A., Courson, R.W., Roberts, W.O., Mosesso, V.N., Link, M.S., and Maron, B.J. 2007. Inter-association task force recommendations on emergency preparedness and management of sudden cardiac arrest in high school and college athletic programs: A consensus statement. *Journal of Athletic Training* 42(1): 143-158.

Hainline, B., Drezner, J., Baggish, A., Harmon, K.G., Emery, M.S., Myerburg, R.J., Sanchez, E., Molossi, S., Parsons, J.T., and Thompson, P.D. 2016. Interassociation consensus statement on cardiovascular care of college student-athletes. *Journal of Athletic Training* 51(4): 344-357.

Kary, J.M., Lavallee, M. 2007. Travel medicine and the international athlete. *Clinics in Sports Medicine* 26(3): 489-503.

Kinderknecht, J. 2016. Roles of the team physician. *Journal of Knee Surgery* 29(5): 356-363.

Martin, D.E. 1994. Emergency medicine and the underage athlete. *Journal of Athletic Training* 29(3): 200-202.

Motyka, T.M., Winslow, J.E., Newton, K., Brice, J.H. 2005. Method for determining automatic external defibrillator need at mass gatherings. *Resuscitation* 65(3): 309-314.

Rehberg, R. 2013. *Sports emergency care.* 2nd Ed. Thorofare, NJ: Slack.

Rubin, A.L. 2004. Safety, security, and preparing for disaster at sporting events. *Current Sports Medicine Reports* 3(3): 141-145.

Vasquez, M.S., Fong, M.K., Patel, L.J., Kurose, B., Tierney, J., Gardner, I., Yazdani-Arazi, A., and Su, J.K. 2015. Medical planning for very large events: Special Olympics World Games Los Angeles 2015. *Current Sports Medicine Reports* 14(3): 161-164.

Walsh, K.M., Cooper, M.A., Holle, R., Rakov, V.A., Roeder, W.P., and Ryan, M. 2013. National Athletic Trainers' Association position statement: Lightning safety for athletics and recreation. *Journal of Athletic Training* 48(2): 258–270.

Index

Note: The italicized *f* and *t* following page numbers refer to figures and tables, respectively.

About the Authors

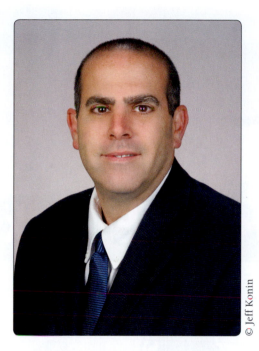

© Jeff Konin

Jeff G. Konin, PhD, ATC, PT, FACSM, FNATA, is chair of the physical therapy department and a Ryan Research professor of neuroscience at the University of Rhode Island (URI) as well as an adjunct professor in the department of family medicine at Brown University. Dr. Konin is a founding partner in The Rehberg Konin Group, which provides scientific investigation, research, and litigation support services for incidents involving sports, physical activity, and rehabilitation. He is the author of the textbooks *Clinical Athletic Training*; *Special Tests for Orthopedic Examination*; *Documentation for Athletic Training*; *Reimbursement for Athletic Training*; *Sports Medicine Conditions—Return to Play: Recognition, Treatment, Planning*; *Rehabilitation from the Perspective of the Athletic Trainer/Physical Therapist*; *Working as a Team Physician*; *Practical Kinesiology for the Physical Therapist Assistant*; and *Sports Emergency Care*. He is a coauthor of the NATA position statement *Preparticipation Physical Examinations and Disqualifying Conditions*, a contributing writer to the NATA's *Best Practice Guidelines for Athletic Training Documentation*, and a contributor to the NATA's *Sports Medicine Legal Digest* newsletter.

Konin is a fellow of both the National Athletic Trainers' Association (NATA) and the American College of Sports Medicine (ACSM). He is a recipient of the NATA Service Award (2008), the NATA Continuing Education Excellence Award (2008), the Southeast Athletic Trainers' Association Education/Administration Athletic Trainer of the Year Award (2010), and the NATA Most Distinguished Athletic Trainer Award (2011).

Konin received his doctorate in physical therapy from Nova Southeastern University, a master of physical therapy from the University of Delaware, a master of education from the University of Virginia, and a bachelor of science from Eastern Connecticut State University.

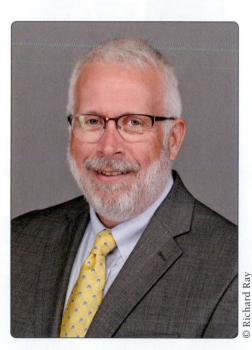

© Richard Ray

Richard Ray, EdD, ATC, is provost emeritus and a professor of kinesiology at Hope College. He has been a member of the Hope College faculty since 1982 and previously served as the college's chief academic officer, dean for the social sciences, and chair of the department of kinesiology. He was the college's head athletic trainer, and he developed the academic program in athletic training at Hope. He is the author of more than 40 peer-reviewed journal articles and three books on sports medicine, leadership in higher education, and health care management.

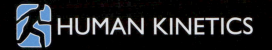
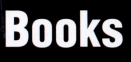